HEALTHCARE LIBRARY

THE NORTH HAMPSHIRE HOSPITAL

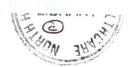
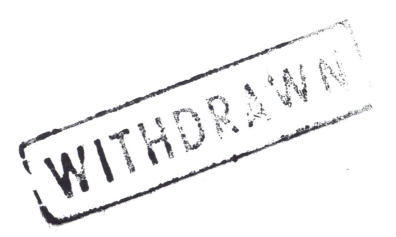

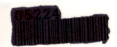

Skeletal Trauma in Old Age

Skeletal Trauma in Old Age

Edited by

David I. Rowley

Professor of Orthopaedic and Trauma Surgery
University of Dundee
Dundee
UK

and

Benedict Clift

Lecturer in Orthopaedic and Trauma Surgery
University of Dundee
Dundee
UK

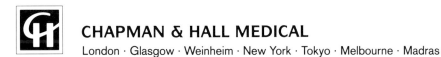

CHAPMAN & HALL MEDICAL

London · Glasgow · Weinheim · New York · Tokyo · Melbourne · Madras

Published by Chapman & Hall,
2–6 Boundary Row, London SE1 8HN, UK

Chapman & Hall, 2–6 Boundary Row, London SE1 8HN, UK

Blackie Academic & Professional, Wester Cleddens Road,
Bishopbriggs, Glasgow G64 2NZ, UK

Chapman & Hall GmbH, Pappelallee 3, 69469 Weinheim, Germany

Chapman & Hall USA, One Penn Plaza, 41st Floor, New York
NY 10119, USA

Chapman & Hall Japan, ITP-Japan, Kyowa Building, 3F, 2–2–1
Hirakawacho, Chiyoda-ku, Tokyo 102, Japan

Chapman & Hall Australia, Thomas Nelson Australia, 102 Dodds
Street, South Melbourne, Victoria 3205, Australia

Chapman & Hall India, R. Seshadri, 32 Second Main Road, CIT East,
Madras 600 035, India

First edition 1994

© 1994 Chapman & Hall

Typeset in 10/12 Palatino by Photoprint, Torquay

Printed in Great Britain at the University Press, Cambridge

ISBN 0 412 48750 0

A catalogue record for this book is available from the British Library

Library of Congress Catalog Card Number: 94–70928

∞ Printed on acid-free text paper, manufactured in accordance with
ANSI/NISO Z39.48–1992 (Permanence of Paper).

Contents

Contents

Contributors

P.L.O. Broos
Head of Department
Traumatology and Emergency Surgery
U.Z. Gashtuisberg
Herestraat 49
3000 Leuven
Belgium

R.P. Clifford
Consultant Orthopaedic and Trauma
  Surgery
The General Hospital
St Helier
Jersey
UK

B.A. Clift
Lecturer
Caird Block
Royal Infirmary
Dundee
DD1 9ND
UK

J.A. Dent
Senior Orthopaedic Lecturer
Royal Infirmary
Dundee
DD1 9ND
UK

M. Dickson
Consultant Plastic Surgeon
Leicester Hospital
Coreys Mill Lane
Stevenage
Herts
SG1 4AB
UK

W. Friedl
Department of Surgery
University of Heidelberg
Im Nueuheimer Feld 110
6900 Heidelberg
Germany

R. Hertel
Orthopedic Trauma and Reconstructive
  Surgery
University of Bern
CH–3010 Bern
Inselspial
Switzerland

D.C. Kennie
Consultant Physician in Geriatric Medicine
Royal Infirmary
Livilands Gate
Stirling
FK8 2AU
UK

S. Larsson
Department of Orthopedics
Uppsala University Hospital
S–75185 Uppsala
Sweden

L. Latta
Director of Research
University of Miami School of Medicine,
Department of Orthopedics and
  Rehabilitation
PO Box 016960 (D-27)
Miami, Florida 33101
USA

N.R. Lestrange
Orthopedic Surgeon
4800 North Federal Highway
Fort Lauderdale
Florida 33308
USA

W.J. MacLennan
Department of Medicine
Geriatric Medicine Unit
City Hospital
Greenbank Drive
Edinburgh EH10 5SB
UK

W.A. Macrae
Consultant Anaesthetist
Ninewells Hospital
Dundee DD1 9SY
UK

M.E.T. McMurdo
Senior Lecturer
Ageing and Health
Department of Medicine
Ninewells Hospital
Dundee DD1 9SY
UK

M.M. McQueen
Senior Lecturer
Department of Orthopaedic Surgery
Clinical Research Unit
Princess Margaret Rose Hospital
Fairmilehead
Edinburgh EH10 7ED
UK

F.A. Millar
Senior Registrar
Department of Anaesthetics
Ninewells Hospital
Dundee DD1 9SY
UK

E.R.S. Ross
Consultant Trauma and Orthopaedic
  Surgeon
Hope Hospital
Salford M6 8HD
UK

D.I. Rowley
Caird Block
Royal Infirmary
Dundee DD1 9NN
UK

P.G. Stableforth
Orthopaedic Department
Bristol Royal Infirmary
Malborough Street
Bristol BS2 8HW
UK

C.P.U. Stewart
Associate Specialist
Dundee Limb Fitting Centre
133 Queen Street
Broughty Ferry
Dundee DD5 1AG
UK

Foreword

The birth rate in the developed countries of the world has decreased steadily, particularly during the second half of the twentieth century. Parallel to that reduction has been the increased longevity of their citizens. The anticipated continuation of those patterns will inevitably result in an enormous challenge to the human and financial resources of the various countries. This may either bankrupt the economies of the less affluent nations or force them into adopting health care rationing of unprecedented proportions. Needless to say, the victims of such measures will be those on the societal ladder who are already finding it increasingly difficult to benefit from the advances that the medical sciences have so dramatically wrought in recent decades.

Even at this time, most western countries are finding it difficult to cope with the demands created by the large number of elderly people suffering from the diseases that afflict them. Disorders of the musculoskeletal system, which do not usually lead to death, but can and frequently do produce disability and incapacitation, account for a disproportionately large percentage of the cost of medical care. Osteoporosis, fractures and arthritis constitute the lion's share of the costs.

This book appears at the appropriate time. The message that it delivers is germaine to the crisis at hand and it is written in such a manner that it permits the reader to appreciate the significant uniqueness of the medical conditions of the elderly, the manner in which their diagnoses are often clouded with uncertainties and the difficulties in making a prognosis of the final outcome.

The contributors to this text have consistently maintained a healthy and pragmatic approach to the general topic and avoided indulging in esoteric dissertation unnecessary in a book of this nature. I found the contributions of Loren Latta particularly valuable because his discussion of the biomechanical implications of the various disorders made the subjects easier to understand and placed them in the proper perspective.

The editors of the book and the contributing authors have made a very worthwhile contribution to the medical literature.

Augusto Sarmiento M.D.
Chairman, Department of Orthopaedics and Musculoskeletal Disorders
Health Care International Medical Centre
Glasgow, Scotland
1994

Preface

This is a multi-author textbook dealing with the problems posed by the continuing growth of the proportion of old people within the population, not only in the West but throughout the world. One thing that emerges from the text is that environmental factors such as falls, activity and diet have much to do with the incidence of fractures and that being old is not the sole reason for breaking bones. Many of us still talk about the 'elderly population' as almost a different species rather than something we will join if we are fortunate. Our priorities should not be to look forward to making us live longer unless we can accompany such aspirations with the desire to ensure we also live well in old age. This book is as much about encouraging high quality of life as to do with survival in the elderly population. For this reason we have encouraged contributors to address the issues of prevention and rehabilitation as well as interventive management of the 'crisis' of the fracture event.

Most of the chapters are confined to joint-related fractures rather than those affecting long bones. This is because the principles applying to long bone fractures in the elderly are generally identical to those in younger people and, therefore, special attention in this area is not so important. It was felt more worthwhile to use the space available in the book to deal with more specialized areas of interest. Details of treating diaphyseal fractures can be found in any textbook. It may seem strange, on the other hand, to find a chapter on amputation surgery in a book that is dealing otherwise with fractures. The reasons for this are to take advantage of the considerable expertise available in Dundee and also to deal with a subject that is often not addressed particularly well in practice in general. This is usually because amputation is all too often seen as a negative end point of treatment rather than as being the positive start of rehabilitation to an often improved lifestyle, relative to the one suffered under the conditions of the disease that led to the amputation. We therefore make no apologies for this slight digression.

An innovation in this book has been to convert individual contributions from authors into integrated chapters. Rather than chapters solely on epidemiology, biomechanics, prevention or rehabilitation, for example, we have taken contributions from these experts and integrated them into the text where we feel their expertise is most relevant. You will therefore find multi-author chapters as well as a multi-author book. We hope this will encourage the reader to think from a thematic and systematic perspective which should be of particular use to the surgeon or physician in training, who currently addresses the patient from a problem-orientated viewpoint, to see the person behind the fracture. Teams are essential and good teamwork from many disciplines is required if an old person is to return to a full life back in the community. We hope physiotherapists, social workers and others in community and primary care will find this a useful text, giving them insight into the epidemic of fractures in old people.

David I. Rowley and Benedict Clift
Dundee
1994

Acknowledgements

We would like to acknowledge the patience and forbearance of our wives, who like many 'surgical widows' are all too used to not seeing their husbands. We are eternally grateful to Margaret Aitken, Departmental Secretary, who has patiently typed manuscript after manuscript and we also acknowledge the expertise of the sub editorial and production staff at Chapman & Hall.

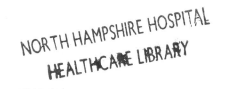

1

Prevention of injuries in elderly people

MARION McMURDO

Injuries in the elderly may be prevented by preventing accidents, preventing falls or by strengthening bone, thus making fracture less likely. The chapter will discuss these in turn.

ACCIDENTS

EPIDEMIOLOGY

Death by accident accounts for a very small proportion of the total deaths in the elderly. However, the death rate from accidents is still considerably greater in the over-75s than in any other age group (OPCS, 1990).

Road traffic accidents account for 20% of accidental deaths in males over 75 years and just over 10% of female deaths. Over 85% of all the road traffic accident fatalities in the elderly are pedestrians, and are often due to confusion with traffic and poor eyesight (Automobile Association Foundation for Road Safety Research, 1989).

STRATEGIES FOR PREVENTION

Scope exists) to prevent such accidents, including educational measures and environmental improvements to streets and the design of cars. Uneven or rough paths are an unnecessary and common cause of falls. Those involved in house design should realize that some of the guidelines developed with children in mind, such as avoiding halfway landings, would benefit old people.

In all accident prevention, the environment is influenced more easily than behavior. The goal should be to make products and environments as safe as possible, even for the frailest old person.

FALLS

Falls in old age are a major cause of morbidity and mortality, and often signify the presence of a serious underlying disorder. The grave prognostic significance of falls has been clearly shown in a comparative study of 125 fallers versus age matched controls. After 2 months, 11 fallers had died compared to one control. At 1 year the comparable figures were 32 and eight (Wild, Nayak and Isaacs, 1981). Even without causing fractures, falls can still have a devastating psychological effect on the quality of life of old people.

Falls are always the result of a failure to adjust to, and correct for, a displacement of the body. It is evident that a major degree of

Skeletal Trauma in Old Age
Published in 1994 by Chapman & Hall, London
ISBN 0 412 48750 0

displacement on the football field will result in falling even in a young and healthy person, while quite a minor displacement may be sufficient in an older and less fit person (Williamson, Smith and Burley, 1987).

NEUROMUSCULAR CONTROL OF POSTURE

The maintenance of good postural control requires a well organized homeostatic mechanism which comprises input, processing, and output functions. The vestibular, proprioceptive and visual systems constitute the sensory inputs which relay information about the external environment. The vestibular apparatus is probably the least important part of the system (Martin, 1967). Internal anticipatory reflex pathways are also important, as they serve to stabilize the individual by activating proximal postural muscles in response to specific tasks. Processing and integration of these sources of information occur at a subconscious level, producing a complex output of postural responses to the head, neck and limbs.

Clear distinctions exist between static and dynamic balance mechanisms. Whereas static balance during standing consists of low frequency, predictable movements, dynamic balance, occurring during walking, results in higher frequency stimulation of the head and vestibular systems.

AGING EFFECTS ON NEUROMUSCULAR CONTROL OF POSTURE

Postural sway can be measured either by assessment of the angular body displacement, or by assessment of the center of foot pressure, using a force platform (Murray, Seireg and Sepic, 1975; Nayak *et al.*, 1982). There is an increase in postural sway with advancing age, and females tend to sway more than males. Sway in elderly fallers as a group tends to be higher than non-fallers

(Overstall *et al.*, 1977). However, absolute measures in individual cases have little predictive value because of the inherent variability of sway scores.

Stretch reflexes are thought to be important mediators of postural adjustment. These reflexes are subject to modulation from higher centers, and age-related alterations in these postural muscle responses have been described. Coexisting orthopedic disabilities in an individual are significant because they impair the ability to use appropriate motor strategies for balance. The patient with painful arthritis of the knees or hips may have difficulty in correcting a displacement because the sudden movement required causes severe and inhibiting pain.

EPIDEMIOLOGY OF FALLS

The incidence of falls increases with age, and surveys of elderly people living at home show that about 20% of men and 40% of women have fallen during the previous twelve months (Prudham and Evans, 1991). Surveys of falls in old people's homes show an even higher prevalence. The majority of falls go undetected since less than 3% a year of the elderly who fall injure themselves sufficiently to require medical attention (Gray, 1966).

Among non-institutionalized old people, the majority of serious falls occur during the day and at home, often descending the stairs. In hospitals, in contrast, getting in or out of bed or hurrying to the toilet is associated with a fall (Overstall, 1985). Women fall more often than men. Other characteristics associated with a high likelihood of falling are living alone, and the presence of chronic illness, impaired mobility, and postural instability.

COMPLICATIONS OF FALLS

Most falls do not result in serious injury, and only 6% of falls are thought to result in fracture. Injury and death are obvious complications of falls. Other physical complications include bruising and lacerations, fractures, hypothermia, pressure sores, dehydration and bronchopneumonia.

It is important to emphasize, however, that even if a fall does not result in physical injury, the psychological implications may be devastating. The shock of falling, together with a fear of future falls, may lead to a debilitating loss of confidence. After experiencing a fall, an older person is less likely to go outside and may be less active within the home.

The psychological consequences of falling may also extend beyond the patient to involve relatives and neighbours. Old people who fall and lie on the floor unable to get up cause pronounced anxiety in carers and friends. This is frequently translated into feelings of guilt and demands that the patient be put into hospital.

CAUSES

Environmental factors and vision

Various environmental hazards including loose rugs and carpets, poor lighting, highly polished surfaces, trailing flexes and telephone cords, and doorsteps have been found to be responsible for accidental falls (Lucht, 1971). Trips and accidents are thought to account for 45% of falls (Overstall *et al.*, 1977). Studies on gait have shown that elderly fallers have gait characteristics different from elderly non-fallers. Slow speed, short step length, narrow stride width, wide range of stepping frequency and large variability of step length have all been identified as gait characteristics of hospitalized fallers (Guimares and Isaacs, 1980).

Significantly reduced visual acuity has been described in elderly fallers, compared to non-fallers, although there is no difference in their use of spectacles (Prudham and Evans,

1991). This is a significant factor since undetected visual disability is common in the elderly (McMurdo and Baines, 1988). Lighting conditions in the homes of elderly people attending a Low Visual Aid clinic were shown to be woefully inadequate (Cullinan, 1986), and impairment of dark adaptation has been demonstrated in elderly fallers (McMurdo and Gaskell, 1991). The significance of poor dark adaptation is that an old person may be virtually blind for a full minute or more on moving from a bright room to a darker area. The provision of adequate lighting may offset the influence of impaired dark adaptation.

Cardiac and hemodynamic factors

Postural hypotension

This should be considered in patients who fall after rising from a chair or getting out of bed. In practice diagnosis and monitoring is achieved by measuring the blood pressure in both the lying and standing position. A fall in systolic blood pressure of 20 mmHg or more on standing establishes that the patient has impairment of postural blood pressure control. The etiology is generally multifactorial, and is usually a combination of age-related defects in homeostatic regulatory activity and extrinsic factors, such as an unduly warm environment or drug-induced hypotension (Lye and Vargas, 1983).

Drugs

Fallers are more likely than non-fallers to have taken drugs within 24 hours of the fall, especially hypnotics, tranquilizers and sedatives (Lye and Vargas, 1983). Long-acting, centrally-acting drugs appear to be particularly hazardous, and it is now acknowledged that such compounds are over-prescribed for old people. Although an American study reported that alcohol played a contributory

3

part in 8% of elderly fallers, in the United Kingdom fallers do not differ from non-fallers in their consumption of alcohol.

To minimize the effects of postural hypotension, elderly patients should be advised to rise from bed in stages – for example, sitting upright in bed for 5 minutes, then 5 minutes with the legs over the side of the bed before standing. This will often prevent the more serious falls following a night's recumbency (Bradshaw and Edwards, 1986). Correction of hypotension may require measures such as bed-head tilt, pressure stockings or, rarely, fludrocortisone.

Cardiac dysfunction

Transient cerebral hypoperfusion due to both structural valve lesions and cardiac arrhythmias is an important cause of falls (Livesley and Atkinson, 1974). This effect is enhanced in old age because cerebral autoregulation may be inefficient, so the complex compensatory mechanisms which serve to protect and preserve cerebral perfusion are sometimes impaired.

Tachyarrhythmias and bradyarrythmias may be implicated, the latter often the result of digoxin or beta-adrenoreceptor blocking drugs. Cardiac pacing can be so effective in suitable patients that the relevant arrhythmias should be sought, and a standard 12-lead ECG may be as helpful as a 24-hour ambulatory recording (Taylor and Stout, 1983).

Neurological factors

Neurological diseases which affect the balance, sensory input and muscle strength are likely to result in falls. Epilepsy is responsible for only a minority of falls in the elderly, although the diagnosis is often missed, and the condition is eminently treatable. Suggestive clues are urinary incontinence and a period of confusion after the fall.

The most frequently implicated conditions are Parkinson's disease, stroke, cognitive impairment and cervical spondylosis. The aging patient who falls may be unable to give a coherent account of the episode, partly as a result of the unexpected and sudden nature of the event. It should also be remembered that patients may unwittingly mislead the enquirer through their attempts to explain what caused the fall. A skilled and careful approach from the person taking the history is necessary to avoid putting words into the patient's mouth (Isaacs, 1985).

All synovial joints possess receptor nerve endings, and the mechanoreceptors in the apophyseal joints of the cervical spine contain receptors which provide both 'static' and 'dynamic' information (Wyke, 1979). These receptors send information to the brain via the propriospinal tracts, and also relay to the external ocular muscles. They are responsible for a number of fundamentally important reflex mechanisms concerned with postural control and movements such as walking and running. Cervical spondylosis is known to cause a variety of symptoms including dizziness, vertigo, nystagmus and deafness. Typically the symptoms are provoked on head turning. This is due to an imbalance in the inflow of stimuli from damaged mechanoreceptors in the apophyseal joints of the cervical spine (Murray, Seirag and Sepic, 1975).

Some cervical spondylosis is present in all old people. Radiologically demonstrated skeletal changes may be severe in the absence of any neurological or skeletal symptoms. This can make the diagnosis of the neurological complications of cervical spondylosis, especially the myelopathy, difficult. It also may cast doubt on the indications for surgical intervention.

Symptomatic improvement undoubtedly occurs in some patients while wearing a cervical collar, although there is little evidence to indicate that the collar itself is responsible. It is important that the collar adequately immobilizes the neck in the neutral or slightly flexed position. The collar should be worn for as long as the patient is mobile. It is important to ensure that the patient or carer knows how to put the collar on, and that the collar is sufficiently comfortable to be worn continuously during the day.

Rarely, falls may be associated with normal pressure hydrocephalus, a syndrome characterized by dementia, incontinence of urine, and an abnormal gait (Hakim and Adams, 1965). There may be a precipitant, for example head injury, spontaneous intracranial hemorrhage, or meningitis. The diagnosis is suspected on clinical grounds and confirmed by a characteristic CT scan showing enlargement of the ventricles and periventricular lucency. The natural history of the condition is not known, but insertion of a cerebrospinal fluid shunt may prove helpful. However, the results of shunting have been disappointing, and much more information is required about the selection of patients most likely to benefit from the procedure (Garfield, 1992).

CLINICAL EVALUATION AND MANAGEMENT

All patients who have experienced two or more unexpected falls should have a complete physical examination and appropriate investigation. It is important to obtain an accurate history of the fall, and the events immediately preceding it. A falls evaluation checklist includes the following:

- History – from patient and witness (if available), noting events leading up to fall, time to recovery, and frequency of falls.
- Physical examination – check lying and standing blood pressure, pulse rate and regularity, and visual acuity.
- Investigation – intercurrent infection in chest or urine, electrocardiogram.

- Drug therapy – review and if possible discontinue any therapy which may be precipitating falls.
- Gait assessment – need for, and use of, walking aids; evidence of specific disorders like Parkinson's disease or cervical myelopathy.
- Home assessment – to assess lighting levels, loose carpets, chair and bed heights.

As with any diagnosis in the elderly, it is important not merely to look for a single cause, but to acknowledge the likelihood of multiple pathology, and possibility that several causes may coexist. Another difficulty is that virtually any acute illness in the elderly may predispose to, and present with, a fall.

STRATEGIES FOR PREVENTION OF FALLS

- Appropriate design of public buildings and private housing with particular attention to railings, step heights, color contrast and lighting.
- Encouraging regular healthy exercise. Lack of physical activity and poor muscle strength are associated with an increased risk of falling. Muscle strength and physical activity levels are important determinants of bone density, so maintenance of physical activity may decrease the likelihood of fracture both by an effect on the bone and by decreasing the risk of a fall (Pocock *et al.*, 1986). Increasing muscle bulk may also produce useful effects by enhancing protective reflexes and increasing the bulk of soft tissue padding. To add further strength to the argument for increasing physical activity to prevent falls, some workers have reported improvements in balance after participation in exercise programs (Overstall, 1980), although other studies contradict this finding (McMurdo and Burnett, 1992).
- Better education of health professionals

on drug prescribing for the elderly, aimed at minimizing polypharmacy (Cartwright and Smith, 1988), and reducing the number of prescriptions for hypnotics and tranquilizers.

• Better education of health professionals on the presentation and management of disease in old age, and the role of rehabilitation in the care of the elderly (Campbell, 1992).

BONE STRENGTH

INTRODUCTION

Osteoporosis is defined pathologically as a decreased amount of bone. Osteoporotic bones are weaker than average, and the importance of osteoporosis lies in its predisposition to fractures. Risk factors for the development of osteoporosis are:

• early menopause
• White or Asian race
• lean build
• high alcohol intake
• current or recent corticosteroid therapy
• smoking
• inactivity

The three main fracture sites associated with the condition are hip (proximal femur), wrist (distal forearm) and spine (vertebral bodies). By extreme old age, one of every three women and one of every six men will have sustained a fracture of the hip. Fractures can produce considerable pain and disability; fracture of the proximal femur leads to death in 12 to 20% of cases. In addition to the social costs, the economic costs of fractures are considerable. For example, figures from the United States estimate that the cost of care for hip fracture patients is $5 billion per year.

For patients with clinically overt osteoporosis, it has proved difficult to provide therapy which restores bone mass to a degree sufficient to significantly reduce the risk of recurrent fractures. Early prevention of bone loss seems the most rational approach to fracture prevention in the older population. The tendency to fall does, of course, ensure that fractures will continue to occur among the elderly despite any increases in bone strength. However, there are a number of measures which, if introduced widely in the population, would substantially reduce the incidence of fractures due to osteoporosis. These will be discussed in turn.

EXERCISE

Inactivity, such as prolonged bed rest and exposure to zero gravity, will result in excessive loss of bone mass. This is due both to a reduction in bone formation and to an increase in resorption. Very active individuals on the other hand, such as athletes or workers in physically demanding jobs, have a greater bone mass than sedentary people. The mechanical stresses of weight-bearing stimulate osteoblast function, so load-bearing is an important stimulus to the skeleton. As muscle mass and bone mass are directly related, it is tempting to propose that increasing muscle mass might prevent postmenopausal osteoporosis (Doyle, Brown and Lachance, 1970).

Exercise can increase the bone density in premenopausal women. One study grouped healthy premenopausal women according to high and low calcium intakes, and high and low customary physical activity levels. A higher vertebral body bone density was demonstrated in the high exercise and high calcium group (Kanders, Dempster and Lindsay, 1988). This interesting finding has not been replicated elsewhere (Stevenson *et al.*, 1989). It is not established whether altering habitual physical activity levels in favour of increasing exercise levels in premenopausal adults will increase their bone density. On the other hand, extreme exercise programes in female athletes may produce amenorrhea reflecting hypothalamic hypogonadism. Such women have considerably lower bone density values than athletes with regular menstrual periods.

Several trials of exercise programs in postmenopausal women have increased bone density, reversing the normal postmenopausal loss seen in control groups. As little as 30 minutes daily walking, jogging or dancing reduces bone loss (Chow, Harrison and Notarius, 1987). One hour of walking twice a week for 8 months led to a 3.5% increase in mineral content of the lumbar spine compared with a decrease of 2.7% in controls. This is about half the effect reported with estrogens (Munk-Jensen *et al.*, 1988). Physical fitness is also related to bone density in both the spine and the femoral neck (Pocock *et al.*, 1986).

The methodological difficulties of studying exercise interventions should not be underestimated. 'Exercise' is a broad term which covers a multitude of activities, only some of which stimulate bone formation. Although weight-bearing exercise is preferable, it has still to be established precisely which types of exercise programs will have the greatest benefit to the skeleton. Of course, there are other benefits of exercise for older individuals, including increases in muscle strength, postural stability, flexibility and cardiovascular fitness (McMurdo and Burnett, 1992; Shephard, 1990).

Reduction in habitual physical activity levels are considered by some to be the reason for the doubling of the age-related rates of hip fracture over the past 30 years. Although no evidence yet exists, it has been estimated that regular exercise could reduce the risk of hip fracture by half (Law, Wald and Meade, 1991).

HORMONE REPLACEMENT THERAPY

Peak bone mass is attained during the third decade and is a major determinant of bone mass in later life. Following the attainment of peak bone mass, there may be a period of some years during which bone mass is maintained until the onset of age-related bone loss. During and after the menopause, increased rates of bone loss occur, particularly in trabecular bone. Although there is considerable biological variability in rates of bone loss among normal women, the question of whether there is a distinct subpopulation of 'fast losers' is controversial.

The precise effect of estrogen deficiency on bone is unclear. It may modulate the actions of calcitonin and parathyroid hormone, in addition to having a direct influence on bone cells via bone estrogen receptors.

Bone mass is but one of several factors influencing fracture risk, but hormone replacement therapy (HRT) is associated with a major reduction in fracture risk. Trials of up to ten years duration have shown that estrogen substantially prevents postmenopausal bone loss (Munk-Jensen *et al.*, 1988). Observational studies have also shown that estrogen protects against hip fracture, with a median reduction in fracture rate of 50%. Combined preparations of estrogen and progestogen have not been in use long enough to provide information on the risk of hip fracture, but it is anticipated that a preventive effect is likely (Hunt and Vessey, 1987).

It remains controversial whether the period of say five or ten years of HRT results in a long-term advantage in diminished risk. However, on the available evidence, HRT is the most effective means of preventing postmenopausal osteoporosis.

Concerns about its safety have discouraged many patients and doctors from using HRT. Endometrial cancer has attracted the widest publicity, but breast cancer must also be considered. Further studies are in progress but any increase in risk of breast cancer appears to be small (Mack *et al.*, 1976). An increased risk of endometrial cancer has been shown to exist if unopposed estrogen is used, and this has led to the introduction of cyclical progestogen-opposed estrogen therapies. Balanced against these fears must be placed growing evidence for a protective effect of estrogen against cardiovascular disease (Bush *et al.*, 1983).

STOPPING SMOKING

Female cigarette smokers tend to have an earlier menopause, and a lower bone density than their non-smoking counterparts. Smoking accelerates the rate of postmenopausal bone loss and increases the risk of osteoporosis two-fold (Krall and Dawson-Hughes, 1991). Both high alcohol intake (see below) and cigarette smoking appear to have a direct toxic effect on bone cells.

As the prevalence of cigarette smoking has increased among older women in the past few decades, smoking is likely to have been a contributory factor to the doubling of the incidence of hip fracture. The relative risk for vertebral body fractures is threefold in cigarette smokers (Cooper and Wickham, 1990).

The potential for doctors to advise about smoking is considerable. Only one-third of smokers acknowledge having been advised by doctors to stop smoking, but most claim that they would make a serious attempt to do so if advised by their doctors (Marsh and Matheson, 1983). Powerful motivating factors to stop smoking include pressure from the mass media, public campaigns, tobacco tax increases, restriction on smoking in public places and other social pressures. Advice and support from health professionals is also a key element.

ALCOHOL

High or even moderate alcohol intake is associated with reduced bone density and a considerably increased risk of hip fracture (Rico, 1990). Moderate alcohol consumption is associated with an increased risk of hip fracture, although this may simply be due to alcohol making a fall more likely (Law, Walde and Meade, 1991).

Education about alcohol faces a difficult challenge (Cust, 1990). Consumption of alcohol is widely enjoyed, and is successfully portrayed as attractive and glamorous by the advertising industry. General advice to reduce intake to safe levels (14 units per week for women, 21 for men) is met with indifference and incredulity by many. It is possible that the present promotion of low alcohol beverages may succeed in reducing consumption in some people.

CALCIUM SUPPLEMENTATION

The major source of dietary calcium in the United Kingdom is dairy produce, which contributes 60–70% of the total intake. Other important sources are cereals, sardines, broccoli and spinach.

The relative importance of dietary calcium in the pathogenesis of osteoporosis is controversial. The most widely quoted work purporting to show a relation between calcium intake and bone mass and fracture has, many believe, been misinterpreted. Two village communities in Yugoslavia were compared, one with a relatively high calcium intake, and the other a lower calcium intake (Matkovic *et al.*, 1979). A dramatically lower femoral fracture rate in the high intake village suggested that lifelong high calcium consumption might reduce the fracture increase with age. There was no difference in the rate of forearm fractures between the two communities. Clearly shown in the paper, but not commented upon by the authors was the finding that where calcium intake was higher the energy intake was also higher. Lower energy intake in a population with similar body weight indicates less physical activity, and diminished physical activity is a factor affecting skeletal mass.

Another study examined the relationship

between calcium intake, physical activity and bone mass in young women (Kanders, Dempster and Lindsay, 1988). Physical activity and a high calcium intake were independently associated with a higher lumbar spine bone mass, and calcium intake also had a significant effect on radial bone mass. It appears therefore that dietary calcium during bone growth is a determinant of peak bone mass.

Dietary calcium is thought to have little effect on the rapid bone loss seen in the decade following the menopause. The efficiency of calcium absorption from the bowel declines with advancing age, and if uncompensated may lead to further bone loss. Elderly people not only have a reduced calcium absorption, but also an impaired ability to increase the calcium absorption in response to a low calcium diet. Calcium requirements for middle-aged and older women may therefore be substantially higher than those for young adults.

Calcium supplements are the most widely used medication prescribed for symptomatic osteoporosis. Calcium supplementation appears to have a beneficial effect on reducing the rate of cortical bone loss in older women (Smith, Reddan and Smith, 1981), although the role of calcium supplementation in prevention of fractures is unclear. Some studies have suggested that they may reduce the incidence of vertebral deformation, although the design of the trials has been criticized (Kanis, 1984). No information is available on the effects of calcium supplementation on femoral fracture rates in osteoporotic women. Calcium may have a protective role as cortical bone mass is a predictor of the risk of femoral fracture

Dietary calcium supplements are no substitute for HRT, but may be useful in the treatment of established osteoporosis (Francis, 1989). It is recommended that postmenopausal women not receiving HRT should have a total calcium intake from diet and supplement of 1500 mg daily.

STRATEGIES FOR PREVENTION OF OSTEOPOROSIS

- Promotion of physical activity. There is a need for health professionals to take a lead in promoting physical activity in middle-aged and older people. In old age, exercise helps to make the most of diminishing physical capacity. The provision of appropriate information and facilities has resource implications for the community.
- Hormone replacement therapy. HRT delays the onset of the accelerated rate of bone loss at the menopause, and reduces the risk of subsequent fracture.
- Smoking and alcohol. Stopping smoking cigarettes before the menopause should reduce the risk of subsequent fracture by about a quarter. Moderate alcohol consumption is associated with an increased risk of hip fracture. Controls on the cost, availability, and advertising of alcohol and tobacco products together with vigorous public education programs may reduce consumption.
- Calcium intake. Dietary calcium intake may be an important factor in the attainment of peak bone mass, but only a minor determinant of the subsequent rate of bone loss. As the efficiency of calcium absorption declines with age, an adequate intake of calcium should be maintained in older patients with established osteoporosis.

REFERENCES

Automobile Association Foundation for Road Safety Research (1989) *Motoring and the Older Driver*, A.A. Basingstoke.
Bradshaw, M.J. and Edwards, R.T.M. (1986)

Postural hypotension-pathophysiology and management. *Q. J. Med.*, **60**, 643–57.

Bush, T.L., Cowan, I.D., Barrett-Connor, E. *et al.* (1983) Estrogen use and all-cause mortality. *J. Am. Med. Assoc.*, **2498**, 903–6.

Campbell, A.J. (1992) Role of rehabilitation in fall recovery and prevention. *Rev. Clin. Gerontol.*, **2**, 53–65.

Cartwright, A. and Smith, C. (1988) *Elderly people, their Medicines and their Doctors*, Routledge, London.

Chow, A., Harrison, J.E. and Notarius, C. (1987) Effect of two randomised exercise programmes on mass of healthy postmenopausal women. *Br. Med. J.*, **63**, 780–7.

Cooper, C. and Wickham, C. (1990) Cigarette smoking and the risk of age-related fractures, in *Smoking and Hormone-Related Disorders* (eds N.J. Wald and J. Baron), Oxford University Press, Oxford, pp. 93–100.

Cullinan, T. (1986) *Visual Disability in the Elderly*, Croom Helm, London.

Cust, G. (1990) Health education about alcohol in the Tyne Tees area, in *Aspects of Alcohol and Drug Dependence* (eds T.S. Madden *et al.*), Pitman Medical, Turnbridge Wells.

Doyle, F.H., Brown, J. and Lachance, C. (1970) Relation between bone mass and muscle weight. *Lancet*, **i**, 391–3.

Francis, R.M. (1989) *The Calcium Controversy. Osteoporosis 1990*. Royal College of Physicians, London.

Garfield, J. (1992) Issues in neurosurgery. *Rev. Clin. Gerontol.*, **2**, 21–30.

Gray, B. (1966) *Home Accidents and Older People*, Royal Society for the Prevention of Accidents, London.

Guimares, R.M. and Isaacs, B. (1980) Characteristics of the gait in old people who fall. *Int. Rehab. Med.*, **2**, 177–80.

Hakim, A. and Adams, R.D. (1965) The special clinical problem of symptomatic hydrocephalus with normal cerebro-spinal fluid pressure. *J. Neurol. Sci.* **2**, 207–310.

Hunt, K. and Vessey, M. (1987) Long-term effects of postmenopausal hormone therapy. *Br. J. Hosp. Med.*, **38**, 450–3, 456–60.

Isaacs, B. (1985) Falls, in *Practical Geriatric Medicine* (eds A.N. Exton-Smith and M.E. Weksler), Churchill Livingstone, Edinburgh.

Kanders, B. Dempster, D.W. and Lindsay, R. (1988) Interaction of calcium nutrition and physical activity on bone mass in young women. *J. Bone Min. Res.* **3**, 145–9.

Kanis, J.A. (1984) Treatment of osteoporotic fracture. *Lancet*, **i**, 27–33.

Krall, E.A. and Dawson-Hughes, B (1991) Smoking and bone loss among post-menopausal women. *J. Bone Miner. Res.*, **6**, 331–7.

Law, M.R., Wald, N.J. and Meade, T.W. (1991) Strategies for prevention of osteoporosis and hip fracture. *Br. Med. J.*, **303**, 453–9.

Livesley, B. and Atkinson, L. (1974) Repeated falls in the elderly. *Mod. Geriat.*, **11**, 458–67.

Lucht, U. (1971) A prospective study of accidental falls and resulting injuries in the home among elderly people. *Acta. Soc. Med. Scand.*, **2**, 105–20.

Lye, M. and Vargas, E. (1983) Postural hypotension, in *Geriatric Heart Disease* (ed. E.L. Coodley), PSG Publishing, Littleton, Massachusetts, pp. 189–200.

Mack, T.M. Pike, M.C. Henderson, B.E. *et al.* (1976) Estrogens and endometrial cancer in a retirement community. *N. Eng. J. Med.*, **294**, 1262–7.

Marsh, A. and Matheson, J. (1983) *Smoking Attitudes and Behaviour*, HMSO, London.

Martin, J.P. (1967) Role of the vestibular system in the control of posture and movement in man, in *Myotatic, Kinesthetic and Vestibular Mechanisms* (eds A.V.S. de Reuck and J. Knight), Ciba Foundation Symposium, Churchill, London, pp. 92–6.

Matkovic, V., Kostial, K., Simonovic, I. *et al.* (1979) Bone status and fracture rates in two regions of Yugoslavia. *Am. J. Clin. Nutri.*, **32**, 540–9.

McMurdo, M.E.T. and Baines, P.S. (1988) The detection of visual disability in the elderly. *Health Bull.*, **46**, 327–9.

McMurdo, M.E.T. and Burnett, L (1992) A controlled trial of exercise in the elderly. *Gerontol.*, **38**, 292–8.

McMurdo, M.E.T. and Gaskell, G (1991) Dark adaptation and falls in the elderly. *Gerontol.*, **37**, 221–4.

Munk-Jensen, N., Nielsen, S.P., Obel, E.B. and Eriksen, P.B. (1988) Reversal of postmenopausal osteoporosis by oestrogen and progestogen:

a double blind placebo controlled study. *Br. Med. J.*, **296**, 1150–2.

Murray, M.P., Seireg, A.A. and Sepic, S.B. (1975) Normal postural stability and steadiness: quantitative assessment. *J. Bone Joint Surg.* **57A**, 510–6.

Nayak, U.S.L., Gabell, A., Simons, M.A. and Isaacs, B. (1982) Measurement of gait and balance in the elderly. *J. Am. Geriatr. Soc.*, **30**, 516–20.

Office of population census and surveys (1990) *Deaths from Accidents and Violence*, OPCS Monitor Series DH4, London.

Overstall, P.W. (1980) Prevention of falls in the elderly. *J. Am. Geriatr. Soc.*, **30**, 516–20.

Overstall, P.W. (1985) Balance and falls, in *Neurological Problems in the Elderly* (ed. M. Hildick-Smith), Baillière Tindall, London.

Overstall, P.W., Exton-Smith, A.N., Imms, F.J. and Johnson, A.L. (1977) Falls in the elderly related to postural imbalance. *Brit. Med. J.*, **1**, 261–4.

Pocock, N.A., Eisman, J.A., Yeates, M.G. *et al.* (1986) Physical fitness is a major determinant of femoral neck fracture and lumbar spine bone mineral density. *J. Clin. Invest.* **78**, 618–21.

Prudham, D. and Evans, J.G. (1991) Factors associated with falls in the elderly: a community study. *Age Ageing*, **10**, 21–33.

Rico, H. (1990) Alcohol and bone disease. *Alcohol*, **25**, 345–52.

Shephard R.J. (1990) The scientific basis of exercise prescribing for the very old. *J. Am. Geriatr. Soc.* **38**; 62–70.

Smith, E.L. Reddan, W. and Smith, P.E. (1981) Physical activity and calcium modalities for bone mineral increase in aged women. *Med. Sci. Sports Med.* **13**; 60–4.

Stevenson, J.C., Lees, B., Devenport, M. *et al.* (1989) Determinants of bone density in normal women: risk factors for future osteoporosis? *Br. Med. J.* **298**; 924–8.

Taylor, I.C. and Stout, R.W. (1983) Is ambulatory electrocardiography a useful investigation in elderly people with 'funny turns'? *Age Ageing*, **12**; 211–16.

Wyke, B (1979) Cervical articular contributions to posture and gait: their relation to senile disequilibrium. *Age Ageing*, **8**; 251–8.

Wild, D., Nayak, U.S.L. and Isaacs, B. (1981) Prognosis of falls in old people at home. *J. Epid. Commun. Health*, **35**; 200.

Williamson, J. Smith, R.G. and Burley, L.E. (1987) Falls; in: *Primary Care of the Elderly. A Practical Approach*, John Wright, Bristol T, pp. 36–54.

FURTHER READING

Muir-Gray, J.A. (ed.) (1985) *Prevention of disease in the elderly*, Churchill Livingstone, Edinburgh.

Royal College of Physicians (1991) *Preventive Medicine*, a report of the Royal College of Physicians, London.

Royal College of Physicians (1991) *Medical Aspects of Exercise. Benefits and Risks*, a report of the Royal College of Physicians London.

Smith, R. (ed.) (1989) *Osteoporosis 1990*, Royal College of Physicians London.

2

Assessment and anesthesia

FERGUS MILLAR and WILLIAM MACRAE

INTRODUCTION

As the population of the developed world ages, anesthetists will find that their workload increasingly involves elderly patients. This is especially true for orthopedic services, whose patients will range from the frail and cachectic person with a pathological fracture, to those who, although old, are still very active members of society. Looking after this group of patients, and giving them the very highest standard of care, is both interesting and rewarding.

The elderly patient does present special problems to the health care team. The process of aging affects all systems, and therefore all the staff who look after old people should be aware of the main changes that occur. This chapter starts by reviewing the changes that principally affect the conduct of anesthesia. Next, pharmacology in the elderly is dealt with and then concurrent illness and medication is discussed. Preoperative assessment and investigations are obviously important and are covered next. The choice of anesthetic technique and its conduct is discussed briefly. Finally postoperative care and analgesia are considered.

Skeletal Trauma in Old Age
Published in 1994 by Chapman & Hall, London
ISBN 0 412 48750 0

PHYSIOLOGICAL CHANGES OF AGING RELEVANT TO ANESTHESIA

CARDIOVASCULAR SYSTEM

Aging affects both the heart and the peripheral circulation. The heart contains fewer active myocardial fibres and an increased amount of fat, collagen and elastin. The collagen itself changes with time to become less elastic. There may also be amyloid deposits. The effect on the heart is to make it stiffer, therefore less easy to fill during diastole and to empty during systole. The sino-atrial node loses cells with age and the conducting system from the sino-atrial node to the ventricles is prone to fibrosis. This makes dysrhythmias more common, in particular sick sinus syndrome and heart block. Valvular disease increases with age, although the decline in the incidence of rheumatic fever means that fewer cases may be seen in the future. The mitral valve is most commonly affected, either because of degeneration of the valve ring or papillary muscle dysfunction. Aortic sclerosis is common, but of little functional importance. Aortic stenosis however can be serious, as it imposes a limit on cardiac output. The coronary arteries are liable to both atheroma and sclerosis. This reduces coronary blood flow which is further reduced by a stiff ventricle's inability to relax fully during diastole.

These changes are reflected in a reduction of both resting and maximal cardiac output with age. A reduced resting cardiac output may not cause problems, but a reduced maximal cardiac output will limit exercise tolerance. With a reduced myocardial reserve, it takes little further reduction in myocardial performance to produce symptoms at rest or on mild exertion. This has implications for anesthesia, as many anesthetic agents depress myocardial function.

In the peripheral circulation, aging is accompanied by a reduction of smooth muscle, degeneration of elastin and an increase in calcium ions in the blood vessel walls. This leads to fibrotic, inelastic arteries, which neither constrict nor dilate. This can interfere with baroreceptor function and therefore the control of blood pressure. The administration of intravenous fluids may increase blood pressure due to the inelastic nature of the vessel walls. Blood pressure normally increases in the elderly to around 160/90.

RESPIRATORY SYSTEM

The respiratory system becomes less efficient with age. The chest wall is less compliant and the muscles of inspiration (diaphragm, intercostals and accessory muscles) are weaker. The lung parenchyma loses some of its elastic recoil and the whole system is less compliant. These changes affect lung dynamics. The vital capacity decreases, the residual volume increases, functional residual capacity rises slightly but the tidal volume is unchanged. There is therefore a reduction in inspiratory and expiratory reserve volumes. Probably the most significant problem is that the closing capacity increases. When this equals functional residual capacity (FRC), small airways start to close during normal breathing. When the closing capacity exceeds FRC, air trap-

ping occurs, which causes intrapulmonary shunting of blood. The closing capacity equals the FRC in the supine position at 45 years of age and in the upright position at 65 years. Both the physiological and anatomical dead spaces increase, so that there is reduced alveolar ventilation for a given tidal volume.

These changes have several deleterious effects. The ability to cough is reduced and the possibility of atelectasis increases as the closing capacity increases. Although $PaCO_2$ remains unchanged, arterial PaO_2 falls with advancing age. By the age of 80 the PaO_2 may have fallen to around 10.7 kPa (80 mmHg).

NERVOUS SYSTEM

From the age of 25 we start to lose nerve cells in our brains and spinal cords, so that by the age of 70 the brain weighs 7% less. The amount of myelin is reduced, the rate of neurotransmitter production falls and the cerebral blood flow decreases. Nerve conduction velocity is reduced. The special sense organs become less efficient. Cataracts impair vision, hearing is less acute and there is a diminished ability to smell and taste. Brain function may be affected by dementia, Parkinson's disease, cerebrovascular disease, drugs and hypoxia. A lack of sensory and intellectual stimulation will accelerate any functional deterioration, so that a dreary hospital ward may be the final insult to an old and tired brain. It is important to seek and treat any reversible cause in a confused elderly patient, and not just to label them as 'a demented old dear'.

RENAL SYSTEM

Renal function deteriorates with age. By the age of 70, the weight of the kidneys has fallen by 30%, and the glomerular filtration rate is 70% of that of a young adult. The cortex is affected more than the medulla. The total number of nephrons falls and this, combined with a thickening of Bowman's capsule and a reduced renal blood flow, leads to a reduced glomerular filtration rate and creatinine clearance. There is a reduction in tubular function and the collecting ducts are less responsive to anti-diuretic hormone.

Despite these changes there are sufficient reserves of renal function to cope with the normal metabolic demands of the elderly patient. The stress of a fracture or intercurrent illness will impose demands that reveal inadequate renal function. Hypovolemia, hypoxia, fat embolus and drugs such as non-steroidal anti-inflammatory drugs (NSAIDs)) can all cause renal damage.

ENDOCRINE AND METABOLIC SYSTEMS

The elderly patient tends to lose weight, with lean body mass being most affected, causing a proportional increase in fat. A reduction in basal metabolic rate (BMR) of about 20%, combined with reduced activity means that the calorific requirements of the elderly are less. A combination of a reduced BMR and a reduced ability to vasoconstrict leads to an increased risk of hypothermia. Despite a reduced BMR and a slightly negative nitrogen balance, it is important that these patients receive a proper balanced diet with enough calories, protein, fatty acids, vitamins and minerals. Dehydration is common in the elderly and adequate fluid intake is essential. The elderly have a reduced sense of smell and taste, so food is less appetizing and they can become cachectic. Gastrointestinal tract function is reduced, with an increased incidence of malabsorption. Liver functional reserve is reduced, therefore any liver damage may have grave consequences.

Diabetes mellitus is commoner in the elderly and is characterized mainly by insulin resistance. The renal threshold for glucose appearing in the urine is unpredictable, often higher, so that urine testing in the elderly is not a reliable diabetes screen. Thyroid dysfunction is common and often presents atypically.

LOCOMOTOR SYSTEM

Muscle fibres waste, the skin atrophies and loses collagen. A combination of nervous system dysfunction, muscle wastings and arthritis reduces the mobility and co-ordination of the elderly patient. Reduced mobility and strength may prolong post-operative recovery. The skin is prone to pressure sores and to damage during anesthesia. Some diseases of the locomotor system, like rheumatoid or osteoarthritis, can make the conduct of anesthesia difficult, especially if these cause cervical spine pathology.

CONSEQUENCES OF PHYSIOLOGICAL CHANGES FOR OLD PEOPLE WITH FRACTURES

Tissue oxygenation is dependent on three factors: cardiac output, hemoglobin and oxygen saturation. From the above sections it will be seen that in elderly people, the ability to maintain both an adequate cardiac output and oxygen saturation is compromised. At rest and in normal health, the patient may be well oxygenated, but because they have very little or no reserve, any stress which increases the body's oxygen demands can result in hypoxia.

Fractures produce several important physiological changes. First there will be blood loss, which may vary from the trivial to the life-threatening. Blood loss has two important effects. It reduces circulating volume, which by diminishing venous return will cause a decrease in cardiac output. Fit young people can, to some extent, compensate for this by increasing heart rate and constricting peripheral vasculature. Old patients will not be able to compensate as well. The second effect of blood loss is to cause a fall in hemoglobin. This will decrease the oxygen carrying capacity of the blood.

Major fractures are often associated with fat embolism. Although the full clinical picture of fat embolism may not be present, pulmonary and renal function may well be affected. Pain produces a cascade of physiological changes that we are only now beginning to understand. As a result of their fracture many patients will be confined to bed for a period. This brings with it the risks of deep venous thrombosis, hypostatic pneumonia and pressure sores.

It will be seen therefore that old people with fractures need to be treated in the same way as all victims of trauma, however, because of the changes in their physiology, special attention must be focused on their particular problems. Although the orthopedic surgeon will be, quite appropriately, focusing attention on the management of the broken bones, this must not compromise the care of the whole patient. The administration of oxygen, analgesics and the replacement of fluid, possibly with blood, must be seen as priorities. It is for these reasons that investigations such as full blood count, urea, electrolytes and creatinine are important and the results must be acted upon. Appropriate investigations will be discussed later.

PHARMACOLOGY

As noted above, there are some physiological changes of age which will alter the way drugs affect the elderly. The reduction in hepatic and renal efficiency and changes in total body water, fat and muscle all contribute to changes in drug handling. As these physiological changes vary from patient to patient, there is immense variation in drug response and incidence of side-effects in the elderly population. Reduced renal function can cause accumulation of renally excreted drugs, for example digoxin and some muscle relaxants. Reduced hepatic function causes similar problems, for example diazepam has a half-life up to four times longer in the elderly. Reduced hepatic blood flow prolongs and increases the action of drugs which have extensive first-pass metabolism, for example popranolol.

It would appear that the elderly can also have altered pharmacodynamics (response to a drug). For example there is reduced adrenergic receptor density and sensitivity and this reduces the response to catecholamines and sympathomimetic drugs.

Elderly patients are often taking several drugs and, as a result, they may not only suffer from the unwanted effects of individual drugs, but also from drug interactions. It is important that those caring for the elderly prescribe drugs carefully and rationally and review current medication to avoid unnecessary drug prescription. A wise precaution is to give small incremental doses until the desired effect is obtained.

THE ANESTHETIC IMPLICATIONS OF COMMON DISEASES AND THEIR TREATMENT

CARDIOVASCULAR DISEASES

Hypertension is common (30–40%) and is usually defined as a BP greater than 160/90 mmHg. Any patient with hypertension is at increased risk of ischemic heart disease (IHD), renal damage and peripheral and cerebro-vascular disease. If the diastolic pressure is more than 100 units advice should be sought, and anti-hypertensive therapy considered, at least for the period of surgery. The blood pressure should be controlled adequately before elective surgery takes place. ECG abnormalities may be found in approximately half of patients over age 75 and 9.1% of elderly surgical patients suffer from congestive heart failure, myocardial infarction or angina. Ischemic heart disease is common amongst the elderly but may be asymptomatic. Patients with ischemic heart disease are at increased risk of perioperative myocardial infarction, which carries a high mortality.

Valvular heart disease is becoming less common with the reduced incidence of rheumatic fever. It has important implications for the anesthetist, as valve lesions significantly alter the heart's function. Diastolic murmurs are likely to be functionally important. Systolic murmurs may be functionally important, particularly that of aortic stenosis. Aortic stenosis has severe implications for patient management and may be distinguished from aortic sclerosis by ECG and BP. If there is doubt about a murmur then a cardiological opinion may be of value. Patients with heart failure have an increased perioperative mortality and any failure should be treated preoperatively if possible.

Dysrhythmias, especially atrial fibrillation, are commoner in the elderly and this can be either a result of IHD or the physiological process of aging causing fibrosis of the conducting system. Most dysrhythmias cause a reduction in cardiac efficiency and may cause congestive cardiac failure (CCF). Some patients have pacemakers and the type should be identified and its function checked by ECG. Changes in acid–base balance and potassium can alter the myocardial response to the pacemaker. Advice from a cardiologist should be sought if there is any doubt about pacemaker function.

Peripheral vascular and cerebro-vascular disease are common and it is important to maintain blood flow to essential organs, especially the brain. Blood flow, already compromised by vessel disease, can be reduced even further if the cardiac output falls, for example due to hemorrhage or anesthetic drugs.

Cardiovascular drugs

The drugs used to treat cardiovascular disease can have important implications for the anesthetist. Diuretics are used to treat hypertension and CCF. As a consequence of their action, dehydration and electrolyte imbalance can occur. Dehydration can cause hypotension especially in conjunction with anesthesia, whilst electrolyte imbalances can cause dysrhythmias and alter muscle relaxant effects.

Beta blockers are used for angina and hypertension. They are myocardial depressants and in the presence of some anesthetic agents, a profound reduction in cardiac output can occur. They may also worsen chronic obstructive airways disease (COAD), peripheral vascular disease and CCF.

Nitrates are used for the treatment of angina and CCF and work by causing vasodilatation (especially veins) and thereby reducing ventricular filling and work. However, blood pressure may fall causing postural hypotension.

Calcium channel blockers, for example verapamil and nifedipine, are used for angina and dysrhythmias. They cause vasodilatation, act on the atrio-ventricular node and are negatively inotropic. Verapamil and beta blockers together can precipitate CCF and heart block.

Digoxin is commonly prescribed in the elderly, usually to treat atrial fibrillation. It has a low therapeutic ratio, so toxicity can be a problem, particularly in patients with renal impairment. Digoxin toxicity causes anorexia, nausea, vomiting, diarrhea and dysrhythmias, including ventricular tachycardia. It is important to check digoxin levels and to avoid hypokalemia (c.f. diuretics) which potentiates digoxin toxicity.

Warfarin and other oral anticoagulants may be encountered in patients with a history of deep venous thrombosis, pulmonary embolism or valvular disease. Anticoagulation has implications for both surgery and anesthesia. Clotting activity must be measured before any decisions can be made. Patients who are fully anticoagulated and require urgent surgery can have their clotting partially corrected by administration of fresh frozen plasma. The use of vitamin K to reverse warfarin effects cannot be recommended, as it makes subsequent anticoagulation difficult.

RESPIRATORY DISORDERS

The elderly, with impaired respiratory function and reduced mobility, are prone to chest infections. General anesthesia and pain, with depression of respiration and reduced ciliary function, will make matters worse. It is important therefore to treat any chest infection, with antibiotics and chest physiotherapy.

Chronic obstructive airways disease (COAD) is common and can be detected clinically and confirmed using simple spirometry. COAD impairs lung function resulting in hypoxia and possibly hypercarbia.

Carcinoma of the lung is relatively common and may present as hemoptysis or recurrent chest infections. More rarely it presents with ectopic hormone production such as ACTH or ADH. Impaired respiratory function, altered electrolytes and the effects of the tumor and its metastases can influence the timing and type of anesthesia.

It is important to remember that left ventricular failure can cause respiratory problems and this should be looked for in any elderly patient with respiratory symptoms. Many other diseases, e.g. rheumatoid arthritis, can also cause respiratory disease. Tuberculosis is relatively rare but is more common in the elderly and should not be forgotten. Further information can be obtained from pulmonary function tests – principally a distinction between a restrictive (e.g. pulmonary fibrosis) and an obstructive (asthma) defect and the response of an obstructive defect to bronchodilator therapy. An assessment of exercise tolerance and blood gases give further valuable information.

Respiratory drugs

Bronchodilators are commonly used to treat respiratory disease and can be classified into two broad groups, sympathomimetics and corticosteroids.

Sympathomimetic drugs can be further divided into the adrenergic agonists and the theophyllines. The adrenergic agonists act at the receptor to cause bronchodilation. These drugs can be given orally, parenterally and by inhalation. At higher doses, they can cause toxicity, namely tachycardia and tremor, especially if given intravenously. Theophyllines are sympathomimetics but do not act via the adrenergic receptor. These drugs are given orally or parenterally. Being sympathomimetic they can cause tachycardia, nausea, palpitations, arrhythmias, convulsions and hypokalemia.

Corticosteroids probably work by reducing inflammation of the bronchial mucosa. Steroids have serious side-effects, which include osteoporosis, adrenal suppression, immune depression, hypokalemia, altered protein metabolism with myopathy, sodium and water retention and diabetes. The systemic effects of inhaled steroids are less, but adrenal suppression can occur with high-dose inhaled steroids. Due to their effect on metabolism and electrolytes, appropriate investigations are required. However, the most important aspect is the adrenal suppression. During the stress of the perioperative period there is normally a surge in glucocorticoid secretion which will be absent in the presence of adrenal suppression. This can result in an Addisonian crisis with hypotension, hyponatremia and hypoglycemia. Steroid replacement therapy is required.

NERVOUS SYSTEM DISORDERS

There are many intra- and extra-cranial causes for CNS dysfunction. Some are sadly iatrogenic. It is important therefore to rule out easily reversible causes, e.g. hypoxia, drugs, infection and electrolyte disturbance.

Cerebrovascular disease is common in the elderly and can cause a varying degree of dysfunction ranging from a stroke to transient ischemic attacks. It is important to maintain a supply of oxygenated blood to the brain and therefore hypoxia and hypotension must be avoided.

Parkinson's disease occurs in 1 in 200 of patients older than 70 years. The disease is characterized by tremor, rigidity, akinesia, and emotional lability. Fractures amongst these patients are common. Treatment is with either anticholinergics (benzhexol, orphenadrine) or by levodopa. The anticholinergics pose few anesthetic problems but levodopa can cause nausea, vomiting, hypertension and tachycardia.

The sudden cessation of therapy in a Parkinson's patient can lead to rebound symptoms with increased rigidity, including chest wall rigidity. Therapy should not be stopped for any longer than necessary. Some drugs can exacerbate Parkinson's disease, particularly dopamine antagonists such as major tranquilizers (chlorpromazine) and the antiemetics (metoclopramide and prochlorperazine). Deleterious effects may last for several months. Cyclizine is an alternative antiemetic.

Dementia is common in the elderly, occurring in about 10% of those over 65 and 20% of those over 80. Most of the causes are irreversible but it is important to realize that there are some reversible causes, for example, hypothyroidism, anemia, hypoxia.

About 25% of the elderly suffer from some sort of psychiatric disturbance, usually anxiety and depression. Hospitalization for a fracture may worsen this. The drugs used for anxiety, usually benzodiazepines, will potentiate anesthesia but can also cause confusion and a dementia-like state. Antidepressants may have important effects during anesthesia and the perioperative period. Monoamine oxidase inhibitors (MAOI) for example, phenelzine and tranylcypromine are now rarely used but can cause serious side-effects and drug interactions – for example with pethidine. The tricyclic antidepressants are more frequently used for depression and cause fewer problems than MAOIs, but may still cause an exaggerated response to sympathomimetic drugs.

RENAL DISEASE

Chronic renal failure (CRF) can be due to a number of causes especially hypertension, diabetes mellitus, prostate disease and drugs (e.g. NSAIDs). CRF is often asymptomatic and may not require treatment. Patients with CRF are often hypertensive and have ischemic heart disease. It is important that any therapy they are prescribed is continued through the perioperative period. Fractures may reduce remaining renal function, because of hypotension caused by hypovolemia, and fat embolism. The aim of treatment should be to prevent any further loss of renal function. This is best achieved by preventing or treating hypovolemia and hypoxia. In patients with long standing CRF, anemia is common and blood transfusion preoperatively should only be given after consultation with a renal physician and the anesthetist. The urea and electrolytes are usually deranged, often with a raised potassium which may need lowering either by hemodialysis or by a dextrose and insulin infusion. A high urea can cause confusion, clotting problems, nausea and vomiting.

NSAIDs can cause renal dysfunction, either acute renal failure (especially if there is some pre-existing renal disease), or chronic renal failure (analgesic nephropathy).

Dehydration can provoke NSAID-induced renal dysfunction. The combination of blood loss from a fracture and chronic dehydration may put patients taking NSAIDs at risk from pre-renal failure. If the fluid deficit is not quickly reversed, then acute tubular necrosis and renal failure can ensue.

METABOLIC AND ENDOCRINE DISEASE

The incidence of thyroid disease amongst the elderly is 1–1.5% with either hypo- or hyperthyroidism. Hyperthyroidism can cause atrial fibrillation, tachycardia, diarrhea, weight loss, angina and heart failure. If possible, hyperthyroidism should be treated prior to surgery. Hypothyroidism causes bradycardia, weight gain, cold intolerance, poor memory, constipation, anorexia and fatigue. Patients with hypothyroidism are more susceptible to anesthetic drugs and should, if possible, have replacement therapy prior to surgery.

Diabetes is of importance to the anesthetist not only for its effect on glucose metabolism but also its effects on other systems. Diabetes is a significant factor in atheroma formation with an associated increase in the incidence of ischemic heart disease. Diabetes also causes microvascular disease leading to retinopathy, nephropathy (a common cause of death) and neuropathy. Diabetics are prone to foot ulcers which are resistant to healing and may become infected or gangrenous. Since in maturity onset diabetes there is some endogenous insulin production, there may be no need for exogenous insulin. Diet can successfully control many such cases of diabetes especially if the patient is overweight.

The oral hypoglycemics can be split into two groups:

1. Sulphonyl ureas, which act by stimulating endogenous insulin release. There are a number of these available, each with a different duration of action. Chlorpropamide lasts for 36 hours and can have important implications for anesthesia and surgery and should ideally be changed to a shorter-acting drug.
2. Biguanides act by increasing the peripheral uptake of glucose. They can however cause lactic acidosis.

Insulin therapy is sometimes required for those patients who do not respond to the above. Diabetic patients presenting for surgery require close attention to their glucose control. This is best done by regular blood glucose monitoring. Non insulin dependent diabetics undergoing minor surgery should have their oral hypoglycemics withheld on the morning of surgery, their operation performed as early on the list as possible and their medication restarted with lunch. Those on insulin undergoing minor surgery should have their insulin withheld in the morning and, when eating lunch, a small dose of soluble insulin given. If eating has returned to normal, in the evening, insulin can be resumed at the usual dose.

Those patients undergoing major surgery are likely to require perioperative insulin even if they are normally diet-controlled. The stress of surgery is enough to cause hyperglycemia. For elective surgery the patient should be scheduled early on the list, and an insulin and glucose regimen commenced. There are a number of regimens available and it is best to discuss the case with the anesthetist.

Emergency surgery presents a different problem, as diabetic medication may have recently been given. It is important to prevent hypoglycemia, so a close watch on the blood glucose is essential and an infusion of glucose is required. Hyperglycemia should also be avoided as it causes a diuresis and can delay wound healing. A drowsy patient may be hypoglycemic and not suffering from an anesthetic hangover. If there is a problem with any patient, help from the anesthetist and diabetologist should be obtained.

Hypercalcemia is occasionally encountered and has many causes, the commonest ones being malignancy (breast, lung, myeloma), sarcoidosis, hyperparathyroidism, renal failure and Paget's disease. It is not surprising that hypercalcemia could be encountered in the elderly patient with a fracture. The symptoms are general malaise, depression, dehydration, nausea, vomiting, thirst, polyuria, confusion, constipation, muscle fatigue and hypotonicity. If serum calcium is above 3.5mmol/l then there is imminent danger of a cardiac arrest. Treatment includes rehydration with intravenous isotonic saline and biphosphonates. Mild hypercalemia does not require special anesthetic considerations.

DISORDERS OF THE LOCOMOTOR SYSTEM

As mentioned earlier the elderly are likely to have degenerative changes in their joints, skin, bone and muscle. Osteoarthritis is the commonest type of arthritis (and is a degenerative disease of old age) (10% of the population, 50% of those older than 60). Rheumatoid arthritis (RA) does not typically present much after age 50 but, as it often lasts for many years, there are many elderly patients who suffer from it. The degenerative changes in the neck can make intubation difficult, with a risk of spinal cord damage. Cervical spine X-rays in flexion and extension are needed to assess such cases. Locomotor system disease can make regional anesthesia difficult, positioning the patient for surgery awkward and subsequent mobilization slow. The elderly often have thin, fragile skin (excerbated by RA) making them more prone to pressure sores. Care must be taken to preserve the skin, to move joints carefully without force and to avoid compression of peripheral nerves.

INVESTIGATIONS

The history and clinical examination are the most important part of the assessment. There are many invasive and non-invasive investigations available and only the important ones will be discussed.

All elderly patients should have a chest X-ray in order to detect cardiac and lung pathology, fractured ribs, carcinoma and metastases. An electrocardiogram is required because the incidence of ischemic heart disease is high. It will also evaluate treatment of dysrhythmia and pacemaker function.

Full blood count, urea and electrolytes, and creatinine should be done routinely on all elderly patients. Many will be receiving medication which can alter electrolytes, e.g. diuretics and steroids. Asymptomatic hypercalcemia or renal failure may also be present. Anemia is common in the elderly and if found should be investigated and treated. Further investigations may be required and these should be based on the history and clinical examination. Abnormal findings must be followed up by appropriate further investigations. Investigations should be seen as an aid to optimizing perioperative care and not an attempt by the anesthetist to delay or cancel the case.

ANESTHESIA

Safe anesthesia for these patients is based on an understanding of the physiological changes in old age and a thorough pre-operative assessment. The aims of anesthesia are to provide the best possible operating conditions for the surgeon, with the minimum physiological disturbance to the patient. Modern anesthesia provides a balance of analgesia, relaxation and sleep or sedation. This can be achieved by either general anesthesia or regional anesthesia.

Anesthesia starts with the administration of drugs for pre-medication. As mentioned previously, most concurrent medication should be continued into the preoperative period. In addition sedative and analgesic drugs are often prescribed. Patients with fractures are usually in pain and analgesic drugs should not be withheld in the preoperative period. Benzodiazepines are commonly used as sedatives preoperatively to allay anxiety. A reassuring talk with the anesthetist may be more effective. The use of psychotropic drugs in the elderly can be fraught with difficulties, in particular dementia and confusional states tend to be made worse by sedative drugs.

The choice of anesthetic technique is controversial. However the outcome is influenced more by the skill with which an individual technique is used than the choice of technique itself. General anesthesia has the advantages of being reliably effective, providing an unconscious patient and being a safe technique in experienced hands. Any anesthetic is a physiological trespass, and in elderly patients, who already have reduced physiological reserves, general anesthesia is not without risk. The main problems relate to the cardiovascular and respiratory systems. Most drugs used to produce general anesthesia depress myocardial function or produce peripheral vasodilation. This results in a fall in cardiac output and a reduction in vital organ perfusion.

Respiratory problems include airways obstruction, depressed respiration, bronchospasm, altered matching of ventilation and perfusion, depressed ciliary function and altered lung dynamics (e.g. fall in FRC). All these factors, often in combination, can lead to hypoxemia, with consequent vital organ damage.

Regional anesthesia provides the necessary conditions for surgery and is ideally suited for many orthopedic procedures. It is not just confined to spinal and epidural anesthetics but includes nerve plexus blocks, peripheral nerve blocks, intravenous regional anesthesia and local infiltration. Details of individual techniques can be found in appropriate textbooks (Wildsmith and Armitage, 1987).

The effect of local anesthesia can last up to 24 hours and therefore provides excellent early postoperative analgesia. A regional technique does not require any sedative or hypnotic drugs (although these can be useful) and local anesthetics, correctly used, do not depress cardiac or respiratory function. However, regional anesthesia does require a good working knowledge of anatomy.

Simpler techniques such as fracture hematoma injection and Bier's block are often used to provide anesthesia for manipulation of fractures. Bier's block merits special mention, as it is a potentially lethal technique and should only be done by those experienced in the block and capable of dealing with the potential problems – there have been fatalities. Local anesthetic drugs are toxic if an overdose is given or there has been inadvertent intravascular injection. The signs and symptoms of toxicity include peri-oral tingling, dizziness, convulsions, coma and cardiac and respiratory arrest. For this reason any local technique must be carried out in an environment where resuscitation can be carried out. Reference to Lonsdale, Buckley and Macrae (1991) will give further information. Some methods of regional anesthesia have well-known side effects, e.g. spinals and epidural anesthetics can result in hypotension, supraclavicular and intercostal blocks can result in a pneumothorax.

There are a number of studies which suggest that spinal or epidural anesthesia for a fractured neck of femur reduces both early mortality and the incidence of deep venous thrombosis.

POSTOPERATIVE CARE AND PAIN RELIEF

Diligent work-up, assessment and intraoperative care will all be wasted if the same attention to detail is lacking in the postoperative care. This can be the most dangerous time for any patient undergoing surgery. The elderly are at greater risk as a result of their increased likelihood of systemic disease. All patients who have undergone anesthesia and surgery require close supervision. This need not entail expensive monitoring equipment but frequent recordings of pulse, BP, respiratory rate, temperature, pain intensity, wounds and drains should be charted. There is nothing to be gained by close observation if no appropriate action is taken. Hypovolemic, hypotensive patients tend to be cold and have a tachycardia (elderly patients may not be able to increase their heart rate much). Blood loss should be replaced with colloid or crystalloid initially and then blood (most patients can sustain loss of a 10–20% blood volume before requiring blood). Patients who have a spinal or epidural anesthesia can become hypotensive as result of their anesthesia (sympathetic block). In contrast with hypovolemia the patient will have warm, well perfused lower limbs, and should be treated with a sympathomimetic such as ephedrine.

If there has been prolonged surgery, significant blood loss or pre-existing renal disease then the urine output should be measured hourly. Falling urine volumes can indicate hypovolemia which can be confirmed with a fluid challenge. Not all oliguria is secondary to hypovolemia and renal failure may be present.

The elderly are not only likely to have a degree of respiratory dysfunction but are also more sensitive to anesthetic drugs and opioids. This can lead to hypoxia with potential multi-organ failure. All elderly patients should be given supplementary oxygen postoperatively. As the hypoxia can last for several days, oxygen should be given for at least twenty four hours and ideally 2–3 days.

Postoperative fluid therapy depends on the length and type of surgery, blood loss, route of administration and concurrent disease. If a patient can manage oral fluids then this is physiologically the best method. Intravenous fluid therapy can cause serious biochemical abnormalities and fluid overload, so it must be administered with care and its effects monitored. Patients on an intravenous infusion should have their biochemistry checked and a fluid balance calculated daily.

Adequate analgesia in the elderly fracture patient is essential and humane. The medical profession's failure in adequately treating acute postoperative pain is rightly criticized in the recent report by the College of Anaesthetists and the Royal College of Surgeons (September, 1990). Pain is disheartening, unpleasant, stressful and it reduces mobility. Its adequate treatment may reduce morbidity and the length of hospital stay.

There are three major groups of drugs used to treat pain – these are NSAIDs, opioids and local anesthetics. They are often used singly but can be more effective if combined. NSAIDs have anti-inflammatory, anti-pyretic and analgesic properties. They can be taken orally or parenterally and have a significant morphine sparing effect. NSAIDs are especially useful for soft tissue and bone pain, and can be effective enough to be the sole analgesic agent. They have several benefits over opioids, namely a lack of respiratory depression, nausea and constipation which make them useful agents in the elderly. They are not without problems however, causing gastric bleeding and ulceration, possible inhibition of platelet function and renal damage. These side-effects are more common in the elderly, so care must be exercised when prescribing these drugs.

Opioids are very effective at treating pain. There are a large number of opioid drugs available with parenteral and oral preparations. Of all the available opioids, none has been shown to be superior to morphine, which should probably be the drug of choice. Opioids have side-effects which include res-

23

piratory depression, nausea and vomiting, constipation, urinary retention and euphoria. There is a large inter-patient variation in the opioid requirement for analgesia. Liver and renal disease also influence opioid requirements. The elderly are more sensitive to opioids than young, fit patients and the incidence of side-effects, especially respiratory depression, is higher. There are a number of ways in which to administer opioids. The oral route is convenient but apart from the sublingual route, not always appropriate for the perioperative patient. The intramuscular (IM) route of opioid administration is commonly used. It entails multiple injections, relies on an adequate local muscle blood flow for drug uptake and is of a fixed dose. This, combined with a 'PRN' or 'as required' prescription makes the IM route far from perfect. Fixed rate infusions either subcutaneously or intravenously avoid the multiple injections and the peak and trough drug concentrations of the IM route. However with the fixed rate infusions comes the risk of gradual overdose and respiratory depression and therefore they must be closely supervised. Patient controlled analgesia (PCA) is an attempt to match opioid supply with patient demand. It comprises a patient activated, computerized infusion pump connected to the patient via an intravenous cannula. A maximum hourly rate is set by a doctor and the patient can self-administer up to that maximum. Although this is at present probably the best way to administer opioids, it is not without problems. The infusion pumps are expensive; they require patient understanding of how to use them (they are not suitable for demented or confused patients) and side-effects still occur.

Opioid side-effects can be unpleasant and dangerous, so close monitoring of patients receiving opioids by any route is mandatory. Nausea and vomiting due to opioids is common and can be treated with metoclopramide, prochlorperazine or cyclizine. Respiratory depression is dangerous and should be treated with oxygen and naloxone.

Local anesthetic techniques are a very useful and under-utilized method of providing analgesia. Spinal and epidural anesthetics are used primarily for operative anesthesia but they can provide postoperative analgesia. Spinal anesthesia provides limited postoperative analgesia as it is a single shot technique and is not usually repeated postoperatively. Epidural anesthesia can incorporate a catheter placed in the epidural (extradural) space. This can be topped up at regular intervals with local anesthetic and/or opioids. It can provide excellent postoperative analgesia in lower limb and pelvis fractures. Peripheral nerve and plexus blocks can provide operative anesthesia and good analgesia in the postoperative period. This analgesia can be prolonged by using catheter techniques, for example in the femoral nerve and brachial plexus.

Recently, there has been an upsurge of interest in acute pain and some hospitals have set up an acute pain service. This comprises a small team of doctors (usually anesthetists) and nurses who take responsibility for the relief of postoperative pain using the methods discussed above. Surgeons should never be reluctant to involve their anesthetic colleagues in the management of postoperative pain.

SUMMARY

The success of any operation depends on adequate assessment and preoperative treatment, the skill of the surgeon and anesthetist and good postoperative care. The Report of the Royal College of Physicians on fractured neck of femur (1989), in its recommendations, stressed the importance of the assessment of coexisting medical problems, mental function and social circumstances. It suggested that almost all patients should receive operative treatment within 24 hours of admission to hospital. The operation should be carried out by day, by senior orthopedic and anesthetic staff.

Elderly patients with fractures have suffered one injury and it is our duty to prevent a second injury, for example, from hypoxia or hypovolemia.

REFERENCES

Lonsdale, M. Buckley, J.R., Macrae, W.A. (1991) Local anaesthesia for the non anaesthetist. *Hospital Update*, **17** (3), 229–35.

Royal College of Physicians (1989) Fractured neck of femur. Prevention and management. Summary and recommendations of a report of the Royal College of Physicians. *J. Roy. Coll. Physic. Lond.*, **23** (1) 8–12.

The Royal College of Surgeons and The College of Anaesthetists (1990). Commission on The Provision of Surgical Services. Report of the Working Party on Pain After Surgery. September 1990.

Wildsmith, J.A.W and Armitage E.N. (1987) *Principles and Practice of Regional Anaesthesia*, Churchill Livingstone, Edinburgh.

FURTHER READING

Davenport, H.T. (1986) *Anaesthesia in the Elderly*, William Heinemann Medical Books Limited, London.

Davis, F.M. and Laurenson, V.G. (1981) Spinal Anaesthesia or General Anaesthesia for Emergency Hip Surgery in Elderly Patients. *Anaesthesia and Intensive Care*, **9** (11), 352–8.

McKenzie, P.J., Wishart, H.Y., Gray, I. and Smith, G. (1985). Effects of anaesthetic technique on deep vein thrombosis. A comparison of subarachnoid and general anaesthesia. *Br. J. Anaes.*, **57**, 853–857.

Waldmann, C. (1992) Anaesthesia for the Elderly, Chapter 11, in *Anaesthesia Review 9* (ed. L. Kaufman), Churchill Livingston, Edinburgh, pp. 194–211.

Perioperative care: The tunnel of rehabilitation

DAVID C. KENNIE

INTRODUCTION

Demographic changes within the population, the rising prevalence of many orthopedic disorders with age and the increase in age-specific incidence rates of some conditions, such as hip fracture, indicate a burgeoning workload on orthopedic departments in the years ahead. The limit to existing resources, the current stringency on health care funding and financial incentives linking payment to case volume indicate that this workload must be met, in part at least, by more rapid throughput and shortened lengths of stay.

This chapter therefore examines early discharge in the light of these concerns and discusses them with particular reference to elderly hip fracture patients who occupy a fifth of all orthopedic beds in the United Kingdom (Department of Health and Social Security, 1981).

CONFOUNDING FACTORS WHEN CONSIDERING LENGTH OF STAY

A number of factors may confound interpretation of lengths of stay. Some of the more important are as follows:

1. Reliability of the data: The first consideration must be the trustworthiness of the data. Often admission and discharge data are entered wrongly and there are even greater problems with the accuracy and completeness of diagnostic coding on which the length of stay may be based.

2. Multiple episodes of care: Lengths of stay in an orthopedic ward can be shortened by a high rate of interspecialty transfers, by transfer to 'second line' orthopedic beds or by transfer to other wards for boarding out purposes when orthopedics is full. These apparent early discharges give the appearance of efficiency when the converse may be the case.

3. The degree of segregation of elderly patients: Some orthopedic departments have a policy of segregating or partially segregating particularly frail elderly patients from their younger counterparts. Certain orthogeriatric services demonstrate this. The average length of stay in the sector dealing with the frail elderly may appear inappropriately long whilst it will be considerably foreshortened elsewhere.

4. Exclusion of data from long-term care facilities: Although most attention has focused on early discharge from hospital, the true impact of various management

Skeletal Trauma in Old Age
Published in 1994 by Chapman & Hall, London
ISBN 0 412 48750 0

policies cannot be evaluated without consideration of the additional duration of stay required for rehabilitation and long-term care. This usually takes place in other wards or facilities that, at times, have poorly developed long-term care information systems resulting in incomplete data on the totality of care required for a particular orthopedic problem. This caveat is more appropriate in health care systems that rely heavily on transference to nursing homes for ongoing care.

5. Exclusion of short stay accident and emergency cases: the average length of stay of orthopedic inpatients will be higher if some elderly patients with very short stay conditions (for example minor fractures) are admitted separately to beds attached to an accident and emergency department.
6. Population bias: Very short lengths of stay may merely reflect a high initial mortality rate or a bias towards an intake of particularly fit patients. The presence of bias is a major factor to consider when analysing results from research trials aimed at early discharge.
7. Premorbid psychosocial disorders: The source of admission (e.g. a nursing home), which influences length of stay, often merely reflects comorbidities in that population. Other factors such as the prefracture level of functioning and the social support available in the community have a considerable component that is immutable. Nevertheless, length of stay can often be shortened by active rehabilitation and the imaginative use of community services.

PATIENT FACTORS INFLUENCING LENGTH OF STAY

AGE

Although average length of stay increases with age for many orthopedic conditions, age itself may only reflect other health problems that may have a more direct effect on the duration of hospitalization. For example, median length of stay following fracture of the femur does not show a direct correlation with age (Evans, 1979), suggesting that the rising mean length of stay is determined by a small group requiring long-stay care (and who are usually suffering from dementia).

TYPE OF ORTHOPEDIC CONDITION

Length of stay obviously varies depending on the type of orthopedic problem yet may in part only reflect the characteristics of the patient group at risk of sustaining the condition. For example, the prolonged lengths of stay of patients with intertrochanteric versus intracapsular fractures of the femoral neck (Beringer, McSherry and Taggart, 1984) may merely reflect the advanced age of those afflicted and their predisposition to dementing illness.

SEVERITY OF ILLNESS

Although there is an obvious association between an orthopedic patient's length of stay and the severity of their illness, the latter is both difficult to define and measure. Severity of illness may range from the nature of the main diagnosis (e.g. a fracture may be simple or comminuted), to the impact of the main diagnosis on other organ systems (e.g. shock secondary to hemorrhage), to other comorbidities (e.g. pneumonia) or to functional disability. Numerous proprietary measures are marketed for assessing 'severity of illness'. Iezzoni (1991) provides a comprehensive review and illustrates 'severity of illness' in a case study of a fractured hip patient using eight different ratings (AIM, APACHE, Body Systems, CSI, Disease Staging, Medisgroups, PMCs and R-DRGs). Nevertheless, severity standardization results are not intended to apply at the individual case level but merely serve as statistical screening tests for substandard care. Unfortunately, little scientific information is yet available about their performance as screening instruments. Their routine use also demands a resource intensive quality assurance program beyond the reach of many hospitals and the implementation of some severity rating measures would likely lead to a change in the extent, timing and recording of diagnostic tests.

It is therefore reassuring that despite the relative lack of sensitivity to illness severity of Diagnosis-Related Group (DRGs), the Health Care Financing Administration in the USA in late 1990 concluded that 'The Department does not believe that any system to measure clinical severity of illness is currently an administratively feasible major improvement or to substitute for DRGs'.

COMORBIDITIES

In the absence of a formal rating for the severity of illness, the accurate recording of comorbidities goes a long way towards explaining length of stay. One of the advantages of orthogeriatric collaboration is the increased recognition and treatment of these problems (Gilchrist et al 1988).

A comorbidity of particular importance is dementia (Baker, Duckworth and Wilkes, 1978) which is common and usually explains the major part of the need for long-stay care. Two studies have therefore attempted to reduce acute confusional states in elderly patients with femoral neck fractures (Williams *et al.*, 1985; Gustafson *et al.*, 1991). One of these (Gustafson *et al.*, 1991) used a package of interventions consisting of pre and postoperative geriatric assessments, oxygen therapy, early surgery, prevention and treatment of perioperative hypotension and

treatment of postoperative complications. There was an incidence of acute confusional states of 47.6% compared with 61.3% in a retrospective control group without such interventions. Moreover, the intervention program appeared to shorten time in the orthopedic ward, the mean duration of stay being 17.4 days in the control group and 11.6 days in the intervention group ($p < 0.001$).

CLINICAL POLICIES INFLUENCING LENGTHS OF STAY

PERIOPERATIVE CARE

Patients with wound infections, thromboembolic disease or pressure sores are likely to have longer than average lengths of stay. Although the number of patients with these problems is likely to be sufficiently low not to significantly affect median lengths of stay, it only takes a few such 'outliers' with prolonged duration of stay to seriously jeopardize the admitting capacity of an orthopedic department. An active strategy with prophylactic antibiotics, antithrombotic therapy and meticulous attention to skin pressure areas is therefore indicated.

It is also claimed that postoperative nutritional status may influence the rate of recovery. Following femoral neck fractures, reductions in length of hospital stay have been shown with oral dietary supplements (Delmi *et al.*, 1990), supplementary nasogastric feeding (Bastow Rawlings and Allison, 1983) and parenteral nutrition (Giacaglia *et al.* 1986).

Although there has been considerable debate surrounding the relative advantages of spinal and general anesthesia for elderly orthopedic patients, a major study of the two types of anesthesia that compared lengths of stay in fractured hip patients found no significant difference between the two groups (Valentin *et al.*, 1986).

FUNCTIONALLY ORIENTATED NURSING CARE

Possibly the key factor in successful rehabilitation and early discharge is the implementation of functionally orientated nursing care whereby patients are increasingly encouraged to carry out everyday activities for themselves. This is a reversal of the 'caring' model of nursing practice traditionally applied in an acute orthopedic ward setting where staff have to carry out personal care tasks for very ill patients. Orem's self-care deficit theory (Orem, 1990) is a functionally orientated model of nursing care appropriate for the rehabilitation environment. Some principles of functionally orientated care are as follows:

DO

- prepare patients adequately with clothes and personal aids;
- promote mobility and independence in self care by giving both the time and the encouragement necessary;
- make instructions slow, simple, clear and audible;
- teach patients to use the simplest method for each task;
- teach patients to repeat a task in the same manner;
- ensure patients walk (at least part of the way) on every visit to toilets or day rooms;
- communicate; establish psychological support with counseling and feedback on progress.

DON'T

- help patients if they can help themselves, even to save time;
- use any chairs with wheels unless the same chair will be used in the same way after discharge;
- allow routine use of bedrooms during the day;
- use formal or informal restraints;
- create undue anxiety among staff about patients falling;
- allow unnecessary nursing tasks; sacrifice them to allow time to concentrate on patients' mobility.

INTENSITY OF THERAPY

As in many other areas of rehabilitation it is extremely difficult to make categorical statements about the optimal frequency and intensity of therapy required to achieve early discharge. Of the little research that has been undertaken, one trial showed that a group of hip fracture patients who received intensive rehabilitation probably had a better functional outcome than a non-rehabilitated group (Katz *et al.* 1962) and one of the few factors associated with hip fracture patients achieving prefracture ambulatory status has been shown to be the amount of physical therapy received (Barnes, 1984). It seems reasonable therefore to argue that the intensity of therapy received by orthopedic patients does make a difference to the length of stay. However, there is probably a 'ceiling' effect with increasing therapy input (rarely reached in British hospitals at the present time) and undoubtedly there is a 'floor' effect or minimum requirement beyond which orthopedic patients suffer and lengths of stay increase. The problem at the present time is that no one can accurately quantify this.

THE NATURE OF SOCIAL WORK INPUT

The intensity, style and administrative base of social work input can also play a major part in facilitating the discharge of elderly orthopedic patients. In an interesting study carried out on behalf of the Social Work Services Group of the Scottish Office (Connor and Tibbit, 1988), preparation for discharge was handled in 'starkly different ways' in units with hospital-based social workers and those who could only refer to community-based social work teams. A difference was also found between those hospitals with high and low intensities of social work staffing.

Many key areas of social care were likely to be missed, picked up very late or dealt with inadequately when the on-site social work contribution was missing or of low intensity. In particular checking home circumstances at the time of admission, early discharge planning, involving the client and his or her carers in those plans, and following up after the person had been discharged to ensure that the community arrangements were functioning as planned. This resulted in unnecessary readmissions because of lack of coordination amongst community services and serious delays in obtaining residential care placements. With regard to the latter it is also important that the social workers consider not only the patients' rights and desires but also accord a degree of priority to their prompt discharge thus enabling the hospital, within which they work, to use its beds effectively and efficiently.

IMMEDIATE VS. GRADUATED WEIGHT BEARING

A major factor affecting early discharge has been the move towards immediate rather than delayed weight bearing after operation for femoral neck fractures. Prior to the implementation of such a policy, mean hospital stay for such patients was in the region of 5 months (Borgquist, 1974). There are regrettably today, still a number of surgeons who argue against the adoption of such a policy despite there being good theoretical and practical evidence that immediate weight bearing is the superior policy. Except in unusual circumstances, elderly patients and their attendants find non weight bearing or graduated weight bearing regimens difficult to comply with. Even if weight bearing on the affected limb is graduated during formal therapy sessions, for example by using a

weight measuring device in the shoe or a walking stick (Engel *et al.*, 1983), this is likely to be ignored when the patient is taken out of bed or transferred to a chair or commode by other attendants. Furthermore, with a non weight bearing policy, the femoral neck may still be subjected to very considerable stresses simply by using a bedpan or straight leg raising of the unaffected leg. If weight bearing is delayed, complications such as pressure sores, venous thrombosis, muscle wasting and osteoporosis are likely to ensue.

Most residual advocates of graduated weight bearing regimens are concerned about healing complications. However, weight bearing at about two weeks following operation has not been shown to increase the complication rate (Andrews, 1987), rather necrosis of the femoral head has been found to be higher in those who bear weight later (Graham, 1968) and compression of the fracture seems to have a beneficial effect on the union of cancellous bone by enhancing stability (Charnley and Baker, 1952).

OTHER APPROPRIATE MEDICAL POLICIES

Other medical policies in surgical aftercare are of importance in achieving early discharge. These are best considered within the conceptual framework of a 'tunnel of rehabilitation' (Figure 3.1). It is a surgeon's responsibility to ensure that patients enter this 'tunnel', are retained within it, are moved through it and discharged from the other end. If the surgeon abrogates responsibility to other professionals for these tasks (other than the collaborative orthogeriatric care described below), or delegates responsibility to very junior staff or himself assumes responsibility but accords it very low priority, then lengths of stay will be suboptimal and appropriate early discharge will not be achieved.

The specific medical tasks to be accomplished are as follows:

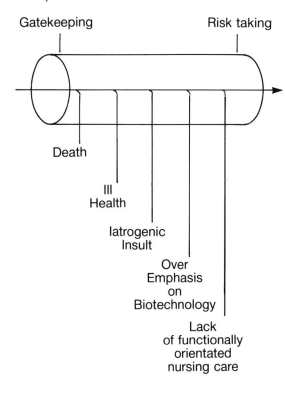

Gatekeeping   Risk taking

Death

Ill
Health

Iatrogenic
Insult

Over
Emphasis
on
Biotechnology

Lack
of functionally
orientated
nursing care

Figure 3.1   The tunnel of rehabilitation.

1. To act as a timely gatekeeper: The first task is to enter the patient into the 'tunnel of rehabilitation' (Figure 3.1) by the doctor's acting as gatekeeper and prescribing rehabilitative therapy. This should be both timely (with little delay after operation) and appropriate (with reasonable goals being set for the therapists). Regrettably, there is evidence that doctors are poor at prescribing rehabilitative services with expectations of successful outcomes being low and therapy being prescribed only after significant unnecessary delays.

2. To keep the patient in good health: The doctor's main role postoperatively is to keep the patients alive and well and fit enough for undergoing rehabilitation. Otherwise they 'fall out of the tunnel of rehabilitation' (Figure 3.1), progress slows and the length of stay increases. This requires regular clinical review of patient status and the prompt treatment of pneumonia, arrhythmias, anemia, cardiac failure and other common complications.

3. To avoid overemphasis on biotechnology: An undue emphasis on the biotechnological aspects of care can result in the orthopedic patient 'falling out of the tunnel of rehabilitation' (Figure 3.1) thus jeopardizing early discharge. It is therefore important that the elderly patient should not be prevented from receiving physiotherapy by being anchored to the bedside by an intravenous infusion set or by being unavailable to go to the gymnasium because the time has been set aside for some relatively unnecessary activity or research investigation or procedure.

4. To avoid iatrogenic insult: Largely due to the increased homeostatic reserve of various organ systems, the elderly patient in the acute care setting is particularly vulnerable to a range of iatrogenic insults (Patterson, 1986). Whenever this happens the orthopedic patient 'falls out of the tunnel of rehabilitation' (Figure 3.1) and progress towards discharge slows. Patients should therefore be investigated and treated with the minimal of interference to their organ systems and to their way of life. This involves any choice of investigation or procedure being based on a knowledge of the risk–benefit ratio in that particular age group and in anesthetic and analgesic medication being carefully selected to avoid unnecessary sedative or anticholinergic side-effects.

5. To practice care management: Care or case management is a term used primarily by social service providers to imply the commitment by a designated person to coordinate a comprehensive plan of management, geared to the client's needs and wishes that avoids unnecessary gaps or overlap between the variety of health and

social service providers involved. To obtain early discharge, this concept of care management should be transposed to the acute elderly orthopedic patient. One clearly identified senior member of staff should be appointed to sustain interest in the patient after operating and orchestrate the various aspects of care being provided by the multidisciplinary team.

6. To act as pace setter: There is a finite time limit within which it is possible to discharge a frail elderly patient back to the community. After this time, successful discharge becomes increasingly difficult. From the patient's point of view then as well as from the point of view of obtaining early discharge, the surgeon (or geriatrician) must act as pace setter, ensuring that he and his team set brief yet realistic timescales for achieving the goals of care in a continual drive towards discharge.

7. To manage risks appropriately when discharging: The decision to discharge frail elderly orthopedic patients back to their home environment can be a difficult one often involving the patient in a degree of risk (Figure 3.1). Early discharge of such patients also incurs the risk of the doctor being involved in litigation if things go wrong. Appropriate management of these risks may be troublesome if the doctor is inexperienced or if there are strong pressures from the patient or family carers not to discharge. In these circumstances, the familiarity of the geriatrician in the risk management of disabled people living in the community may be valuable in obtaining early discharge. Certainly this skill accounts, in part, for geriatricians' success in reducing lengths of stay of elderly patients in acute medical wards without a concomitant need to increase transfer to long-term care facilities (Burley *et al.*, 1979).

8. To involve family carers: Liaison with families should primarily (though not exclusively) be through the doctor. Families should be interviewed shortly after admission and at regular physician-instigated times thereafter. This permits the dissipation of anxiety and stress. To wait until near the end of a patient's stay before involving the family often results in failure. Positive counseling about the community services available to the patient or respite services available to carers as well as encouraging families to participate actively in the patient's rehabilitation in the ward setting can do much to inculcate a positive approach and facilitate early discharge.

RESOURCE FACTORS INFLUENCING LENGTH OF STAY

THE EXTENT OF RESOURCES

The adequacy, availability and efficient use of theatre facilities all influence the rate of throughput of elderly patients through orthopedic wards but is beyond the scope of the current discussion.

Orthopedic length of stay, within certain limits, is inversely correlated with the number of available hospital beds usually because the longer stay outliers are transferred elsewhere for further care.

Perhaps the most important resource of all is the adequacy of various types of 'outlets' from the hospital to lesser levels of care. These 'outlets' may comprise patients' own homes coupled with supportive community services or a range of institutional places. Within the United Kingdom, the institutional places of the chronic hospital are being replaced by smaller nursing home units with a domestic environment. Whatever types of place are being considered, it is well to remember that the United Kingdom has fewer institutional places per head of its elderly population than almost any other nation (Wagner, 1988).

Adequacy of 'outlets' to nursing home care is, however, not in itself a guarantee of early discharge. Currently, the United Kingdom operates a 'fixed price' payment system for nursing home patients irrespective of their dependency or needs. There is therefore a disincentive for nursing homes to allocate places to the very frail, often demented patients, occupying orthopedic beds. This potential for negative selection bias can at times be a very real problem mitigating against early discharge. A number of solutions are possible:

- In Manitoba, Canada, inter-institutional transfers between hospitals and nursing homes did not improve simply by the provision of more nursing home beds, if each facility to which these patients were referred, retained the right to determine its own criteria for admission. However, a centralized placement agency with an impartial prioritizing system was found to expedite transfers out of hospital (Shapiro, Roose and Kavanagh, 1980).
- In the United Kingdom, the geriatrician and his team, using either explicit or implicit criteria, have traditionally prioritized placements into long-term care facilities as long hospital stays result in a poorer functional outcome, increased mortality and fewer patients being discharged back to independent living in the community (Kennie *et al.*, 1988; Reid and Kennie 1989). It may also block beds in orthopedic or accident and emergency departments, particularly where elderly patients are transferred to 'second-line' orthopedic beds for postoperative care.

ORTHOGERIATRIC COLLABORATIVE CARE

In a 1985 survey of departments of geriatric medicine in the United Kingdom, 43 out of 289 were reported as having special collaboration with orthopedic surgeons in the management of elderly fracture patients, particularly for those with proximal hip fracture (Brocklehurst and Andrews, 1985). A recent, comprehensive evaluation of the impact of these ventures in promoting earlier discharge has been provided by Newman (1992).

A number of descriptive studies and studies using retrospective controls have been conducted over the last thirty years most of which have demonstrated shortened hospital stays (Devas, 1964; Clark and Wainwright, 1986; Devas and Irvine, 1969; Ceder, Linberg and Odberg, 1980; Lefroy, 1980; Boyd *et al.*, 1982; Taggart, 1983; Smith, 1984; Burley *et al.*, 1984; Desai, Shakeel and Safty, 1985; Sainsbury *et al.*, 1986; Murphy *et al.*, 1987; Blacklock and Woodhouse, 1988; Whitaker and Currie, 1988; Harrington, Brennan and Hodkinson, 1988). Geriatricians may collaborate by providing a consultancy service, the patients remaining in orthopedic wards under the day-to-day care of the orthopedic surgeon. Alternatively the patients may be transferred to geriatric or rehabilitation wards (geriatric orthopedic rehabilitation units: GORUs), the day-to-day care largely being taken over by the geriatrician and his team. No comparison between these two models of care has been reported. Recently, a number of prospective randomized trials have been conducted on GORUs. The first, Fordham *et al.* (1986), focusing exclusively on elderly patients with hip fracture, found no difference in the lengths of hospital stay between the rehabilitation and the control group but they experienced considerable difficulties in achieving acceptable transfer times from the orthopedic department to these rehabilitation facilities. The mean length of stay before transfer was approximately 18 days. Just under half of the rehabilitation group patients were not transferred to these beds because they either died or made sufficient progress to allow discharge before transfer.

In contrast, a comprehensive randomized trial by Kennie *et al.* (1988), also focusing on elderly women with fractures of the proximal femur, did show clear benefit. Compared with controls, who remained in the orthopedic admission ward, the median length of hospital stay for the intervention group who were transferred postoperatively to a rehabilitation ward was 17 days shorter (24 vs. 41). Significantly more patients in the intervention group regained independence in the activities of daily living, significantly fewer were discharged to institutional care (10 vs. 32%) and more were discharged to their own homes (63 vs. 38%). These benefits were consistent across a wide range of ages and mental states.

At annual follow up (Reid and Kennie, 1989) significantly fewer women in the intervention group than in the control group were more dependent than before fracture. Of the two groups, 69% and 39% respectively were living in the same place as before fracture and 6% and 13% respectively had moved to institutional nursing care. The earlier discharge and greater numbers of hospital discharges in the intervention group were not detrimental to either the patients' quality of life or the stress perceived by family carers. A third randomized trial (Gilchrist *et al.*, 1988) of a GORU treating hip fracture patients, although showing other benefits, failed to demonstrate a reduction in length of stay. However, they provided a less intense input by the geriatrician and his team to the rehabilitation group and provided a significant consultancy service to their control group.

A further randomized controlled trial (Cameron, Lyle and Quine, 1993) in which the treatment group received 'accelerated rehabilitation' after surgical treatment of a proximal femoral fracture showed a 20% reduction in length of hospital stay, a modest though short-term improvement in the level of physical independence, as measured by the Barthel Index, and a reduction in non-nursing-home patients being discharged to nursing homes.

NURSING HOME CARE

The importance of nursing homes as 'outlets' from orthopedic wards has already been stressed. However, although the increased use of nursing homes for the rehabilitative aftercare of hip fracture patients in the USA allowed for shorter hospital stays, it may have been at the expense of an increased proportion of patients remaining as long-term patients in nursing care rather than eventually returning to their own homes. Certainly the frequency of transfer of community-living hip fracture patients to nursing homes from hospital increased after the introduction of the DRG-based prospective payment scheme (Fitzgerald *et al.* 1987 and Fitzgerald, Moore and Dittus, 1988), and, at least initially, this led to the percentage of patients remaining in nursing homes one year after hospitalization increasing from 9% to 33% (Fitzgerald, Moore and Dittus, 1988). Much of the reason for this lay with the lack of ongoing case management and drive towards discharge in the nursing home environment and the eventual loss, after a prolonged stay of the patients social support within the community. These problems may now be being more effectively countered as a more recent study failed to show an increase in the proportion remaining in nursing homes six months later (Palmer *et al.* 1989). A recent randomized trial of nursing home care in Britain for other elderly patient groups has already raised the possibility that this model of care is less effective in achieving eventual discharge than hospital wards (Bond, Gregson and Atkinson, 1989). The quantity and quality of input from general practitioners to British nursing homes is also extremely variable. One survey found that only 13% of patients received regular or routine review and 19% had not been seen since admission (Hepple, Bowler and Bowman, 1989). If patient outcomes are to be safeguarded after hip fracture, consultant supervision of rehabilitative aftercare would seem necessary.

HOSPITAL AT HOME CARE

A number of schemes emphasizing close links with the hospital orthopedic team, good discharge planning, increased community support and rehabilitation have reported reduced lengths of hospital stay (Cedar and Thorngren, 1982; Sikorski, Davis and Senior, 1985; Pryor *et al.* 1988). A significant number may still achieve hospital discharge by this means.

The impact on the patients' quality of life and the family carers' burden has not yet been evaluated with this technique and there remains debate over the exact percentage of patients that can be managed in this way. Pryor *et al.* (1988) judged 55% of their series as suitable for early discharge though only 28% (average hospital stay 8.2 days) were accepted into the hospital at home scheme because the community support was restricted to only a part of the hospital's geographical catchment area. Sikorski, Davis and Senior (1985) entered an even higher number of patients (72%) into their 'rapid discharge system' with the mean duration of hospital stay for this group being only three nights in hospital.

These estimates are probably optimistic for general extrapolation. This may have been due to their applying the strategy to relatively low risk populations (Warne, 1985). In order to provide further information, this author has retrospectively applied Sikorski's exclusion criteria to 144 consecutive female patients admitted with fractured femoral neck to a Scottish hospital and reported on in their previous study (Kennie *et al.*, 1988). The

hospital had responsibility for a defined catchment of elderly people and the numbers of fractured hip patients admitted elsewhere during the same time frame was negligible. The results are shown in Figure 3.2. They suggest that about 10% of such patients are already discharged from hospital within a few days without the need for a formal rapid transit system but that its introduction would see its being offered to a further 7.6% to 14.5% of patients depending on the criteria used. Whether or not such a system would be acceptable to these patients and their families is unknown.

SPECIAL PROVISIONS FOR 'MINOR' FRACTURES

The focus for this chapter has been on shortening the length of stay after surgery. However, relatively minor fractures that may not require operation, such as those of the wrist and proximal humerus, may still be of sufficient severity to require either hospitalization at the time of presentation, or admission to a longer-term care facility a few days later because of the resultant dependency. Certainly Roberts (1990) noted particular difficulties even for mobile elderly patients after discharge from an accident and emergency department and Nankhonya, Turnbull and Newton (1991) showed significantly lower activities of daily living scores after such fractures. The risk for readmission of these patients has been estimated at 5.6% (Rowland *et al.* 1990) and is a particular problem for those patients with upper limb fractures with a contralateral hemiplegia who require to hold a walking aid in their unaffected hand to achieve balance or for those patients with senile gait patterns who require to use a walking frame for stability. They then become immobile whilst the arm or hand is functionally out of commission

1. Would have to live alone
2. Required prior heavy community support
3. Marked postoperative physical dependency
4. Poor postoperative mental status
5. Poor concommitant medical condition
6. Resides over 15 miles from hospital base

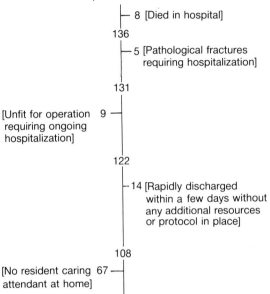

144
Consecutive admissions of women 65 years
and over with proximal femoral fractures

— 8 [Died in hospital]

136

— 5 [Pathological fractures
requiring hospitalization]

131

[Unfit for operation 9 —
requiring ongoing
hospitalization]

122

— 14 [Rapidly discharged
within a few days without
any additional resources
or protocol in place]

108

[No resident caring 67 —
attendant at home]

41

—1 × 5 exclusion criteria
—5 × 4   "   "
—6 × 3   "   "
—8 × 2   "   "
—10 × 1   "   "
—11 no   "   "

Summary: Assuming those with no or only one exclusion criterion and living alone are suitable for rapid transit back home, the total who might be offered this method of management = 35 (11 + 10 + 14) or 24.3% (35/144) of all women 65 + years with proximal femoral fractures. The additional numbers who might benefit from the formal introduction and resourcing of a rapid transit system = 21 (11 = 10) or 14.5% (21/144) in addition to the existing 9.7% (14/144) who are already discharged rapidly. If only those with no exclusion criteria are considered, the additional benefit of rapid transit is 7.6% (11/144).

Figure 3.2 Extent of eligibility for 'rapid transit' care: exclusion criteria for rapid transit back to the community (Sikorsky, Davis and Serios, 1985).

because of immobilization or the application of a splint.

The following measures may therefore be employed either to prevent admission in the first place or to reduce duration of stay:

1. The provision of a care manager in the accident and emergency department:
   Every accident and emergency department should have prompt access to a care manager (social worker, occupational therapist or nurse) provided they either arrange additional informal support for the elderly person from family or friends or they have the responsibility and authority to arrange or purchase the necessary community support services that will enable the patient to remain in their own home.
2. Provision of appropriate aids:
   Alternatively in otherwise fit elderly people the temporary provision of aids (for example a one-handed walking frame) may be all that is required to ensure independent living.
3. Provision of a placement in a continuing care facility:
   Rather than admit 'minor' fracture patients inappropriately to acute trauma or orthopedic beds for the few weeks necessary before the fractured upper limb becomes functional again, alternative placement may be sought through a nursing home for high dependency patients or a residential home for those with only minimal dependency needs. Alternatively in the United Kingdom, the health board may have contract care beds specifically for this purpose or, once cost and volume and per case contracts come into effect, orthopedic directorates may find it more economical to purchase alternative care for these patients directly and to fill the hospital bed with someone requiring surgical care.

THE APPROPRIATENESS OF EARLY DISCHARGE

The foregoing discussion about elderly ortho-pedic patients assumes that there is some-thing inherently difficult about achieving their early discharge. This is not the case. The orthopedic surgeon merely has to ignore the distress and risk to his patients and the inconvenience and burden to their carers and he can discharge at almost any time he wants. This policy can be particularly suc-cessful if readmission to the orthopedic service is made difficult and abrogated to other health or social service departments.

There is unfortunately considerable clinical and research evidence that this frequently happens. For example, several studies in the United Kingdom (Skeet, 1970; Hirst, 1975; Bowling and Betts, 1984; Victor and Vetter, 1988) have shown that approximately half of all elderly patients discharged from hospital leave without any member of the hospital staff discussing with them their needs for assistance once back at home. One recent survey in Wales (Victor and Vetter, 1988) also found that 39% were given less than twenty-four hours notice of discharge.

Irrespective of poorly considered discharge arrangements, it may be difficult to reconcile the drive towards earlier discharge with patient choice and consumer satisfaction for already in the United Kingdom 30% of surgical patients consider their hospital stay too short (Rowland, 1991).

The presence of a prospective payment scheme for health care, where provider or-ganizations are paid an average cost based on DRGs, creates a financial incentive to dis-charge as rapidly as possible from the hos-pital so that another revenue-earning patient can be admitted. This incentive is greatest when payment is made for each case as occurs in the USA but the increasing trend in the British National Health Service towards cost and volume contracts encourages the same goals. It is important to note therefore, that whilst the introduction of prospective payment in the USA shortened hospital stay, it increased the likelihood of patients being discharged home in an unstable condition (Rogers et al 1990). Lastly, the presence of various discharge 'outlets' from hospital with payment for each coming from different public subsidized sources, also encourages rapid placement based on the best way of shifting costs rather than on what is optimal for the patient and their carers.

There must therefore be safeguards set by the purchasers of health care and limitations imposed on the providers of orthopedic or orthogeriatric services to ensure that dis-charges are appropriate and consistent with quality care. The following section therefore considers various ways by which the quality of a service can be maintained despite the drive towards early discharge.

MAINTAINING QUALITY

The following measures may be employed, in full or in part, to maintain the quality of orthopedic or orthogeriatric services and ensure the appropriateness of discharge. They may be included as the purchasers' standards in contracts or as items for multi-disciplinary clinical audit conducted by the providers of health care.

DEFINE STANDARDS OF FITNESS FOR DISCHARGE

There should be an explicit statement of the minimal criteria considered necessary for an appropriate discharge. These should include, surgical items such as the wound being satisfactory; general health items such as pain control being adequate and other medical conditions being stable; functional items which will vary depending on the level of care to which the patient is being discharged (e.g. to go home – to be able to mobilize, attend to basic self-care and to have any incontinence socially contained); and items relating to the support system such as agreement that informal carers are willing to provide necessary support.

Many other items can be added to these. Contrarily, discharge may be effected without all being complied with. The importance lies in having explicit criteria against which discharges can be judged and in the discussion their creation engendered amongst staff.

DEVELOP A PROTOCOL FOR COMMUNICATION

Predischarge planning should include a protocol for communicating patients' needs to the community primary health care team. This protocol should include the necessary data as well as a clear statement as to who has responsibility for communicating the various items. In the United Kingdom, interim discharge summaries reach their general practitioner more quickly if the elderly patients or their carers deliver them by hand (Sandler and Mitchell, 1987). Ideally, the hospital and community services should have sufficiently compatible information technology to permit the computerized inflow and outflow of necessary information (Branger, van der Wounde and Schudel, 1992).

RATIONALIZE MEDICATION

Prescribed medication should be rationalized and, where possible, reduced to a minimum. Hypnotics and anxiolytics with long half-lives, tricyclic antidepressants, certain antipsychotic medication, codeine and propoxyphene all of which have been shown to have an association with falls and hip fracture (Ray *et al.* 1987; Shorr *et al.* 1992) should be substituted with an alternative drug. Predischarge counseling about medication, which has been shown to improve compliance (MacDonald, MacDonald and Phoe-nix, 1977), should be a routine part of the hospital pharmacy service.

ATTEND TO CARERS' NEEDS

Discharge planning should include at least one consultation by a senior member of medical staff with the patient's family carers and detailed attention by other staff to those carers' needs with the creation of a package of support services and respite necessary to promote a reasonable quality of life as judged by the monitoring instruments (see below).

PREPARE THE HOME ENVIRONMENT

Where appropriate, a home visit should be undertaken by the therapy staff to ensure that access around the patient's house is adequate, that hazards in the home, which are implicated in about 17% of non-syncopal falls in elderly people (Tinetti *et al.*, 1988), are eliminated and that various aids and adaptations to counteract the handicap in performing the activities of daily living (Hart *et al.*, 1990) have been considered.

ENSURE SERVICES AND SUPPORTS IN PLACE PRIOR TO DISCHARGE

All aids and adaptations should be in place and fitted prior to the patient's arrival there and community support should be timed to provide some assistance immediately the patient reaches home and at appropriate intervals thereafter.

ENSURE ADEQUATE FOLLOW UP

Times for further outpatient clinic and/or day hospital attendance should be given to the patient prior to discharge.

TIME DISCHARGES OPTIMALLY

Whenever possible, unless informal carers are available and have agreed to provide assistance, the discharge of frail elderly patients to live alone should be avoided at weekends and public holidays when social support services are usually unavailable. Ward rounds conducted in the afternoon with discharge decisions being made late in the day can also result in insufficient time to arrange adequate transport and support services for the following day. Such inappropriately timed discharges should be a subject for regular audit.

ENSURE ADEQUATE MONITORING

The following areas should be included when considering a monitoring package for the quality of orthopedic or orthogeriatric care for elderly patients.

Complications and readmission rates

Certain negative parameters such as death, wound infection rates, thromboembolism, dislocated prostheses and readmission rates should be included as routine data collection for clinical audit.

Discharge functional status

An additional measurement required to assess the quality of orthopedic discharge for an elderly patient is to record functional status around the time of discharge, the functional components of greatest importance being mobility, the personal activities of daily living (e.g. dressing, toileting, etc) and continence. Other functional parameters such as the domestic activities of daily living (e.g. mealmaking) may also require assessment if independent living at home is contemplated.

There are many comprehensive texts (e.g. Kane and Kane, 1985) that provide guidance on the measurement instruments available. In the United Kingdom, the British Geriatrics Society in collaboration with the Royal College of Physicians of London have recently published further information on standardized assessment scales for elderly people (BGS/RCP, 1992).

An unresolved problem is that many of these scales have only been used in the short term for operational research purposes and have not been well integrated into an ongoing long-term monitoring package. An alternative strategy may be to use a measure such as the Functional Independence Measure (FIM) (Granger, Hamilton and Sherwin, 1986). In the United States, FIM is used not only by doctors and other researchers in short-term projects but by therapists, nurses and other members of the multidisciplinary team as part of ongoing quality assurance programmes. FIM is now used in over half the rehabilitation units in the United States; it is supported by a range of training videos and documents; and telephone follow up after discharge is possible using the standardized FONEFIM protocol. Submission of results can if desired be displayed as part of a computerized comparative data set with other departments.

Outcome packages

Purchasers' and payers' interest in the outcomes of health care in the United States has led to the development of rating instruments containing a range of questions about functional status and psychosocial well-being that are administered to patients on discharge from hospital. Some of these, such as the SF-36 Health Status Questionnaire, are general health status measures that would be relevant to elderly orthopedic patients (Interstudy Report, 1991) and it has now been validated for use in the British setting (Brazier *et al.*, 1992). Additionally, condition-specific outcome instruments are also available for hip fracture, hip replacement and osteoarthritis of the knee and rheumatoid arthritis.

Carer burden

With careful attention to the detailed needs of carers, early discharge can be achieved without an increase in the burden they experience. In their randomized controlled trial of orthogeriatric rehabilitative care, Reid and Kennie (1989), using Robinson's Caregiver Strain Index, found no difference one year after trial entry between the carers of those patients treated with orthopedic postoperative management and the carers of those patients managed postoperatively by the geriatrician and his team despite the median stay in hospital of the latter group being seventeen days shorter than the group receiving conventional orthopedic management.

Nevertheless, carers are often expected to continue their role without advanced notification, in the presence of patients' increased dependency and without prior arrangement of the necessary support and respite services. Any outcome monitoring package must therefore include an assessment of the objective and subjective burden imposed on family and other carers.

Recently, Vitaliano, Young and Russo (1991), provided a comprehensive review of ten measures used among caregivers of individuals with dementia, the likeliest comorbidity to induce significant carer stress.

REFERENCES

Andrews, K. (1987) *Rehabilitation of the Older Adult*, Edward Arnold, London.

Baker, B.R., Duckworth, T. and Wilkes, E. (1978) Mental state and other prognostic factors in femoral fractures of the elderly. *J. Roy. Coll. Gen. Practit.*, **28**, 557–9.

Barnes, B. (1984) Ambulation outcome after hip fracture. *Phys. Therapy*, **64**, 317–21.

Bastow, M.D. Rawlings, J. and Allison, S.P. (1983) Benefits of supplementary tube feeding after fractured neck of femur: a randomised controlled trial. *B.M.J.*, **287**, 1589–92.

Beringer, T.R.O., McSherry, D.M.G. and Taggart, H.McA. (1984) A microcomputer based audit of fracture of the proximal femur in the elderly. *Age Ageing*, **13**, 344–8.

Blacklock, C. and Woodhouse, K.W. (1988) Orthogeriatric liaison. *Lancet* i, 999.

Bond, J., Gregson, B.A. and Atkinson, A. (1989) Measurement of outcomes within a multi-centred randomised controlled trial in the evaluation of the experimental nursing homes. *Age Ageing*, **18**, 293–302.

Borgquist, L. (1974) Organisation levels in public health service. A study of fractures of the proximal end of the femur in the elderly. University of Lund Thesis, Lund, Sweden.

Bowling, A. and Betts, G. (1984) Communication on discharge. *Nurs. Times*, **80**, 31–3 and 80, 44–6.

Boyd, R.V., Compton, E. Hawthorne, J. and Kemm, J.R. (1982) Orthogeriatric rehabilitation ward in Nottingham: preliminary report. *B.M.J.*, **285**, 937–8.

Branger, P.J. van der Wounden, J.C., Schudel, B.R. *et al.* (1992) Electronic communication between providers of primary and secondary care. *Bri. Med.*, **305**, 1068–70.

Brazier, J.E., Harper, R., Jones, N.M.B. *et al.* (1992) Validating the SF-36 health survey questionnaire: a new outcome measure for primary care. *B.M.J.*, **305**, 160–4.

Brocklehurst, J.C. and Andrews, K. (1985) Geriatric medicine – the style of practice. *Age Ageing*, **14**, 1–7.

Burley, L.E., Currie, C.T., Smith, R.G. and Williamson, J. (1979) Contribution from geriatric medicine within acute medical wards. *B.M.J.*, **2**, 90–2.

Burley, L.E., Scorgie, R.E., Currie, C.T. *et al.* (1984) The joint geriatric orthopaedic service in South Edinburgh: November 1979–October 1980. *Hlth Bull.*, **42**, 133–140.

Cameron, I.D., Lyle, D.M. and Quine, S. (1993) Accelerated rehabilitation after proximal femoral fracture: a randomised control trial. *Disability and Rehabilitation*, **15**, 29–34.

Ceder, L. and Thorngren, K.G. (1982) Rehabilitation after hip fracture. *Lancet* ii, 1097–8.

Ceder, L., Lindberg, L. and Odberg, E. (1980) Differentiated care of hip fracture in the elderly. Mean hospital days and results of rehabilitation. *Acta Orthop. Scand.*, **51**, 157–62.

Charnley, J. and Baker, S.L. (1952) Compression arthrodesis of the knee: a clinical and histological study. *J. Bone Joint Surg.*, **34B**, 187–99.

Clark, A.N.G. and Wainwright, D. (1966) The management of the fractured neck of femur in the elderly female: a joint approach of orthopaedic surgery and geriatric medicine. *Geront. Clin.*, **8**, 321–6.

Connor, A. and Tibbitt, J.E. (1988) Social Workers and Health Care in Hospitals. Research Study by the Central Research Unit for Social Work Services Group, Scottish Office.

Delmi, M., Rapin, C.H., Bengoa, J. *et al.* (1990) Dietary supplementation in elderly patients with fractured neck of the femur. *Lancet*, **335**, 1013–16.

Department of Health and Social Security (1981) *Report of a Working Party. Orthopaedic Services: Waiting time for outpatient appointments and inpatient treatment*, HMSO, London.

Desai, H.N., Shakeel, M.H. and El Safty M.E. (1985) Combined orthopaedic-geriatric care. *Lancet*, i, 349–50.

Devas, M.B. (1964) Fractures in the elderly. *Geront. Clin.*, **6**, 347–59.

Devas, M.B. and Irvine, R.E. (1969) The geriatric orthopaedic unit. A method of achieving return to independence in the elderly patient. *Brit. J. Geriat. Prac.*, **6**, 19–25.

Engel, J., Amir, A., Messer, E. and Caspi, I. (1983) Walking cane designed to assist partial weight bearing. *Arch. Phys. Med. Rehabil.*, **64**, 386–8.

Evans, J.G. (1979) Fractured proximal femur in Newcastle upon Tyne. *Age Ageing*, **8**, 16–24.

Fitzgerald, J.F., Fagan, L.F., Tierney, W.M. and Dittus, R.S. (1987) Changing patterns of hip fracture care before and after implementation of the prospective payment system. *J. Am. Med. Assoc.*, **258**, 218–21.

Fitzgerald, J.F., Moore, P.S. and Dittus, R.S. (1988) The care of elderly patients with hip fracture: changes since implementation of the prospective payment system. *N. Engl. J. Med.*, **319**, 1392–7.

Fordham, R., Thompson, R., Holmes, J. *et al.* (1986) A cost-benefit study of geriatric-orthopaedic management. Centre for Health Economics, University of York, Discussion Paper 14.

Giaccaglia, G., Malagu, U., Antonelli, M. *et al.* (1986) Il supporto nutrizionale negli interventi di fratture dell'anca nell'anziano: esperienze et risultati. *Min. Anest.*, **52**, 397–400.

Gilchrist, W.J., Newman R.J., Hamblen D.L., Williams, B.O. (1988) Prospective randomised study of an orthopaedic geriatric inpatient service. *B.M.J.*, **297**, 1116–8.

Graham, J. (1968) Early or delayed weight bearing after internal fixation of transcervical fracture of the femur. *J. Bone Joint Surg.*, **50B**, 166–71.

Granger, C.V., Hamilton, B.B. and Sherwin, F.S. (1986) Guide for the use of the uniform data set for medical rehabilitation. Uniform Data System for Medical Rehabilitation Project Office, Buffalo General Hospital, New York, 14203, USA.

Gustafson, Y., Brannstrom B., Berggren, D. *et al.* (1991) A geriatric-anesthesiologic program to reduce acute confusional states in elderly patients treated for femoral neck fractures. *J. Am. Geriatr. Soc.* **39**, 655–62.

Harrington, M.G., Brennan, M. and Hodkinson, H.M. (1988) The first year of a geriatric orthopaedic liaison service: an alternative to ortho-geriatric units? *Age Ageing*, **17**, 129–33.

Hart, D., Bowling, A., Ellis, M. and Silman, A. (1990) Locomotor disability in very elderly people: value of a programme for screening and provision of aids for daily living. *B.M.J.*, **301**, 216–20.

Hepple, J., Bowler, I. and Bowman, C.E. (1989) A survey of private nursing home residents in Weston-Super-Mare. *Age Ageing*, **18**, 61–3.

Hirst, H.J. (1975) Elderly patients discharged home from hospital, Department of Social Work, John Radcliffe Infirmary, Oxford.

Hornbrook, M.C. (1989) Nursing home case-mix measurement, in *Health Care of the Elderly* (eds. M.D. Peterson and D.L. White). Sage Publications, California.

Iezzoni, L.I. (1991) Severity Standardisation and Hospital Quality Assessment, in *Health Care Quality Management for the 21st Century* (ed. J.B. Couch), The American College of Physician Executives, Florida.

Interstudy (1991) *Quality Edge: Measurement and Management of Clinical Outcomes*, Interstudy: MN, USA.

Joint Working Group of the Royal College of Physicians and the British Geriatrics Society (1992) Standardised Assessment Scales for Elderly People, The Royal College of Physicians, London.

Kane, R.A. and Kane, R.L. (1985) *Assessing the Elderly: A Practical Guide to Measurement*, Lexington Books,

Katz, S. Jackson, B.S., Jaffe, M.W. *et al.* (1962) Multidisciplinary studies of illness in aged person. VI: Comparison study of rehabilitated and nonrehabilitated patients with fracture of the hip. *J. Chron. Dis*, **15**, 979–84.

Kennie, D.C., Reid, J., Richardson, I.R. *et al.* (1988) Effectiveness of geriatric rehabilitative care after fractures of the proximal femur in elderly women: a randomised clinical trial. *B.M.J.*, **297**; 1083–6.

Lefroy, R.B. (1980) Treatment of patients with fractured neck of the femur in a combined unit. *Med. J. Aust.*, **2**: 669–70.

MacDonald, E.T., MacDonald, J.P. and Phoenix, M. (1977) Improving drug compliance after hospital discharge. *B.M.J.*, **2**: 618–21.

Murphy, P.J., Rai G.S., Lowy, M. and Bielawska, C. (1987) The beneficial effects of joint orthopaedic-geriatric rehabilitation. *Age Ageing*, **16**; 273–8.

Nankhonya, J.M., Turnbull, C.J. and Newton, J.T. (1991) Social and functional impact of minor fractures in elderly people. *B.M.J.* **303**: 1514–15.

Newman, R.J. (1992) Special collaborative rehabilitation schemes following femoral neck fractures, in. *Orthogeriatrics* (ed. R.J. Newman), Butterworth-Heinmann, Oxford.

Orem, D. (1980) *Nursing Concepts of Practice*, McGraw-Hill, New York.

Palmer, R.M., Saywell, R.M., Zollinger, T.W. *et al.* (1989) The impact of the prospective payment system on the treatment of hip fractures in the elderly. *Arch Intern Med.*, **149**, 2237–41.

Patterson, C (1986) Iatrogenic disease in late life, in *Clinics in Geriatric Medicine*, **2**(1) (ed. M.J. Magenheim), Saunders, Philadelphia.

Pryor, G. A., Myles, J W., Williams, D.R.R. and Anand, J.K. (1988) Team management of the elderly patient with hip fractures. *Lancet*, **i**: 401–3.

Ray, W.A., Griffin, M.R., Schaffner, W. *et al.* (1987) Psychotropic drug use and the risk of hip fracture. *N. Engl. J. Med.*, **316**, 363–9.

Reid, J. and Kennie, D.C. (1989) Geriatric rehabilitative care after fractures of the proximal femur: one year follow up of a randomised clinical trial. *B.M.J.*, **299**, 25–6.

Roberts, N.A. (1990) Prospective follow up study of elderly patients discharged from an accident and emergency department. *Clin. Rehab.*, **4**, 37–41.

Rogers, W.H., Draper, D., Kahn, K.L. *et al.* (1990) Quality of care before and after implementation of the DRG-based prospective system: a summary of effects. *J. Am. Med. Assoc.*, **264**, 1984–8.

Rowland, K., Maitra, A.K., Richardson, D.A. *et al.* (1990) The discharge of elderly patients from an accident and emergency department: functional changes and risk of readmission. *Age Ageing*, **19**, 415–18.

Rowland, B. (1991) The human toll of rapid discharge. *Hosp. Doctor*, **C11**, 23–5.

Sainsbury, R., Gillespie, W.J., Armour, P.C. *et al.* (1986) An orthopaedic geriatric rehabilitation unit: the first two years experience. *N.Z. Med. J.*, **99**, 583–5.

Sandler, D.A. and Mitchell, J.R.A. (1987) Interim discharge summaries: how are they best delivered to the general practitioners? *B.M.J.*, **295**, 1523–5.

Shapiro, E., Roos, N.P. and Kavanagh, S. (1980) Long term patients in acute care beds; Is there a cure. *Gerontologist*, **20**, 342–5.

Shorr, R.I., Griffin, M.R., Daugherty, J.R. and Ray, W.A. (1992) Opioid analgesics and the risk of hip fracture in the elderly: codeine and propoxyphene. *J. Gerontol*, **47**, M111–15.

Sikorski, J.M., Davis, N.J. and Senior, J. (1985) The rapid transit system for patients with fractures of proximal femur. *B.M.J.*, **290**: 439–43.

Skeet, M. (1970) Home from Hospital, Dan Mason Nursing Research Committee, MacMillan, London.

Social Services Inspectorate (1991) Care Management and Assessment: Practitioner's Guide. Department of Health in conjunction with the Scottish Office and Social Work Services Group.

Smith, D.L. (1984) The elderly in the convalescent orthopaedic trauma ward: can the geriatrician help? *Hlth Bull.*, **42**, 36–44.

Taggart, H. (1983) Geriatric orthopaedic rehabilitation in Belfast, in *Advanced Geriatric Medicine*, 3rd edn (eds F.I. Caird and J.G. Evans) Pitman, London.

Tinetti, M.E., Speechley, M. and Ginter, S.F. (1988) Risk factors for falls among elderly persons living in the community. *N. Engl. J. Med.*, **319**: 1701–7.

Valentin, N., Lomholt, B., Jensen, J.S. *et al.* (1986) Spinal or general anaesthesia for surgery of the fractured hip? *Brit. J. Anaesth*, **58**, 284–91.

Victor, C.R. and Vetter, N.J. (1988) Preparing the elderly for discharge from hospital: a neglected aspect of patient care? *Age Ageing*, **17**, 155–63.

Vitaliano, P.P., Young, H.M. and Russo, J. (1991) A review of measures used among caregivers of individuals with dementia. *Gerontol.*, **31**, 67–75.

Wagner, G. (1988) Residential care: A positive choice. Report of the Independent Review of Residential Care. National Institute for Social Work.

Warne, R.W. (1985) The rapid transit system for patients with fractures of the proximal femur (letter). *B.M.J.*, **290**, 1076.

Whitaker, J.J. and Currie, C.T. (1988) An evaluation of the role of geriatric orthopaedic rehabilitation units in Edinburgh. *Hlth Bull.* **46**, 273–6.

Williams, M., Campbell, E., Raynor, W. *et al.* (1985) Reducing acute confusional states in elderly patients with hip fractures. *Res. Nurs. Health*, **8**, 329–32.

4

Biomechanics of old bones

LOREN LATTA

INTRODUCTION

There are many controversies about how to clinically assess osteoporosis and its relationship to the biomechanics of orthopedic care. One of the most important considerations related to choosing and implementing orthopedic management involves the mechanical changes in the skeleton related to osteoporosis. This chapter will focus on (1) those detectable factors which relate to the potential mechanical problems the surgeon must face in choosing and implementing orthopedic care, and (2) practical options available to the surgeon to approach the special mechanical problems of fixation in osteoporotic bones.

BONE MEASUREMENTS AND BIOMECHANICS

New technology in recent years has provided the surgeon with a vast armamentarium which was not previously available. Besides plain radiographs (Foltin, 1988; Meema, 1991; Inoue *et al.* 1983; Barth, Williams and Kaplan, 1992; Ostlere and Gold, 1991; Bloom and Laws, 1970; Latta, Zych and Greenbarg, 1988), one can now choose from ultrasonic imaging (Baran *et al.*, 1988; Saha and Albright, 1990), computerized tomography

(CT) (Saha and Albright, 1990) and magnetic resonance imaging techniques (MRI) (Hayes, 1991). Methods for evaluating bone mineral density (BMD) include single photon absorption, SPA (Carter *et al.*, 1990; Van Der Voort *et al.*, 1990; Ostlere and Gold, 1991) dual photon absorption, DPA (Carter *et al.*, 1990; Ross, Wasnich and Vogel, 1988; Meltzer, Lessig and Siegal, 1989; Cornell *et al.*, 1988; Saha and Albright, 1990; Khairi *et al.* 1976; Ostlere and Gold, 1991) dual energy radiography (Saha and Albright, 1990; Ostlere and Gold, 1991) and computed values from CT (Ostlere and Gold, 1991) and MRI (Hayes, 1991) images. One method of bone density measurement which is often overlooked in the literature is a simple step wedge X-ray density scale from plain radiographs. These also have proven to be a very effective and inexpensive means of evaluation (Inoue *et al.*, 1983; Latta, Zych and Greenbarg, 1988). Imaging information provides a qualitative assessment of changes in trabecular pattern in the cancellous bone and changes in cortical thickness and increased diaphyseal diameter on cortical bone. Mineral density measurements provide a quantitative measurement of the density of both trabecular and cortical bone, but is still limited to evaluation of two-dimensional projections of three-dimensional structures. Quantitative CT and MRI techniques provide

Skeletal Trauma in Old Age
Published in 1994 by Chapman & Hall, London
ISBN 0 412 48750 0

the advantage of evaluation of individual slices through the anatomic structure which can be used to reconstruct the full three-dimensional structure. Research on the mechanical properties of both cancellous and cortical bone in both normal and osteoporotic patients clearly shows that quantitative bone mineral density measurements correlate much more accurately with bone strength measurements than do qualitative measurements from images (Goldstein, 1987; Jensen, 1989; Hayes, 1991; Barth, Williams and Kaplan 1992; Roser *et al.*, 1991). Despite these facts from researchers, the clinical and epidemiologic studies have not clearly defined the role of densitometry measurements in the management of injuries in osteoporotic bones (Carter *et al.*, 1990; Cornell *et al.*, 1988; Khairi *et al.*, 1976; Kranendonk, Jurist and Lee, 1972; Ostlere and Gold, 1991). Although most of the research has focused on the role of mineral density measurements in predicting future fractures in osteoporotic bones based on predictions of the strength of the bone (Hirby, Anderson and Gyrtup, 1989; Baran *et al.*, 1988; Van Der Voort *et al.*, 1990; Meltzer, Lessig and Siegel, 1989; Meema, 1991; Khairi *et al.*, 1976), these same measurements can be very useful in evaluating the strength of the bone in which orthopedic implants must achieve fixation for skeletal stabilization.

From plain radiographs, trabecular bone changes can be evaluated in a number of skeletal sites with surprising consistency. The types of changes which occur have certain similarities regardless of the site (Figure 4.1). Normal metaphyses in weight-bearing long bones have major structural columns of trabeculae visible within the plane of maximal bending. In the proximal femur there are two major columns clearly defined in the medial and lateral regions of the trochanter and neck and cross-coupling patterns of trabeculae of less well-defined orientation (Khairi *et al.*, 1976; Kranendonk, Jurist and Lee, 1972). The distal femur has

similar patterns with well-defined medial and lateral columns connected with more randomly oriented cross-coupling trabeculae which provides a clear image of the two well-oriented, structural columns. The next major change which occurs is loss of continuity of one of the two major columns. The first change visible on plain radiographs with osteoporosis is loss of density of these cross-coupling trabeculae. The final stage of bone loss involves both of the major columns and is always associated with gross cortical thinning. All grades of progression of osteoporosis include some description of these patterns of change (Singh, Hagrath and Nairi, 1970; Meema, 1991; Saha and Albright, 1990). Some investigators have proposed that the ratio of cortical thicknesses to cortical diameter in any given projection is the most sensitive measure of cortical bone changes with osteoporosis (Hirby, Anderson and Gyrtrup, 1989; Ostlere and Gold, 1991). However, other investigators have shown that simple measurements of cortical thickness are inadequate to consistently diagnose the changes in mechanical properties of the cortical bone as well as risk of fracture in that and other nearby bones (Meema, 1991; Saha and Albright 1990).

There are many mixed reports on the correlation of qualitative measurements from plain radiographs and bone density in the same bone as well as adjacent bones in the skeleton (Kranendonk, Jurist and Lee, 1972; Khairi *et al.*, 1976). Qualitative measures of cancellous bone changes (such as the Singh Index) have proven to be excellent predictors of bone density in the hands of some investigators but not in others. Both cortical and cancellous bone strength have a direct relationship to bone density regardless of the method of measurement (Roser *et al.*, 1991). What most investigators do agree upon is that qualitative or quantitative measurements in the upper limb do not serve as good predictors of the osteoporotic changes in the

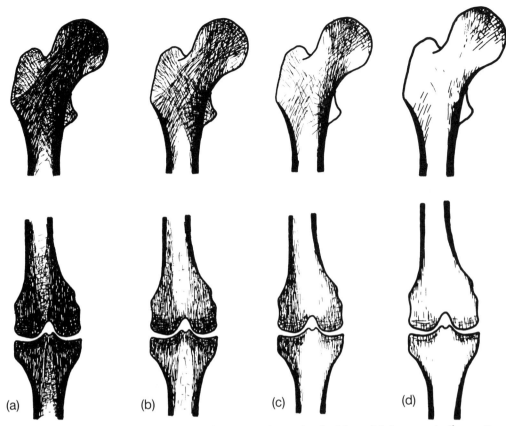

Figure 4.1 The proximal femur, distal femur, and proximal tibia exhibit very similar patterns of trabecular bone changes as osteoporosis progresses. There are two main structural columns of highly oriented trabeculae seen in each of these regions in normal bone, (a), connected by more randomly oriented, cross-coupling trabeculae. The first changes which occur are the loss in density of the cross-coupling trabeculae between the major columns, (b). The most significant event which seems to separate the trabecular changes from clearly 'normal' to clearly 'osteoporotic', involves the loss of one of the major structural columns of trabeculae, (c). In the proximal femur, this loss consistently occurs first in the tension trabecular column which crosses from lateral distal to proximal medial. In the distal femur and proximal tibia, the first structural column to disappear is consistently on the medial side of the knee. In the late stages of osteoporosis all major structural columns of support have this discontinuity and loss of density, (d) (Latta, 1991).

lower limbs and vice versa (Carter *et al.*, 1990; Cornell *et al.*, 1988; Meltzer, Lessig and Siegel, 1989). Measurements in the spine seem to correlate a little bit better with measurements in the lower limb, however, each body region seems to be changing relatively independent of the others, at least in terms of measurable parameters using current diagnostic techniques (Eastell *et al.*, 1989; Carter *et al.*, 1990; Cornell *et al.*, 1988; Meltzer, Lessig and Siegel, 1989). Besides bone mineral loss, there is mineral redistribution which affects osteoporotic patterns of change more than the overall average of BMD (Jensen, 1989). This redistribution is more pronounced between than within limb segments. Using cortical measurements to predict changes in cancellous bone or cancellous measurements to predict changes in cortical bones is also met with mixed success (Van Der Voort *et al.*, 1990; Meema, 1991).

Amidst all of this confusion, however, there seem to be some consistent points of value in utilizing each of these diagnostic techniques in making decisions about orthopedic care:

1. Qualitative and quantitative measurements in the lower limb seem to correlate quite well from femur to the tibia and between regions within the femur or tibia (Jensen, 1989; Latta, Zych and Greenbarg, 1988). Similar measurements in the hand, distal radius, and proximal humerus seem to correlate well with each other but not with measurements with the same individual in the lower limb or the spine (Meema, 1991; Ostler and Gold, 1991; Jensen, 1989; Bloom and Lans, 1970).
2. Bone density measurements provide the best correlations with mechanical strength and can be used to predict the incidence of fractures and strength of fixation of orthopedic devices in both cancellous and cortical bone.
3. Qualitative measures of bone changes do provide consistent useful information for clinical evaluation of bone strength, at least in a relative sense.

MECHANICAL CHANGES WITH OSTEOPOROSIS

Bone yield strength and ultimate strength has a direct relationship to bone density. Bone stiffness (or elastic modulus) is not affected as much as strength (McCalden *et al.*, 1991). The best measure of bone density which correlates with strength, is apparent density, which is a simple calculation from the weight of a specimen divided by its volume (McCalden *et al.*, 1991; Goldstein, 1987, Jensen, 1989; Leichner, 1982; Smith *et al.*, 1992). Obviously

this measure of density is not practical in a clinical setting. One other parameter which is correlated with strength *in vitro* is ash content. The next best parameters, which can be measured in a clinical setting, are BMD and X-ray intensity measured as described previously. The relationship of BMD and strength is roughly geometric with ultimate and yield stress proportional to the curve of the density of the bone (Ciarelli *et al.*, 1991; Goldstein, 1987; Jensen, 1989; Carter and Hayes, 1977). The strength of cancellous bone can be predicted in practice in order to assess the quality and location of fracture fixation by reading plain X-rays and knowing something about what to expect. Since cortical bone increases in diameter and decreases in thickness as osteoporosis progresses, the material strength and stiffness changes are not necessarily related to the structural strength and stiffness changes (Ostlere and Gold, 1991; Hayes, 1991). The geometric properties of the diaphyseal cross section (moment of inertia) controls stiffness and strength in bending and torsion, more than material properties do. This moment of inertia increases with osteoporosis. This means that for a given bending or torsional load, the stress in an osteoporotic bone will be less than that same bone had when it was normal. But for a given amount of bending or twisting distortion, the strain in an osteoporotic bone will be more than in the same bone when it was normal, although material stiffness loss is much less rapid than strength loss with osteoporosis. Thus, 'old bones' tend to be stiffer and weaker than young bones, and behave in a more brittle fashion. Therefore, stress concentration is more of a concern in osteoporotic bones.

PRACTICAL APPLICATIONS OF CLINICAL EVALUATION TECHNIQUES

It is important for the orthopedic surgeon to have a variety of techniques available for evaluation of bone quality when choosing a method of fracture fixation for an individual patient. Unfortunately, the area where fracture fixation is needed is that portion of the bone which is the most difficult to assess by imaging or X-ray density technique because of the distortion of the normal anatomy caused by the fracture. Also certain regions of the body (particularly the hip and the spine) are covered by very thick layers of soft tissue which vary a great deal from one patient to another, which makes it very difficult to obtain consistent image or bone density measurements in these areas. Therefore, the surgeon must have means of evaluating other regions with the knowledge that their evaluation provides a consistent reflection of the problem that one must deal with in the fractured portion of the limb.

Both imaging and bone density measurements are much easier and more consistent in the more distal portions of the limb; and the contralateral limb generally correlates very well in both mineral density and bone quality evaluations. Certain technical features of each X-ray site must be carefully evaluated to provide good consistent X-ray technique when one is using plain radiographs. A simple step wedge can provide consistent relative measures of bone density and help to assure that the X-ray exposure is consistent from one view to another (Inoue *et al.* 1983; Latta, Zych and Greenbarg, 1988). Since measurements in the same or contralateral limb correlate well, the difficulty of reading a Singh Index in a fractured hip can be avoided by reading the opposite hip or the distal femur (Figure 4.2). Problems with measurements of the distal femur and proximal tibia have to do with blockage of full view of the bone by other bones in conventional X-ray views. The fibula obscures the view of the lateral column of the proximal tibia because of its posterior location and overlap to the tibia in a normal front view. Likewise, the patella obscures the central view of the distal

femur when the knee is extended. Thus, special radiographic techniques may be used to help provide better qualitative measures from these views. X-rays of the distal femur with the knee flexed can provide an excellent view of the medial and lateral columns in the central portion of the distal femur in the critical region of assessment. A slightly lateral oblique view of the tibia can provide a reasonable assessment on the medial and lateral columns while reducing the overlap of the proximal fibula on the lateral column.

The proximal humerus, like the hip, is surrounded by a thick layer of soft tissue which is quite variable among individuals. This makes it difficult to obtain consistent X-rays in this region. The distal radius can provide much more consistent plain X-rays because of the very thin layer of soft tissue and lack of other bones which impede the view. The metacarpals provide consistent plain radiographic images which provide an excellent opportunity for consistent measurements of cortical bone changes which relate well to osteoporotic changes in the distal radius and proximal humerus (Meema, 1991). A step wedge can be very important in assessing the exposure in a plain radiograph when measuring cancellous density and cortical thickness, as one must keep in mind that the image of each can be dramatically altered by the X-ray exposure.

FRACTURES IN OSTEOPOROTIC BONES

The most common fractures to occur in osteoporotic bone consistently occur in the cancellous regions of the long bones and spine. The most common sites of fracture are in the vertebral bodies, the proximal humerus, the distal radius, the proximal femur, the distal femur, and the proximal tibia. In subsequent chapters, the specific problems of fracture fixation in the upper and lower limbs will be addressed for those areas of most common fracture incidence. The spine will

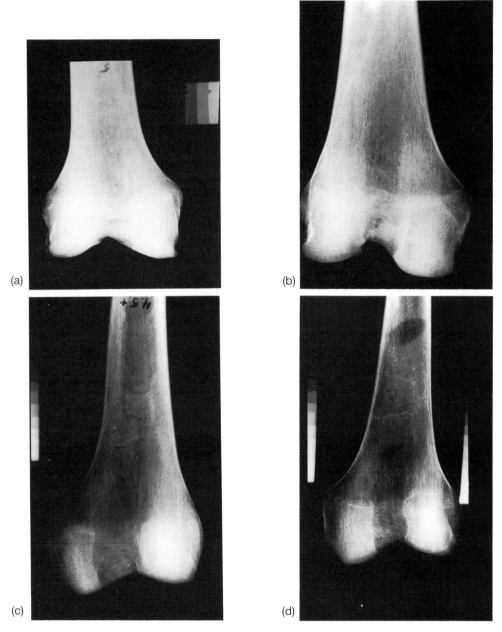

Figure 4.2 Frontal view of the distal end of the femur in normal bone, (a), Grade IV, demonstrates both medial and lateral structural trabecular columns and good cross coupling trabeculae. In the earliest stages of osteoporotic change, the cross coupling trabeculae are the first to disappear leaving the medial and lateral structural columns intact, (b), Grade III. The most significant change which distinguishes the relatively 'osteoporotic' bone from the relatively 'normal' bone can be seen as a loss of continuity of one of the major structural columns, (c), Grade II. Note that the medial column of trabeculae is the first to lose continuity and remains less dense than the lateral column as osteoporosis progresses to Grade I, (d).

not be addressed because spinal fractures generally require minimal treatment and are associated with lower risk of morbidity and mortality (Cohen 1990).

Injuries to the upper and lower limb in patients with osteoporosis are, in most cases, closed injuries of less energy and minimal soft tissue damage. Because of the osteoporosis, however, the bone bleeds profusely when fractured and edema in adjacent limb parts is often extensive. Closed treatment of closed injuries is generally the most acceptable for all types of fractures (Charnley, 1968; Sarmiento and Latta, 1981). However, if the closed treatment requires prolonged bed rest, or prolonged immobilization in elderly patients with osteoporosis, the morbidity can be extensive. Therefore, all treatment techniques should aim at early functional return, long before the fracture has healed. Immobilization during fracture healing can provide a false sense of security, as the X-ray evidence of healing and the fracture stiffness progresses much faster than the strength of the healing callus. Thus healing under conditions of limb immobilization creates muscle atrophy and hard, brittle callus which is weak (Sarmiento *et al.*, 1977b). On the other hand, motion at the fracture site resulting from function causes a large peripheral callus to form which is strong before it is stiff and radiographically dense (Goodship and Kenwright, 1985; Kenwright *et al.*, 1986; Latta, Sarmiento and Tarr, 1980; Panjabi *et al.*, Wardlaw *et al.*, 1981). The motion which causes large peripheral callus to form at a diaphyseal fracture however, may be too much for the healing of a metaphyseal fracture, since the healing process is different (Charnley, 1968; Uhtoff, Goto and Cerckel, 1987). The majority of the fractures which occur in osteoporotic bone are metaphyseal rather than diaphyseal. This poses two problems in the application of aggressive, closed techniques. First, fracture fragments in the metaphyseal region tend to be short

which makes it difficult to control them through soft tissue compression. Functional braces or casts must use soft tissue tension band principles through joint positioning or direct three-point pressure to be effective at controlling most metaphyseal fractures (Sarmiento *et al.*, 1975; Sarmiento, Zagorshi and Sinclair 1980; Zagorski *et al.*, 1987; Oullette *et al.*, 1989; Moir *et al.*, 1991).

Generally the most efficient way of providing early functional return is to provide maximal skeletal stabilization. This often requires extensive surgical procedures and good bone fixation. This group of patients, in general, have poor tolerance for extensive surgical procedures and the poor mechanical quality of the bone makes it difficult to achieve good mechanical fixation. Therefore, one must carefully weight these priorities when evaluating methods of fracture fixation in context with the need to minimize the surgical trauma and maximize early function return. Often the biological disadvantage of good rigid internal fixation outweighs its mechanical advantages in this group of patients (Sarmiento and Latta, 1981). The enthusiastic surgeon must keep in mind that perfect anatomic alignment is not a necessary prerequisite for a good functional result and that early functional activity usually is more important than the anatomic alignment and strength of fracture fixation in obtaining the best possible outcome (Sarmiento *et al.*, 1977a; Sarmiento, Zagorshi and Sinclair, 1980; Sarmiento and Latta, 1981; Zagorski *et al.*, 1987; Kristensen Kiaer and Blicher, 1989; Tarr *et al.*, 1985; Wagner *et al.*, 1984) (Figure 4.3). Often alterations of the methods of fracture fixation specifically designed for normal bone may be necessary in order to achieve adequate fixation in osteoporotic bone. Supplemental methylmethacrylate in specific regions where fracture fixation is critical often provides excellent mechanical advantage with minimal risks to the patient (Tronzo, 1983; Enis, McCollough and

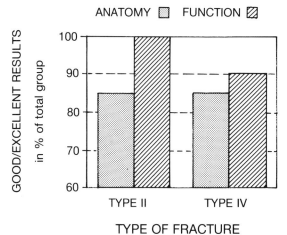

Figure 4.3 Anatomic and functional results for displaced Colles' fractures. With closed functional treatment of fractures, the functional result is usually better than the anatomical result by normal standards of evaluation. In this instance, a comparison was made of the percentage of patients that were judged to have a qualitative result of good to excellent for anatomic alignment vs. function at final follow-up after treatment in a Colles' functional brace, (Sarmiento, 1980). Note that all of the fractures were displaced requiring initial reduction and immobilization in a plaster cast for 1 to 2 weeks.

Cooper, 1974; Hawkins and Kieter, 1987; Struhl *et al.*, 1990; Husband, 1992; Bartucci *et al.*, 1985; Harrington, 1975; Cohen, 1990). Stress concentration in this very brittle bone can be very dangerous and the use of cerclage wires instead of screw fixation is often advantageous (Jensen, 1989; Partridge, 1980). Often, when screw fixation is precarious, the addition of nuts and washers on the cortical surface has proven to be very effective at improving cortical fixation and reducing the stress concentration at the interface (Hohl, 1967; Porter, 1970).

REFERENCES

Baran, D.T., Kelly, A.M., Karellas, A. *et al.* (1988) Ultrasound attenuation of the os calcis in women with osteoporosis and hip fractures. *Calc. Tiss. Internat.*, **43**, 138.

Barth, R.W., Williams, J.L. and Kaplan, F.R. (1992) Osteon morphometry in females with femoral neck fractures. *Clin. Orthop.*, **283**, 178.

Bartucci, E.J., Gonzalez, M.H., Cooperman, B.R. *et al.* (1985) The effect of adjunctive methyl-methacrylate on failures and function in patients with intertrochanteric fractures and osteoporosis. *J. Bone Joint Surg.* **67A**, 1094.

Bloom, R.A. and Laws, J.W. (1970) Humeral cortical thickness as an index of osteoporosis in women. *Br. J. Radiol.*, **43**, 522–7.

Carter, D. and Hayes, W.C. (1977) Compressive behaviour of bone. *J. Bone Joint Surg.* **59A**, 954.

Carter, M.D., Lester, G., DeMasi, M.P.H. and Talmage, R. (1990) Bone mineral content at three sites in normal perimenopausal women. *Clin. Orthop.*, **266**, 295.

Charnley, J. (1968) The Closed Treatment of Common Fractures, 3rd edn, William and Wilkins, Baltimore.

Ciarelli, M.J., Goldstein, S.A., Dickid, J.L. *et al.* (1991) Experimental determination of the orthogonal mechanical properties, density distribution of human trabecular bone from the major metaphyseal regions utilising materials testing and computed tomography. *J. Orthop. Res.*, **9**, 674.

Cohen, L.D. (1990) Fractures of the osteoporotic spine. *Orthop. Clin. N. Amer.*, **21**, 143.

Cornell, C.N., Schwartz, S. Bansal, M. *et al.* (1988) Quantification of osteopenia in hip fracture patients. *J. Orthop. Trauma*, **2**, 212.

Eastell, R., Wahner, H.W., O'Fallen, W.M. *et al.* (1989) Unequal decrease in bone density of lumbar spine and ultradistal radius in Colles' and vertebral fracture syndromes. *J. Clin. Invest.*, **83**, 168.

Enis, J.E., McCollough, N.C. and Cooper, J.S. (1974) Action of MMA on osteosynthesis. *Clin. Orthop.*, **105**, 283.

Foltin, E. (1988) Osteoporosis and fracture patterns. A study of split-compression fractures of the lateral tibial condyle. *Internal Orthop.*, **12**, 299.

Goldstein, S.A. (1987) The mechanical properties of trabecular bone: dependence on anatomic location function. *J. Biomech.*, **20**, 1055.

Goodship, A.E. and Kenwright, J. (1985) The

influence of induced micromovement upon the healing of experimental tibial fractures. *J. Bone Joint Surg.*, **67** (4), 650.

Harrington, K.D. (1975) The use of methylmethacrylate as an adjunct in the internal fixation of unstable comminuted fractures in osteoporotic patients. *J. Bone Joint Surg.*, **57A**, 138.

Hawkins, R.J. and Kiefer, G.N. (1987) Internal fixation techniques for proximal humeral fractures. *Clin. Orthop.*, **223**, 77–85.

Hayes, W.C. (1991) Biomechanics of cortical and trabecular bone: Implications for assessment of fracture risk, in *Basic Orthopaedic Biomechanics* (eds V.C. Mow and W.C. Hayes), Raven Press Ltd, New York, pp. 93–142.

Hirby, J., Anderson, A.P. and Gyrtrup, H.J. (1989) Hip fractures in previously amputated patients. *Acta Orthop. Belgica*, **55**, 35.

Hohl, M. (1967) Tibial condylar fractures. *J. Bone Joint Surg.*, **49A**, 1455.

Husband, J.B. (1992) Fractures of the distal radius (not just another Colles' fracture). *Trans 4th Current Concepts in Trauma Care*, 11–15.

Inoue, T., Kusida, K., Miyamoto, S. *et al.* (1983) Quantitative assessment of bone density on X-ray picture. *J. Jp. Orthop. Ass.*, **57**, 1923.

Jensen, R.K. (1989) Changes in segmental inertia proportions between 4 and 20 years. *J. Biomech.*, **22**, 529.

Kenwright, J., Richardson, J.B., Goodship, A.E. *et al.* (1986) Effect of controlled axial micromovement on healing of tibial fractures. *Lancet*, **2**, 1185.

Khairi, M.R.A., Cronin, J.H., Robb, J.A. *et al.* (1976) Femoral trabecular pattern index and bone mineral content measurement by photon absorption in senile osteoporosis. *J. Bone Joint Surg.*, **58A**, 221–5.

Kranendonk, D.H., Jurist, J.M. and Lee, H.G. (1972) Femoral trabecular patterns and bone mineral content. *J. Bone Joint Surg.*, **54A**, 1472–7.

Kristensen, K.D., Kiaer, T. and Blicher, J. (1989) No arthrosis of the ankle 20 years after malaligned tibial-shaft fracture. *Acta Orthop. Scand.*, **60**, 208.

Latta, L.L., Sarmiento, A. and Tarr, R.R. (1980) The rationale of functional bracing of fractures. *Clin. Orthop.*, **146**, 28.

Latta, L.L., Zych, G.A. and Greenbarg, P. (1988)

Mechanics of distal locking in I.M. Rods – comparison in osteoporotic and normal femurs, in *Femoral Intramedullary Rods: Clinical Performance and Related Laboratory Testing*, ASTM, Philadelphia, PA.

Leichner, L. (1982) Relationship between bone density, mineral content and mechanical strength of the femoral neck. *Clin. Orthop*, **163**, 272.

McCalden, R.W., McGeough, J.A., Barker, M.B. *et al.* (1991) The effect of ageing in the tensile properties of human cortical bone: the relative importance of changes in porosity, mineralization and microstructure. *Orthop. Trans*, **15**, 520.

Meema, H.W. (1991) Improved vertebral fracture threshold in postmenopausal osteoporosis by radiogrametric measurements: its usefulness in selection for preventive therapy. *J.Bone Min. Res*, **6**, 9.

Meltzer, M, Lessig, J.H. and Siegel, J.A.D. (1989) Bone mineral density and fracture in postmenopausal women. *Calc. Tiss. Internat*, **45**, 142.

Moir, J.S., Wytch, R., Ashcroft, G.P. *et al.* (1991) Intracast pressure measurements in Colles' fractures. *Injury*, **22**, 446.

Ostiere, S.J. and Gold, R.H. (1991) Osteoporosis and bone density measurement methods. *Clin. Orthop*, **271**, 149.

Ouelette, E.W., Dennis, J., Milne, E.L. *et al.* (1989) The tension band effect of soft tissues in the bending behaviour of external and internal metacarpal fixation. *Proc 13th Internat. Conf. Hoffman Ext. Fix.*, p 80.

Panjabi, M.M., Lindsey, R.W., Walter, S.D. and White, A.A. (1989) The clinician's ability to evaluate the strength of healing fractures from plain radiographs. *J.Orthop.Trauma*, **3**, 29.

Partridge, M.M. (1980) Nylon cerclage fixation for osteoporotic fractures. *J. Bone Joint Surg.*, **62B**, 123.

Porter, B.B. (1970) Crush fractures of the lateral tibial table. *J.Bone Joint Surg*, **52B**, 676.

Roser, S.E., Keller, T.S., Weisberger, A.M. and Spengler, D.M. (1991) Compressive mechanical properties and the distribution of density and porosity in the human femur. *Orthop. Trans*, **15**, 524.

Ross, P.D., Wasnich, R.D. and Vogel, J.M. (1988)

Detection of prefracture spinal osteoporosis using bone mineral absorptiometry. *J.Bone Min. Res.*, **3**, 1.

Saha, S. and Albright, J.A. (1990) Evaluation of osteoporosis by ultrasound, cat scan and photon absorptiometry. *Rehab,R. & D.*, **27**, 56.

Sarmiento, A. and Kinman, P.B., Galvin, E.G. *et al.* (1977a) Functional bracing of fractures of the shaft of the humerus. *J.Bone Joint Surg.*, **59A**, 596.

Sarmiento, A. and Latta, L.L. (1981) *Closed Functional Treatment of Fractures*, Springer-Verlag, Berlin.

Sarmiento, A., Pratt, G.W., Berry, N.C. and Sinclair, W.F. (1975) Colles' fractures – functional bracing in supination. *J. Bone Joint Surg*, **57A**, 311.

Sarmiento, A., Schaeffer, J., Beckerman, L. *et al.* (1977b) Fracture healing in rat femora affected by functional weight bearing. *J. Bone Joint Surg.*, **59A**, 369.

Sarmiento, A., Zagorski, J.B. and Sinclair, W.F. (1980) Functional bracing and Colles' fractures: A prospective study of immobilisation in supination vs. pronation. *Clin. Orthop.*, **146**, 175.

Singh, M.D., Hagrath, A.R. and Naini, P.S. (1970) Changes in trabeculae pattern of the upper end of the femur as an index of osteoporosis. *J. Bone Joint Surg.*, **52A**, 1970.

Smith, M.D., Cody, D.D., Goldstein, S.A. *et al.* (1992) Proximal femoral bone density and its correlation to fracture load and hip-screw penetration. *Clin. Orthop*, **283**, 244.

Struhl, S., Szporn, M.N., Cobelli, N.J. and Sadler, A.H. (1990) Cemented internal fixation for supracondylar femur fractures in osteoporotic patients. *J. Orthop. Trauma*, **4**, 151.

Tarr, R.R., Resnick, C.T., Wagner, K.S. and Sarmiento, A. (1985) Changes in tibiotalar joint contact areas following experimentally induced tibial angular deformities. *Clin. Orthop. Rel. Res.*, **199**, 72.

Tronzo, R.G. (1983) Augment internal fixation with fenestrated hip screw and cement. *Orthop. Review*, **12**, 59–64.

Uhtoff, H.K,. Goto, S. and Cerckel, P.H. (1987) Influence of stable fixation on trabecular bone healing; A morphologic assessment in dogs. *J. Orthop. Res.*, **5**(1), 14.

Van Der Voort, P.H., Taconis, W.K., Van Schaik, C.L. and Silberbusch, J. (1990) The relationship between densitometry of the radius and vertebral fractures. *Netherlands J. Med.*, **37**, 53.

Wagner, K.S., Tarr, R.R., Resnick, C. and Sarmiento, A. (1984) The effect of simulated tibial deformities on the ankle joint during the gait cycle. *Foot & Ankle*, **5**, 31.

Wardlaw, D., McLaughlan, J., Pratt, D.J. and Bowker, P (1981) A biomechanical study of case-brace treatment of femoral shaft fractures. *J. Bone Joint Surg.*, **63B**, 7.

Zagorski, J.B., Zych, G.A., Latta, L.L. and McCollough, N.C. (1987) Modern concepts in functional fracture bracing – upper limb, in *AAOS Instructional Course Lectures*, Vol XXXVI, Chap 24, AAOS, Chicago, IL.

5

Techniques of osteosynthesis

RALPH HERTEL

PROBLEMS OF INTERNAL FIXATION IN THE ELDERLY PATIENT

GENERAL PROBLEMS

All internal fixation procedures require anesthesia, and many involve significant blood loss and prolonged operating times. The elderly patient is generally less well equipped to withstand this surgical trauma than the younger patient, and the potential hazards of even relatively straightforward surgery must not be underestimated when planning the overall treatment. These matters are discussed in detail elsewhere in this text.

The other difficulty which is often encountered is the need to protect internal fixation postoperatively, whilst still getting the benefits of early mobilization. The elderly are rarely able to comply with the instruction to only partially bear weight on an injured leg. The majority of hip fracture patients are allowed to take as much weight as possible as soon as they are mobilized, but more complex osteosyntheses, such as a supracondylar femoral reconstruction, require protection in the initial stages of healing, to avoid screw cut out and implant fatigue fracture, the two commonest modes of failure, even in a correctly executed fixation. As it is often impossible to predict the patient's ability to comply with restrictions on bearing weight it may be necessary to err on the side of caution in many cases, using casts and functional braces in certain injuries as adjuncts to internal fixation.

PROBLEMS RELATED TO OSTEOPOROSIS

Fracture location and morphology are influenced by the degree of osteopaenia. Metaphyseal fractures with compression of the cancellous bone are frequent, whereas in the diaphysis long torsional fractures are more typical. Fractures in the elderly are usually due to low energy trauma, causing little displacement and leaving the soft tissues intact.

Fractures of osteoporotic bone have impaired healing compared to normal bone (Lane, 1980), although the same biological response occurs in osteoporotic and normal bone and the stages of fracture healing are the same. Hard callus formation and remodeling are less certain in osteoporosis.

Skeletal Trauma in Old Age
Published in 1994 by Chapman & Hall, London
ISBN 0 412 48750 0

Mineralization is dependent on calcium, vitamin D and parathyroid hormone, all of which are altered in osteoporosis. The altered mechanical properties of osteoporotic bone result in a greatly impaired anchorage of any implant. *In vitro* the maximal axial load of standard 4.5 AO screws has a close correlation with cortical radiolucency (Matter *et al.*, 1977), decreasing from normal values of 3000–4000 N, to values below 1000 N. Transpedicular screws used in spinal fixation have only weak anchorage in the presence of osteoporosis. Kirschner wires and cerclage wires tend to cut through the relatively soft bone. Intramedullary rods and pins provide little stability in the metaphyseal area and may cut through atrophic cancellous trabeculae and the subchondral bone plate.

Reduction techniques in porotic bone should be extremely atraumatic. Forcefully applied bone clamps may lead to impression fractures, jeopardizing further implant anchorage. Indirect reduction techniques as described by Mast, Jakob and Ganz (1989), are of great value in this regard.

The implant can act as a stress riser and lead to additional fractures either during the procedure or at any time afterwards. Typical examples are fractures at the end of a plate or a prosthetic stem.

Metaphyseal fractures in osteoporotic bone tend to be highly impacted. Reduction may result in large defects in the bone. Since autologous cancellous bone donor sites, such as the iliac crest, yield relatively little in the elderly, the alternatives, such as allograft, bone substitutes or methylmethacrylate may be required. In some cases it is wiser to accept a degree of deformity than to create a defect with its inherent instability by narrow-minded anatomical reduction. A common example of where disimpaction may well be contraindicated is a fracture at the proximal end of the femur.

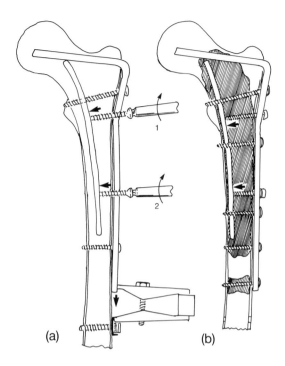

(a)   (b)

Figure 5.1 Use of methylmethacrylate to enhance stability of the compound. (a) After indirect reduction and preliminary fixation of the outer plate, the medullary plate is introduced through the comminuted fracture area or a narrow fenestration. Push screws 1 and 2 are used to medialize the plate as far as possible. (b) The medullary cavity is filled with methylmethacrylate. Cement in the fracture gap is undesirable. The remaining screws are tightened after hardening of the cement.

PROBLEMS RELATED TO PREVIOUS SURGERY

Metal implants are much stiffer than porotic bone. This leads to important stress concentrations at the ends of any implant. The longer the lever arm the higher is the stress. This is especially true in ankylosis or arthrodesis of adjacent joints. The most frequent problem is a fracture at the end of a prosthetic stem (Figure 5.11). If significant osteoporosis is present then fixation becomes a true challenge. In these cases the biological

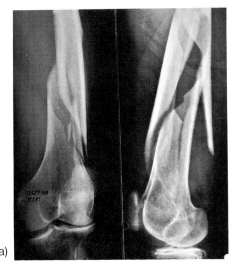

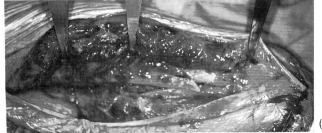

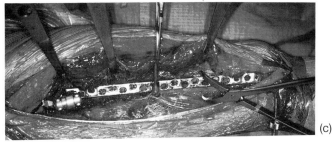

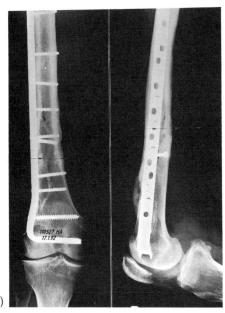

Figure 5.2 Long splintage. (a) Multifragmental spiral fracture in a 64-year-old man. (b) Biological osteosynthesis. Epiperiosteal exposure of the bone. (c) Indirect reduction technique (fixation of the plate to the distal main fragment, gross reduction to the plate, distraction, fine axial alignment, compression). (d) Healed bone without signs of vascular disturbance.

response in the fracture zone is further mitigated by the disturbed endosteal circulation.

Fractures at the ends of plates occur mainly in the diaphysis of long bones. Treatment with replating is followed by another fracture if the plate is not long enough to splint the entire length of the bone.

AIMS OF INTERNAL/EXTERNAL FIXATION IN OSTEOPOROSIS

GENERAL CONSIDERATIONS

The aim of fracture treatment, restoring the best possible function, is the same for any age

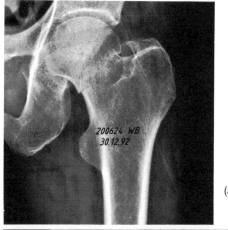
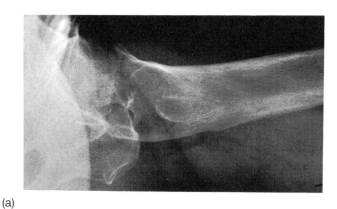

(a)

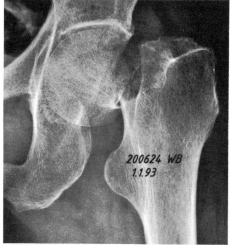

Figure 5.3 Impaction. (a) Valgus impacted femoral neck fracture in a 78-year-old female. (b) Secondary dislocation due to inadvertent full weight bearing. (c) Open reduction, valgus impaction and fixation with cannulated screws.

(b)

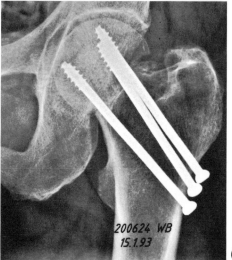
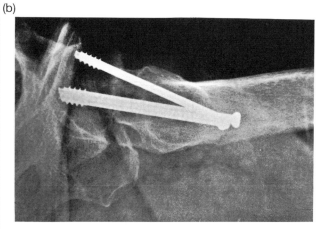

(c)

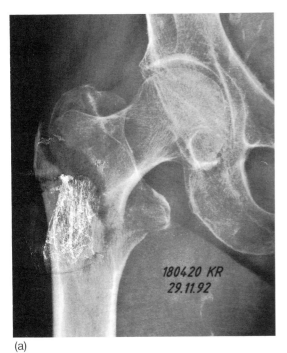

(a)

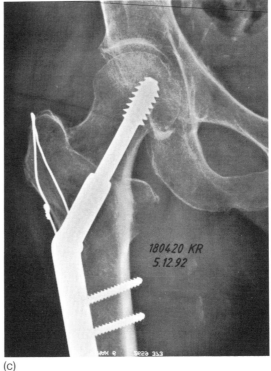

(c)

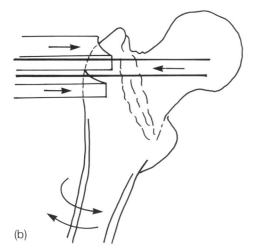

(b)

Figure 5.4 Impaction. (a) Pertrochanteric fracture with typical varus malalignment in a 72-year-old woman. (b) Reduction with slight overcorrection is temporarily held by K-wires. A slotted hammer is placed between the wires and used as a pusher. Impaction of the partially comminuted fracture zone is obtained with a heavy mallet. (c) The selected fixation device is implanted. In this case secondary impaction allowed by screw gliding is expected to be minimal.

group. For the senior population special considerations are given to the possible ways of restoring function. For a similar fracture, treatment can be quite different in a young adult compared to a senior patient, even though both treatments are aimed at best possible function. Before planning, realistic goals should be set.

Rapid restoration of mobility is the most important short-term goal. The relative merits

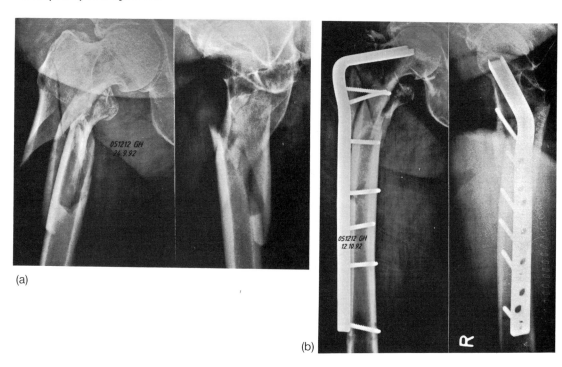

(a)

(b)

Figure 5.5 Controlled impaction. (a) Subtrochanteric fracture in a 80-year-old patient. (b) Condylar blade-plate osteosynthesis with marked controlled shortening. The technical steps were as follows: 1. introduction of a condylar blade-plate in the proximal fragment, 2. gross, indirect reduction of the distal fragment to the plate, 3. distraction with the articulated tension device followed by correct axial alignment, 4. compression with the articulated tension device to 1500 N, accepting a shortening of 2 cm.

of conservative and operative treatment should be evaluated. If operative treatment is chosen, the procedure should be minimally invasive, yielding a low complication rate, and the long-term outcome ought to be comparably good.

In all fracture treatment the correct balance between mechanical stability and preservation of bone perfusion is the key to successful osteosynthesis. This issue is embraced by the term 'biological osteosynthesis'. This concept is highly relevant to porotic bone. The essentials of minimal exposure and indirect reduction techniques are found in Mast's classic work (1989).

AIMS OF OSTEOSYNTHESIS IN THE WEIGHT BEARING EXTREMITY

Since early mobilization is the main concern, fractures in the lower extremity require a fairly stable fixation. Extra-articular fractures that can be stabilized with below knee or Sarmiento (patella tendon bearing) casts do not require operative treatment. Long casts are cumbersome for the patient, restrict mobility and can cause complications. Operative treatment, to avoid restrictive immobilization, is therefore often justified. Internal fixation aims at early mobilization to avoid cardiopulmonary and thromboembolic com-

60

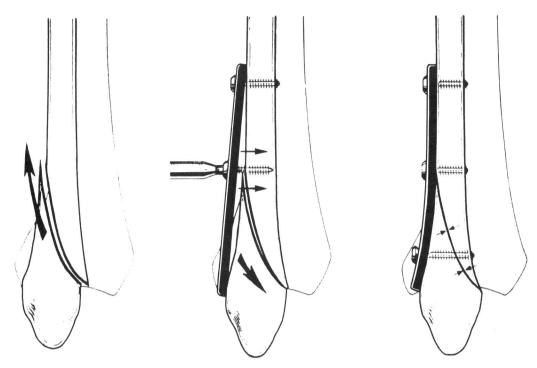

Figure 5.6 Antiglide principle. Wide buttress can be obtained by careful selection of the plate position. Dorsal plate application for type B malleolar fractures is excellent in providing high primary stability (From H. Weber, *Spezielle Osteosynthesen*, Springer-Verlag 1979).

plications. Any osteosynthesis must be stable enough to resist uncontrolled full weight bearing, given the difficulties the elderly may have in complying with restricted mobilization, or the fixation must be externally protected, inevitably losing some of the benefits of early mobilization.

AIMS OF OSTEOSYNTHESIS IN THE UPPER EXTREMITY

In the upper extremity conservative treatment is indicated in the majority of fractures. Splints, casts or bandages do not excessively limit ambulation, provided that the lower extremities are functional, although the marginally autonomous patient may become temporarily or permanently dependent. It may sometimes be necessary to treat upper limb injuries operatively, to allow a multiply injured patient to use crutches and similar devices effectively.

TECHNIQUES OF INTERNAL FIXATION IN OSTEOPOROSIS

IMPACTION

Impaction is a key factor in stability. In some cases impaction is created by the trauma itself. A typical example is the valgus impacted abduction fracture of the femoral neck (Figure 5.3). This primary stability may be sufficient for careful functional treatment, thus allowing immediate mobilization. Compression fractures of the vertebral bodies

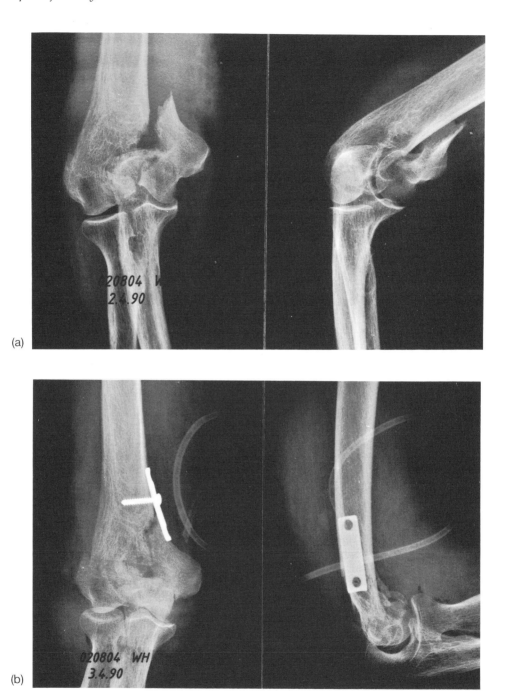

(a)

(b)

Figure 5.7 Wide buttress. (a) Distal, intraarticular fracture of the humerus. (b) Medial antiglide plate as a minimally invasive procedure to obtain reduction. A stable fixation allowing early motion is an unrealistic goal here, and should therefore not be attempted.

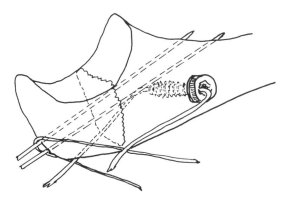

Figure 5.8 Wide buttress. Should the bone be so soft that the wire cuts through, a canulated screw may be inserted. The wire is then passed through the screw and tightened in the usual manner.

generally have sufficient stability for functional treatment in older patients. Taking advantage of impaction is a useful concept in the osteosynthesis of porotic bone. For example, in fractures of the proximal femur impaction can be achieved by the following steps: preliminary reduction of the main fragments (abduction, internal rotation), preliminary fixation with Kirschner wires, impaction with a slotted hammer placed over the trochanteric region (used as a broad impactor) and a heavy mallet (Figure 5.4). Controlled impaction can also be achieved by tensioning a plate (Figure 5.5). In subtrochanteric and supracondylar comminuted fractures, compression of fragments may be necessary to obtain stability. The resultant shortening is usually well tolerated by the elderly patient and may be looked upon as the price paid for stability.

The concept of postoperative gradual and controlled impaction has improved the stability of fixation in proximal femoral fractures. The dynamic hip screw illustrates this concept. The implant acts as a rail on which axial movement is allowed. Weight bearing leads to gradual impaction, thus increased stability

of the fixation. Over impaction is not infrequent, but does not lead to major clinical problems in this population.

WIDE BUTTRESS

The concept of the wide buttress applies to epiphyseal and metaphyseal fractures. Special implants with large surface areas are available, such as the buttress plates for the proximal tibia and distal radius.

Very efficient wide buttressing inside the bone is provided by the blade of an angled blade plate. As far as axial and rotational stability is concerned a blade is far better than a gliding screw. For supracondylar femoral fractures, which in the presence of osteoporosis typically have a long spiral element, the condylar plate is the implant of choice.

The antiglide plate as proposed by Ellis (1965) and Brunner and Weber (1981) is an excellent example of a simple buttress (Figure 5.6). It is used as a means of reduction, taking advantage of the mechanically most favorable position for the given fracture. The reduction is held by the spring-like effect of the protruding plate segment. This principle can be applied to any epiphyseal fracture (Figure 5.7).

The tension band principle can also provide a wide buttress. Two K-wires, connected by a tensioned cerclage wire, provide excellent stability in the epiphyseal and metaphyseal areas, especially when compared to screw fixation. Should the bone be so soft that the wire cuts through, a cannulated screw may be used to increase the strength of the fixation. (Figure 5.8).

LONG SPLINTAGE

Forces acting at the bone-implant interface can be influenced by modification of the lever arms (Gotzen Haar and Rietenstahl, 1983). A

63

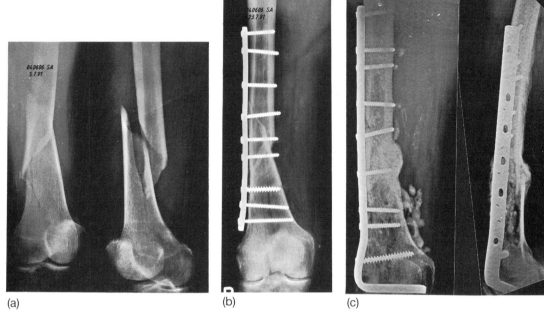

(a)   (b)   (c)

Figure 5.9 Long splintage (a) Long spiral fracture of the femur in a 85-year-old woman. (b) Failed short plate osteosynthesis. In osteoporosis this is a common failure mode. (c) Salvage with a very long plate, the blade acting as an intraosseus extension of the plate. In addition bone cement was used to enhance screw anchorage.

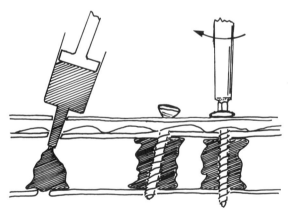

Figure 5.10 Use of methylmethacrylate to enhance screw fixation. 1. Introduction of cement with a 10 cm^3 syringe. 2. Incomplete introduction of the screw. 3. Tightening after the cement has hardened. Cement in the fracture gap is undesired.

long plate with relatively few screws gives greater stability than a shorter plate with the same number of screws (Figure 5.9). Long plates compensate for the reduced holding power of the screws in the osteoporotic bone. A clinical example is the long torsional fracture of the femur, which is typically seen in osteoporotic bone. For those fractures very long plates, often extended with an intraosseous blade, are recommended (Figure 5.2).

Intramedullary nailing represents a very efficient form of a long splintage. If used for the correct indication, it is the best way of achieving early weight bearing. Unfortunately, the ideal fractures for intramedullary nailing, that is short oblique and transverse fractures in the diaphysis, are rare in the elderly patient. The use of nails for meta-

64

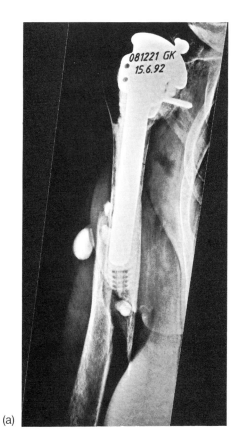

(a)

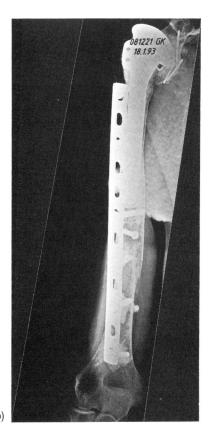

(b)

Figure 5.11 Use of methylmethacrylate to enhance screw fixation. (a) Periprosthetic fracture of the humerus in a 73-year-old woman. (b) Osteosynthesis with a long LC-DCP plate, axial compression of the fracture, use of methylmethacrylate to enhance screw fixation, decortication and autologous bone grafting at the fracture focus.

physeal fractures, using interlocking screws, is often unsuccessful because of their impaired anchorage in the soft bone.

Fascicular nailing is more appropriate in soft bone, especially for metaphyseal stabilization. It is very useful in fractures of the humerus where its indications can be extended to the proximal epiphyseal area. For fractures of the proximal femur fascicular nailing as proposed by Ender (1988) is losing popularity, due to its poor inherent stability. For the nonambulatory patient it remains a viable, minimally invasive, alternative.

The principles of long splintage can be applied to the osteoporotic spine. Fractures of the vertebral bodies that cause neurologic deficit, although rare in osteoporotic bone, need rapid decompression and stabilization. Since transpedicular systems are not suitable because of impaired screw anchorage, stability can be obtained with multisegmental Luque instrumentation. A uniform load distribution through stepwise tightening of the wires is the aim. The high stability of the resulting construct allows early brace-free mobilization.

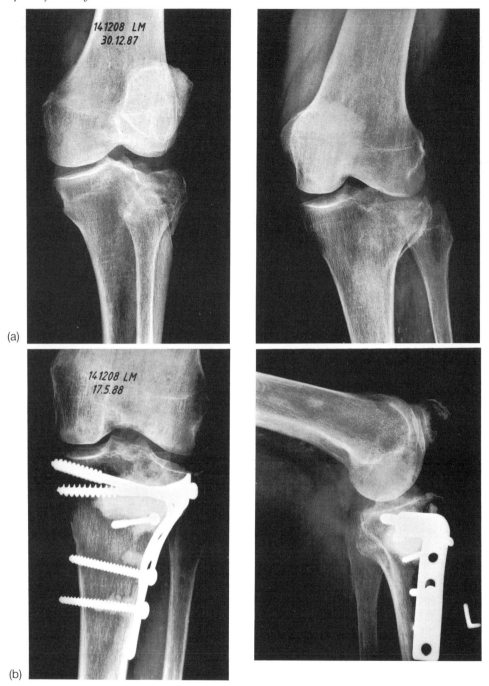

(a)

(b)

Figure 5.12 Use of methylmethacrylate to fill a defect. (a) Impacted fracture of the lateral tibial plateau in a 80-year-old woman. (b) Reduction leaves a huge cancellous bone defect that was filled with methylmethacrylate. Note the use of cement to enhance the holding power of the distal screws. Despite early weight bearing the compound remained stable.

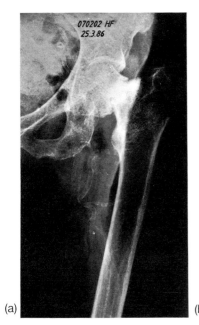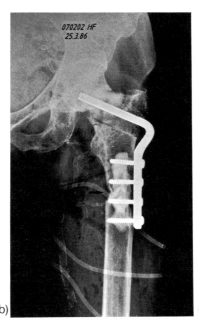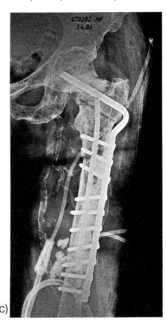

(a)   (b)   (c)

Figure 5.13 Osteotomy and problems of osteoporosis. (a) Spontaneous cervical fracture due to bone insufficiency in a 84-year-old female. (b) Intertrochanteric valgus osteotomy to unload the implant and axially compress the fracture. Fixation with a 120° plate was insufficient, due to the cortical defect that was created by a Verbrügge clamp (black arrow). Eventually a second fracture occured at this weak point. (c) Stabilization with a long plate and an intramedullary plate embedded in bone cement. Screw fixation was enhanced by methylmethacrylate.

USE OF METHYLMETHACRYLATE

Cement can be used to enhance screw fixation or as a mechanical spacer to substitute for missing bone (Figure 5.1).

When screw fixation is insufficient or even nonexistent, the introduction of a limited amount of low viscosity methylmethacrylate in the screw hole, locally filling the medullary cavity, is a very effective technique. After introduction of the cement using a syringe, the screw is incompletely inserted and fully tightened after hardening of the cement (Cameron *et al.*, 1975). (Figure 5.10). The torque that can be obtained is comparable to the torque in normal bone. Fracture healing is essentially undisturbed when using bone cement in this way (Benum, 1977; Levin and Ganz (in press); Mensch, 1987; Schatzker

Haeri and Chapman, 1978), although pouring cement into the fracture zone should be avoided (Figure 5.11).

Metaphyseal and epiphyseal defects due to temporary impaction may become apparent after reduction of a fracture. Bone cement may be used to fill these defects (Figure 5.12), particularly if the availability of good autologous bone graft is limited. If a relevant cortical defect is filled with cement, a thin layer of autologous cancellous bone should be laid on the exposed cement, to encourage bridging consolidation. Again, cement should not be interposed in the major fracture planes, where it would prevent healing.

In larger defects it is preferable to include an intramedullary plate or nail in the cement bolus which enhances primary and long term stability, acting as an armature in the concrete (Ganz, Isler and Mast, 1984) (Figure 5.1). This technique has proven valuable for pathologic fractures in metastatic disease and is increasingly used for pathologic fractures in massive osteoporosis. The main areas of application are the proximal and distal femur and the proximal humerus.

OSTEOTOMY

Osteotomy is a biomechanical approach to the problem of osteoporosis. The impaired mechanical properties of the affected bone are addressed directly. Through modification of the acting force vectors, the bone is given a more favorable mechanical environment.

A typical example is spontaneous fracture of the femoral neck due to insufficient strength of the bone, which then fails due to the normal bending moments. A varus morphology is often associated with this type of failure. Anatomical reduction and stabilization would result in high loading of the implant, without improving the mechanically unfavorable situation. Intertrochanteric abduction osteotomy, fixed with a 120° blade plate, reduces the bending moment on the bone and implant, and increases the axial compression force on the fracture (Figure 5.13). Unfortunately, these procedures are technically demanding and associated with a relatively high complication rate. In recent times the introduction of implants such as the gliding screw has led to a reduction in the number of cases suitable for such an osteotomy.

CONCLUSION

Osteosynthesis of osteoporotic bone is jeopardized by the impaired anchorage of the implants. Poor compliance in many elderly patients potentiates this problem. Solutions are directed toward increasing the stability of the osteosynthesis. Impaction, wide buttressing, long splintage, the use of methylmeth-

acrylate and osteotomy are valuable techniques.

REFERENCES

Benum, P. (1977) The use of cement as an adjunct to internal fixation of supracondylar fractures of osteoporotic femurs. *Acta Orthop. Scand.*, **48**, 52.

Brunner, Ch.F. and Weber, B.G. (1981) *Besondere Osteosynthese-Techniken*, Springer Verlag.

Cameron, H.U., Jakob, R.P., Macnab, J. and Pillard, R.M. (1975) Use of polymethylmethacrylate to enhance screw fixation in bone. *J. Bone Joint Surg. (Am.)*, **57**, 655.

Ellis, J. (1965) Smith's and Barton's Fractures: A Method of Treatment. *J. Bone Joint Surg. (Br.)*, **47**, 724–7.

Ender, H.G. (1988) Ender Nailing of the Femur and Hip, in *Operative Orthopaedics* (ed. M.W. Chapman), J.P. Lippincott, Philadelphia, pp. 379–87.

Ganz R., Isler, B. and Mast, J.W. (1984) Internal fixation technique in pathological fractures of the extremities. *Arch. Orthop. Trauma Surg.*, **103**, 73.

Gotzen, L., Haas, N. and Riefenstahl, L. (1983) Untersuchungen zur Plattenfixation an die Hauptfragmente. *Hefte Unfallheilkd*, **165**, 10.

Kenzora, J.E., McCarthy, R.E., Lowell, J.D. and Sledge, C.C. (1985) Hip fracture mortality: Relation to age, treatment, preoperative illness, time of surgery, and complications. *Clin. Orthop.*, **186**, 45.

Lane, J.M. (1980) Metabolic bone disease and fracture healing, in *Fracture Treatment and Healing* (ed. R.B. Heppenstall), W.B. Saunders, Philadelphia, pp. 946–62.

Levin, L.S., Ganz, R. (in press) The use of methylmethacrylate in the treatment of fractures of the osteoporotic tibial plateau. *J Orthop Trauma*.

Mast, J., Jakob, R.P. and Ganz, R. (1989) *Planning and Reduction Techniques in Fracture Surgery*, Springer, Berlin, Heidelberg, New York.

Matter, P., Rahn, B.A., Cordey, J. *et al.* (1977) Die Beziehung zwischen Rontgendichte und maximal erreichbarer Axialkraft von AO-Schrauben im Knochen. *Monatsschr Unfallheilkd*, **80**, 165.

Mauro, S., Tatekawa, F. and Nakano, K. (1987) Paraplegia infolge von Wirbelkompressionsfrakturen bei seniler Osteoporose. *Z. Orthop.*, **125**, 320.

Mensch, J.S. (1979) Rigid stabilisation of fracture using adjunctive methylmethacrylate. *J. Fla. Med. Assoc.*, **66**, 45.

Muller, M.E., Allgower, M., Schneider, R. and Willenegger, H. (1988) *Manual der Osteosynthese*, AO-Technik 2, Aufl Springer, Berlin, Heidelberg, New York.

Schatzker, J., Haeri, G.B. and Chapman, M. (1978) Methylmethacrylate as an adjunct in the internal fixation of intertrochanteric fractures of the femur. *J. Trauma*, **18**, 732.

FURTHER READING

Ganz, R., Thomas, R.J. and Haemmerie, C.P. (1979) Trochanteric fractures of the femur. Treatment and results. *Clin. Orthop.*, **138**, 30.

Hertel, R. (1984) Beanspruchung von Osteosyntheseplatten mit schraubenfreiem Plattenloch. Dissertation, Universitat Bern.

Hertel, R., Aebi, M. and Ganz, R. (1990) Osteosynthese bei hochgradiger Osteoporose. *Unfallchirurg*, **93**, 479–84.

6

Skin and other soft tissue injuries

MILES DICKSON and PAUL CLIFFORD

INTRODUCTION

Aging can be defined as a decline in the ability of an organism to maintain homeo-stasis under conditions of physiological stress. Put simply, this means a decrease in viability with an increase in vulnerability, and is certainly the situation as far as skin is concerned. Nowhere are the effects of aging more noticeable than in the skin. In fact, the appearance of the skin is often used in assessment of a patient's age. Skin is the primary physical barrier between man and his environment, and environmental factors such as sun exposure, play a major part in the changes that affect the skin with advancing years. Elderly skin is thinner, both at the epidermal and dermal levels. In the dermis there is a reduction in connective tissue and there are changes in collagen cross-linkages and alterations in the elastic fibers leading to reduced elasticity. The overall effect is an alteration of the biophysical properties of the skin which is rendered weaker and less elastic than young skin. Elderly skin is less able to withstand shearing forces and is therefore more prone to extensive lacerations and degloving injuries.

WOUND HEALING

The aging process leads to a reduction in cell turnover and this has an influence on wound repair and the ability of the skin to withstand wear and tear. Wound healing is essentially normal in most elderly but fit people, although healing time, especially in super-ficial wounds, is prolonged. There is often minimal scar tissue formation which can pro-duce esthetically better results than in young people. In many elderly patients who are unfit from systemic disease, such as diabetes, rheumatoid arthritis, arteriosclerosis and who may also be on long term steroid treatment, wound healing is seriously im-paired. In those patients who are unfit, special measures may be needed prior to surgery. These include the control of diabetes, correction of anemia, uremia and the control of hypertension. The effects of long-term steroids on the skin are not revers-ible. In these patients, particular attention must be paid to careful handling of the skin which is unusually fragile and harvesting of skin grafts must be done with extreme caution. Prolonged healing time, coupled with the thinness of elderly skin, can lead to particular problems with skin graft donor

Skeletal Trauma in Old Age
Published in 1994 by Chapman & Hall, London
ISBN 0 412 48750 0

sites. In a fit adult, a normal donor site should be healed within ten days and two weeks but in the elderly, epithelialization may take three or more weeks to occur.

MECHANISMS OF INJURY

As has been stated, elderly skin, because of its loss of elasticity and reduction in thickness, is less able to withstand traumatic forces that in a younger person would not be expected to cause a breach of the integument. This vulnerability is epitomized by the lower limb soft tissue injuries so frequently seen in the elderly. Blunt trauma often leads to a tearing laceration with extensive degloving of the skin. The crushing and tearing forces on the dermis and fat lead to thrombosis of the small vessels and devitalization of the skin edges. The degree of undermining is often far more extensive than would at first be apparent. Injudicious closure of even small degloving wounds often results in marginal necrosis and delay in wound healing. Closed injuries on the lower limb often lead to sizable hematoma formation. This can happen with a relatively trivial knock. The stripping and undermining caused by the hematoma leads to devitalization of the overlying skin. The effect of hyperextension injuries in the elderly can frequently be seen to be more dramatic as a result of the weakness of elderly skin. For example, a fall on the outstretched hand, hyperextending the metacarpophalangeal joints can tear the skin of the palm. Widespread capillary damage from skin trauma is common in the elderly. This often leads to bruising, occurring over much larger areas than would otherwise be expected, and can make the assessment of skin viability very difficult.

PRINCIPLES OF REPAIR

The main aim of surgical repair of wounds in any category, is to create the ideal circum-stances for quiet primary healing. In general terms, this involves the debridement of all dead and devitalized tissues and scrupulous cleansing of contaminated wounds. Should circumstances allow for the wound to be closed primarily, then this should be carried out. The difficulties arise with the elderly patient when there is doubt about skin viability and when the general condition of the patient does not allow for extensive surgery. The vast array of modern reconstructive surgical techniques that are available, has lead to a situation where, in theory at least, there is no wound that cannot be closed primarily, but such closure may require extensive and complex maneuvres such as microvascular free tissue transfers. The most common soft tissue injuries in the elderly however, do not require such extensive procedures and the vast majority of wounds can be treated, either by direct closure, or with the judicious use of skin grafts. The degloving injury on the anterior aspect of the lower leg is perhaps the best example and one of the most common of all skin injuries seen in the elderly. Under certain circumstances, these types of injuries can be treated conservatively by carefully approximating the skin edges and holding them in place with steristrips. However, where there is a particularly large laceration with extensive undermining of the skin flap, the viability of the skin is undoubtedly compromised. Under these circumstances, it is often better to excise the devitalized skin and replace it with a split skin graft. A decision to undertake a skin graft must be taken in the context of the patient's general health and desires. Conventional postoperative regimes in the management of skin grafts on the lower limb call for a period of between five days and one week of bed rest to allow a good 'take' of the graft. A prolonged stay in a hospital bed to allow this adequate take may not be in the patient's best interests. It is possible in many circumstances to carry out a meshed split skin graft of these wounds and allow early mobilization of the patient (Sharpe, Cardoso and Bahetti, 1983; Wood and Lees, 1994). The alternative is to treat the wound as a leg ulcer, and allow secondary healing with regular out-patient dressings. It should be remembered that for a split skin graft to 'take' the bed that the graft is placed on must be vascular. Skin grafts will not take on an avascular bed such as bone denuded of its periosteum, or tendons denuded of the paratenon. Wounds where such circumstances prevail will require more extensive flap cover. The essence of a skin flap as compared to a skin graft is that it has its own blood supply and is not dependent for its survival upon the tissues which it is covering. However, a local flap will not provide a new blood supply to an avascular area and must be sutured to healthy tissues around its margin. The importance of adequate wound debridement when undertaking flap repair is paramount.

Skin flaps are classified by their blood supply (random or axial patterned, fasciocutaneous, myocutaneous or microvascular free) and/or by their shape or design (advancement, rotation, transposition). In principle, skin flaps are designed to ensure a good blood supply and to utilize lax skin in one site to provide for a skin shortage elsewhere. Where there is sufficient lax skin in one site, direct closure of the resulting secondary defect is often possible. Where it is not possible, the secondary defect will need to be skin grafted. Local skin flaps in the presence of trauma may be unsafe due to the degloving effects of the injury. This is particularly the case in the injuries of the lower limb, especially when there is an underlying fracture. Under these circumstances, utilization of more complex flap cover such as local muscle transposition or even a free microvascular tissue transfer should be considered. When dealing with a severe compound injury of the lower limb, the goal should be the attainment of primary healing of all the tissues involved. Primary bone union is unlikely to occur in the absence of stable and well vascularized soft tissue cover and such injuries often call for a joint approach from orthopedic surgeons and plastic surgeons.

TECHNIQUES OF REPAIR

PRIMARY CLOSURE

Before attempting primary closure, wounds must be thoroughly cleaned and all dead and devitalized tissues removed. Elderly skin requires careful handling because of its relative fragility. Because of the laxity of elderly skin, it is frequently possible to close wounds primarily with little tension. Care should be taken to obliterate the dead space deep to the wound in order to prevent hematoma formation and the possibility of subsequent infection. Closure of the dead space may require the use of buried absorbable sutures such as Vicryl, Dexon, Maxon, PDS or chromic catgut. The author prefers the use of modern monofilament absorbable sutures (PDS, Maxon) as these are less likely to cause tissue reaction. The use of cutting needles rather than round-bodied needles enables the approximation of the dermis by taking a bite of the deeper layers of the dermis. This helps to relieve the tension in the upper dermis and epidermis making the skin closure neater and easier. It is advisable to bury the knot of a subcutaneous absorbable suture so that it does not penetrate through the skin wound. Closure of the skin itself is best carried out with monofilament, nonabsorbable sutures such as nylon or proline of a size suitable for the particular anatomical region. On the face, this will be 5/0 or 6/0 whilst in other parts of the body, 3/0 or 4/0 will be required. Delayed primary closure may sometimes be indicated if there is gross swelling or contusion of the wound and where there is uncertainty about the degree of devitalization of the tissues. It is usually not necessary to delay this closure for more than three to four days.

SKIN GRAFTS

There are many different types of skin grafts (pinch grafts, full thickness grafts, composite grafts, split thickness grafts) but in cases of large skin wounds with skin loss, split thickness skin grafts are usually indicated. For a split skin graft to take, the wound must be clean. Excess bacterial colonization may prevent the early fibrin linkage between the underside of the graft and the bed that is required for a good take. The infective organisms which trouble the plastic surgeon most include hemolytic streptococci, especially Lancefield group A and some of the pathogenic staphylococci. Old dirty wounds will require regular dressings to clean them and swabs should be taken to ensure that there are no hemolytic streptococci. Clean fresh wounds require adequate removal of any devitalized tissues prior to grafting. If there are areas of exposed tendon or bone in the wound, then a split skin graft is unlikely to succeed and alternative forms of skin cover may be required.

Split skin grafts are best harvested using either a special skin graft knife such as a Watson knife, or if available, a power dermatome. Ideal donor sites are the thigh and upper arm. The author's preference in the elderly is for the postero-lateral aspect of the thigh where the skin tends to be slightly thicker and where the wound is less likely to be rubbed by the opposite thigh. Because of the thinness of elderly skin, it is vital to set the cutting thickness of the knife to cut a very thin graft. If in doubt, it is best to cut too thin a graft to begin with. The appearance of the donor site once the skin has been harvested is a good indication of the thickness of the graft. Small punctate bleeding indicates the graft of the correct thickness leaving a good proportion of the dermis behind. Any evidence of fat in the donor site indicates that the graft is too thick. It is possible to harvest skin grafts under a local anesthetic. In the lower limb, this can be achieved either with regional anesthesia, direct infiltration of the skin with 1/2% lignocaine with adrenalin or application of local anesthetic cream (Emla). When using direct infiltration of the skin with lignocaine, it is a good idea to mix the local anesthetic with hyaluronidase as this allows the anesthetic solution to spread for a considerable distance in the subcutaneous tissues. Once the skin graft is harvested, the donor site should be dressed. There are many different methods described for dressing donor sites. These include the use of Opsite, paraffin gauze, or calcium alginate dressings. The author's preference is for sheets of calcium alginate (Kaltostat) that have been lightly soaked in saline. Several layers of gauze should be placed on top of this to absorb any exudate and the donor site dressing should be left undisturbed for at least ten days unless there is evidence of donor site infection. It is frequently a good idea to mesh or fenestrate the skin graft prior to applying it to the wound. The meshing or fenestration allows tissue fluid and blood to seep out through the interstices of the graft thereby limiting the risk of blood or fluid lifting the graft away from the bed. Meshing also allows the skin graft to conform to irregularities in the wound bed and appears to increase the chance of a 'good take'. Meshing is best carried out using a skin graft mesher which cuts a precise pattern in the graft. Many meshers allow for different proportions of mesh to be cut. For general purposes, a 1:1.5 mesh is best. A bigger mesh such as 1:3 enables the skin graft to be expanded, thereby allowing for a larger area to be covered. The alternative is to fenestrate the graft with the tip of a number 10 blade. This is best carried out by spreading the graft on a wooden board and then making multiple cuts through the graft onto the board with the tip of the blade. When the patient's skin is particularly thin, there is often delay in donor site healing. It is frequently a good idea when harvesting the skin graft, to take more skin than is required for wound coverage. The extra skin can be meshed, expanded and reapplied to the donor site (Fatah and Ward, 1984). Re-epithelialization of the donor site will be greatly improved with this technique. Any spare skin graft can be stored in a fridge at about 3°C for up to 10 days. The skin should be spread on a moist saline gauze which can then be rolled up and placed in a sterile container.

Once the wound has been cleaned and any excessive hemorrhage controlled, the graft should be carefully spread with care being taken to ensure that the graft makes good contact throughout the bed of the wound. Skin grafts have a certain hemostatic effect and once the graft has been spread, careful milking of any blood collected under the graft may be required until any residual bleeding ceases. In most circumstances, the graft sticks quite firmly to the bed as a result of fibrinous exudate from the bed. Under these circumstances, it may not be necessary to use any additional form of graft fixation but if in doubt, some tacking sutures between the graft and the skin edges can be employed. An alternative is to use histoacryl glue, carefully applied to the edges of the graft. Most skin grafts should be dressed with a carefully applied, lightly padded, dressing. The author's preference is to use a layer of paraffin gauze followed by a layer of cotton wool soaked in saline or acroflavin to fill the irregularities of the bed then a layer of Orthoband and a firm elasticated bandage. An alternative to the use of soaked wool is to cut a piece of sponge to the shape of the wound and place this on top of the paraffin gauze then continue the bandaging over the top of the sponge. The sponge provides a constant light compression of the graft

against the bed. If the wound is in an area where movement will cause shearing of the graft against the bed, then a plaster of Paris splint may be required. Postoperatively, the graft should be inspected between three and five days. Where there has been 'good take' the graft will appear pink and will not move on the wound bed. With grafted wounds on the lower limb, it is safe to mobilize at this stage provided there is a firm dressing with good toe to knee bandaging.

There is good evidence that when a meshed skin graft has been applied to a wound on the lower limb, and sponge has been used as part of the dressing with firm compression bandaging, that immediate mobilization can be undertaken in the early postoperative period. Wounds in awkward sites that are difficult to dress, may benefit from the delayed exposed application of a skin graft. The skin graft, once harvested, is stored in the fridge. Once the patient has been returned to the ward, the wound dressings are removed and the skin graft applied directly. Such skin grafts require frequent attention from the nursing staff to remove any exudate and to ensure that the graft has not been dislodged.

FLAPS

The principles of governing the use of flaps for repairing skin wounds have already been discussed. Details of the various techniques of flap repair are beyond the scope of this chapter and the reader is encouraged to refer to the relevant plastic surgery texts or preferably to a plastic surgeon.

FURTHER READING

Behrens, F. (1992) Fractures with soft tissue injuries, in *Skeletal Trauma* (eds B.D. Browner, J.B. Jupiter, A.M. Levine and P.G. Trafton), W.B. Saunders Company, Philadelphia, pp. 311–36.

Fatah, M.F. and Ward, C.M. (1984) The morbidity of skin graft donor sites in the elderly: the case for mesh grafting the donor site. *Brit. J. Plastic Surg.*, **37**, 184–90.

Nerlich, M.L. and Tscherne, H. (1992) Biology of soft tissue injuries, in *Skeletal Trauma* (eds B.D. Browner, J.B. Jupiter, A.M. Levine and P.G. Trafton), W.B. Saunders Company, Philadelphia, pp. 77–94.

Sharpe, D.T., Cardoso, S. and Bahetti, V. (1983) The immediate mobilization of patients with lower limb skin grafts: a clinical report. *Brit. J. Plastic Surg.*, **36**, 105–8.

Stevenson, T.R., Whetzel, T.P. and Chapman, M.W. (1993) Soft tissue wound management, closure and complications, in Operative Orthopaedics, 2nd edn (ed. M.W. Chapman), J.B. Lippincott Company, Philadelphia, pp. 109–22.

Wood, S.H. and Lees, V.C. (1994) A prospective investigation of the healing of grafted pre-tibial wounds with early and late mobilization. *Brit. J. Plastic Surg.*, **47**, 127–31.

7

Non-operative treatment and early management of trauma

BENEDICT CLIFT and DAVID ROWLEY

INTRODUCTION

There is a large group of fractures in the elderly population which are similar in their bony anatomy to the kind of injury encountered in younger patients, but require a less aggressive management protocol. This is primarily due to the fact that much less energy is required to break osteoporotic bone, and such injuries, which are often due to 'trivial' trauma, consequently have less displacement of bone fragments and less associated soft tissue injury. Healing therefore tends to be uncomplicated and predictable. This group includes most of the vertebral, pelvic and acetabular fractures seen in the elderly. There is a much smaller group of patients whose fractures would usually be treated operatively who will nevertheless obtain an acceptable result treated conservatively, when surgery is precluded for any reason. These include fractures around the elbow and the knee. Lastly, there are many injuries, such as fractures of the clavicle, in which the primary treatment would be non-operative in any age group. The following chapter is concerned with the first and second of the above groups. The term 'non-operative' is used in the sense of requiring neither surgery, nor any other procedure which would entail general or regional anesthesia.

VERTEBRAL FRACTURES

Elderly people are not exempt from high-energy spinal injuries with the potential for instability and associated damage to neural structures. However, by far the commonest vertebral fractures seen in this age group are those occurring in the thoracolumbar spine in association with osteoporosis. Although patients with these injuries frequently present following a fall, it is now thought that atraumatic loading of the vertebrae – as occurs in bending forward, lifting objects and climbing stairs – is the primary cause of the majority of these injuries (Cooper and Melton, 1992).

There are a number of terms employed to describe these fractures – crush, compression, collapse and wedge being the main ones – but they all refer to one basic mechanism of injury. Reduced bone density within the vertebral body decreases the capacity of the vertebra to absorb forces, be they small and repetitive as in the activities of daily living, or one-off larger loads such as

Skeletal Trauma in Old Age
Published in 1994 by Chapman & Hall, London
ISBN 0 412 48750 0

might occur in a fall. The internal architecture of the body collapses, and the subsequent radiological picture of wedging, biconcave collapse or a complete crush simply reflects the net direction of these forces.

EPIDEMIOLOGY

There have been several problems in calculating the incidence of these injuries. Firstly, what is the definition of a vertebral fracture? Using the lateral radiograph of the spine it has been suggested that loss of height of the vertebral body by at least three standard deviations from the mean (Eastell *et al.*, 1991), or a decrease in area of the body by at least 35% (Ross *et al.*, 1991) are defining criteria. Using either method, it must be borne in mind that each successive vertebra has unique dimensions, and clearly neither technique is of great value in normal clinical practice. In addition, recent work suggests that even so-called objective criteria like those mentioned are open to considerable subjective bias (Armstrong *et al.*, 1992). The second problem is that a large number of these injuries, probably the majority, are asymptomatic. It is thought that only about one-third of people with these fractures seek medical advice for the condition. Large-scale screening of the population is therefore the only likely way to obtain true figures for incidence and prevalence. Thirdly, it is becoming clear that the incidence probably varies widely, even between countries in the developed world with broadly similar lifestyle and health patterns.

Bearing in mind these provisos, it has been estimated that among white women over fifty years old in the United States the age-adjusted incidence is 15.1 per 1000 person years (Cooper and Melton, 1992). The prevalence increases steadily with increasing age, so that by seventy years the figure is 21.9%, and by eighty years it is 37.4%. The rate in Britain may well be much less than this, in keeping with the observed transatlantic difference in incidence of fracture of the hip, although a Danish population-based study found that the prevalence of these fractures in 70-year-old women was also 21% (Jensen *et al.*, 1982). Another way to look at it is that the overall incidence of vertebral fractures, both silent and symptomatic, is about twice that of hip fracture.

CLINICAL PRESENTATION

The dominant feature is pain. This is felt over a fairly wide area of the back, but the fracture may be localized to some extent by the site of maximum tenderness, and by pain referred along the corresponding dermatomes, usually symmetrically. The vertebrae most commonly involved are between T8 and L3, and pain may therefore be referred over a wide distribution from the chest to the legs. More than one level is frequently involved, but the single most affected vertebra is T12. The pain is of variable severity, but in the acute situation may be excruciating. The slightest movement tends to exacerbate this, bed rest is therefore beneficial and thus forms the basis of treatment. Apart from age, there may be other risk factors for osteoporosis evident, such as alcohol abuse or the use of systemic steroids. A relatively small number of patients will accurately relate the onset of their pain to a specific episode of trauma, usually a fall.

On physical examination there may be a noticeable kyphosis centered over the vertebral collapse. Local tenderness over the involved vertebrae is usual, as is a variable amount of paraspinal muscle guarding and restriction of spinal movement. In cases of multiple fractures these features are more diffuse. The absence of certain signs is also valuable. Lack of tenderness can help to distinguish old from new fractures, as seen on the radiograph, and a normal neurological examination is necessary before one can safely treat these injuries with early mobilization.

INVESTIGATIONS

Antero posterior (AP) and lateral radiographs are required of the relevant areas of the spine. Further imaging is rarely needed except to investigate those cases where another underlying pathology is suspected. The differential diagnoses are vertebral collapse secondary to metastases, multiple myeloma and Paget's disease, and more rarely, infection. In such circumstances coned views and tomograms of affected vertebrae can reveal useful detail. Limited skeletal screening is also helpful if these potentially systemic conditions need to be excluded. Isotope bone scanning will aid diagnosis in these circumstances and is occasionally useful to determine whether or not a fracture is recent in patients with back pain of uncertain origin. Using the grading systems currently in vogue it has been shown that there is no correlation between back pain and the presence of minor vertebral fractures and this symptom is only present when there is loss of more than 35% of the area of the vertebral body on the lateral radiograph. Caution is therefore advised when ascribing severe back pain to such injuries, particularly in the elderly where multiple pathologies are rife.

Hematological and biochemical tests have a role in the above differential diagnosis but with a simple osteoporotic vertebral fracture the results are normal. Nevertheless it is prudent to perform the simplest screening tests, notably the erythrocyte sedimentation rate (ESR), full blood count (FBC), urea and electrolytes (U&Es) and basic bone biochemistry.

Further investigations such as CT scanning, bone aspiration and so on are very rarely required and will not be discussed.

MANAGEMENT

The acute management of these injuries consists of rest, analgesia and early mobilization. There are no published clinical trials to support this line of action, although one reported survey of orthopedic surgeons has shown a universal consensus in support of it (Woolf and Dixon, 1988). If the patient's home circumstances permit, it is possible to manage such patients at home, and indeed, one presumes that the majority who never seek medical advice must follow this path. Those that do present usually require admission. Most patients get adequate pain relief from simple analgesics such as paracetamol, the cautious use of non-steroidal anti-inflammatories and occasionally a small dose of diazepam to relieve muscle spasm. The need for more powerful drugs, such as opiates, suggests the possibility of more sinister pathology. Within a few days most patients are able to sit out of bed and begin to mobilize, although they usually need the help of walking aids and physiotherapists in this early period. Once mobilization is established, the help of the rehabilitation team may be required to return the patient to their previous environment. A number of patients benefit from wearing a well-fitted orthosis although care is required to prevent the development of pressure sores, particularly over the spinal prominence and the iliac crests.

Anabolic steroids, sodium fluoride and a number of other agents have been used in an effort to present further fractures in this condition with somewhat mixed results. The most promising agent based on current evidence may be oral etidronate, a diphosphonate compound, in combination with calcium and vitamin D supplements. Over a three-year period the incidence of further fracture was significantly reduced in a prospective trial, with no adverse side-effects (Storm *et al.*, 1990). No single agent has yet been adopted on a widespread basis in the United Kingdom, and a cost–benefit analysis has yet to be performed. There is some epidemiological evidence that fractures with a crush, rather than wedge configuration, are the group more likely to be associated with further osteoporotic vertebral collapse, and this group in particular may benefit from secondary preventive measures (Jensen *et al.*, 1982).

COMPLICATIONS

The main complications are those of recumbency. Chest infection, deep vein thrombosis (DVT), confusion and pressure sores are all risks. Renal tract stone formation is moderately common due to the temporary elevation in plasma calcium as a consequence of bed rest and skeletal injury. The pain of thoracic vertebral fractures may reduce a patient's vital capacity and tidal volume, thereby increasing the chances of chest infection and hypoxia. A prominent kyphosis must be carefully watched for signs of pressure necrosis of the overlying skin. As with most complications, the key to management is prevention.

There are a few reports in the literature describing the late onset of paraplegia following osteoporotic vertebral collapse. The gradual development of leg weakness, bladder and bowel disturbance and variable sensory changes are the usual findings in such cases. In this very rare situation surgical decompression and immobilization is reported to be beneficial (Shikata *et al.*, 1990).

In the longer term some patients will complain of backache for which symptomatic treatment only is required.

ACETABULAR FRACTURES

The acetabular fractures of the elderly tend to be regarded as relatively benign injuries that do well with simple conservative measures. While this is true in most cases, there is a significant subgroup that may require more aggressive management, the problem being to identify such patients as early as possible.

Isolated acetabular fractures constitute about 8% of all fractures of the pelvic bones in the elderly (Melton *et al.*, 1981), and of this group, about 70% have minimally displaced or undisplaced fractures at the time of presentation. The remainder show displacement of greater than five millimetres of the fragments. One would correctly expect this latter group to fare badly with non-operative management as with any displaced intra-articular injury. The difficulty lies with the initially undisplaced group, as in about a quarter of these patients there will be subsequent fragment displacement (Spencer, 1989).

Clinical presentation

Most of these fractures result from a simple fall, although displaced fractures are more likely to be due to higher energy trauma, such as a road traffic accident. The main complaint is pain, mainly around the groin and thigh. Hip movement is restricted and nearly always very painful. Weight bearing is usually not possible. With a displaced fracture the leg may appear shortened.

Radiography

An AP radiograph of the pelvis (Figure 7.1) will usually show that an acetabular fracture is present. Full assessment of the injury is only possible with 45 degree oblique views as well, known as the obturator oblique and the iliac oblique views. The former shows the anterior column of the bony pelvis particularly well, and the latter demonstrates the posterior column and iliac wing. Many acetabular fractures extend beyond the confines of the acetabular dome and this, along with unsuspected displacement of the fracture,

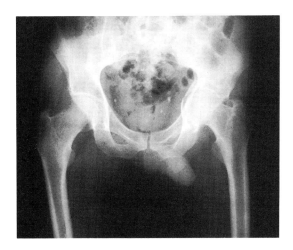

Figure 7.1 A minimally displaced acetabular fracture, following a simple fall.

may only be apparent on the oblique films. On the AP radiograph one usually sees a crack in the dome, sometimes with extension along the ilio-pubic line. Using all three views one finds that in the elderly about half of the fractures are transverse fractures, with the remainder split into three roughly equal groups of posterior column, anterior column and both-column fractures. Beyond this, further imaging is usually unnecessary in the elderly, as only a few of these patients will require surgery. In this small group, a CT scan of the pelvis is usually advisable as it provides detailed information on the state of the articular surface, the presence of loose fragments, and any associated injuries, particularly femoral head fractures and damage to the posterior elements of the bony pelvis.

MANAGEMENT

It is important to establish as soon as possible whether or not the injury is a result of high energy trauma or not. This is usually obvious from the mode of injury, for example being hit by a car rather than a simple fall, whether or not the patient is in shock, the presence of

associated injuries, and the radiographic appearance of the fracture. Such patients are at risk of death from internal hemorrhage and require very careful assessment and resuscitation. It is an established fact that elderly adults are less able to withstand any delay in resuscitation (Smith, Enderson and Maull, 1990). The definitive management of these patients will be discussed below.

The majority of patients with low energy trauma require only simple measures. Inpatient care is advisable. In posterior wall fractures it may be necessary to reduce an associated posterior displacement of the femoral head, under sedation or general anesthesia. Bed rest is necessary initially and most patients benefit from a variable period of skin traction. Even in undisplaced fractures this may give valuable pain relief, while allowing passive and active joint movement. After about two weeks, depending on pain, most patients begin to sit in a chair and mobilize without bearing weight on the affected side. Bony union is well advanced by about six weeks, but the risk of asymptomatic displacement is present in the preceding period. For this reason it has been recommended that traction be maintained for the full six weeks, but as most fractures will not displace, and given the risks of prolonged recumbency, it is reasonable to mobilize relatively early, while monitoring the situation with repeat radiographs. There are few reported studies on this 'benign' fracture, but there is evidence that poor functional results relate to such late displacement (Spencer, 1989).

Until recently the accepted management of displaced acetabular fractures of the elderly, whether due to high energy trauma or not, has been to stabilize the fracture on traction, and hopefully reduce the displacement to some extent in the process. This generally yielded poor results, if the patients eventually returned to weight bearing activity, due to the rapid onset of post-traumatic arthritis. The solution to this was to perform a total hip replacement (THR). However, although early reports were encouraging, longer-term studies have shown a very high rate of cup loosening in this situation, about half being radiologically loose at seven-and-a-half years, and half of this group being symptomatic. This is nearly five times the incidence following primary joint replacement. In addition, this operation on a traumatized acetabulum is considerably more difficult than a THR performed for primary osteoarthritis, usually requiring bone grafting either as a single or two-stage procedure (Romness and Lewallen, 1990). In younger patients this situation rarely arises as current practice is to perform open reduction and internal fixation of displaced fractures. This branch of trauma surgery is both hazardous and technically very demanding and it was widely regarded as inappropriate in the elderly, because of their inferior bone quality and the high physiological toll of prolonged anesthesia and major surgical trauma. Recent work has show, however, that in carefully selected elderly patients, such surgery can be highly successful. The crucial selection criterion was that the patient was an independent walker before injury. Out of 18 patients over 60 years old, only one had a functionally poor result, and the operative morbidity was no higher than in younger adults. The patients are able to mobilize early, avoiding the dangers of prolonged recumbency, and having minimized the chances of requiring a difficult THR subsequently (Helfet *et al.* 1992). It must be stressed that acetabular surgery of this kind requires special skills and equipment, and where these are unavailable the wiser course is to opt for conservative treatment (Figure 7.2).

COMPLICATIONS

It has been suggested that iliofemoral DVT is virtually inevitable in any pelvic fracture, due

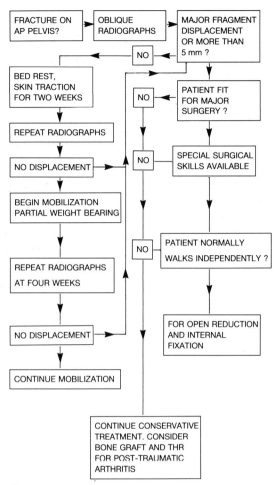

Figure 7.2 Clinical algorithm. A suggested scheme for the management of acetabular fractures in the elderly.

to a combination of post-traumatic hypercoagulability, venous stasis and direct trauma to these vessels. The reported incidence of fatal pulmonary embolus (PE) following such injuries, treated conservatively, varies between 1 and 10%. Decisions on anticoagulation are therefore best made by treating each case on its merits, rather than adopting a blanket policy.

In patients confined to bed the usual risks of recumbency are present, as mentioned elsewhere in this text.

Displaced fractures are associated with a risk of sciatic nerve injury which has been estimated at up to 30%, although most of these are effectively subclinical. Surgery increases this risk. Heterotopic bone formation occurs rarely, the risk again increased by surgery.

The problem of malunion and post-traumatic arthritis in displaced fractures has already been referred to above.

PELVIC RING FRACTURES

As with acetabular fractures a distinction must be drawn between high and low energy trauma. The high morbidity and mortality of the former group has been outlined above. High energy fractures constitute a distinct group of injuries which frequently require operative stabilization, and they will not be discussed further here. Single breaks in the pelvic ring on the other hand although relatively benign are very common and present great difficulties in terms of management where a dilemma between the need to hospitalize patients for pain relief and the urgency of rapid rehabilitation back to a familiar environment always faces the clinician.

CLINICAL PRESENTATION

The traumatic event is nearly always a simple fall. Pain, maximal on weight bearing, is the predominant feature. It is felt around the hip region, usually in the groin. There may be local tenderness over the pubic rami, and 'springing' the pelvis by compressing it from both sides, then releasing it, may be very painful. Also it should be remembered that pubic and ischial rami are easily palpated and tenderness may be well localized and easy to elicit to the point of being diagnostic of fracture.

Unlike acetabular fractures, hip movement is often unimpaired. After a few days bruising may develop around the groin.

RADIOGRAPHY

An AP film of the pelvis will show most fractures. They are often minimally displaced and further more localized views are occasionally helpful. If the fracture is not visible on the admission radiographs, repeating them in a few days will often show it, as minor degrees of late displacement commonly occur. About 85% of these injuries are fractures of one or both ipsilateral pubic rami (Figure 7.3); the remainder consist of acetabular fractures of the kind described above, fractures adjacent to the symphysis pubis, and rarely fractures of all four rami (Rossvoll and Finsen, 1989). In a few cases isotope bone scan will be needed, when the plain radiographs are normal and particularly if metastatic disease or myeloma is suspected, the pelvis being a common site for both. In such cases further laboratory investigations are indicated.

MANAGEMENT

This is similar to the other lower energy fractures of the axial skeleton. These fractures do not lead to instability of the pelvic ring, and the only functional impairment they produce is due to pain in the early stages. Patients therefore only require bed rest, analgesia and mobilization when the pain is settling, usually within a few days of injury.

COMPLICATIONS

These are the same as for acetabular fractures. The mortality of all low energy pelvic fractures at one month has been reported as being 5% (Rossvoll and Finsen, 1989).

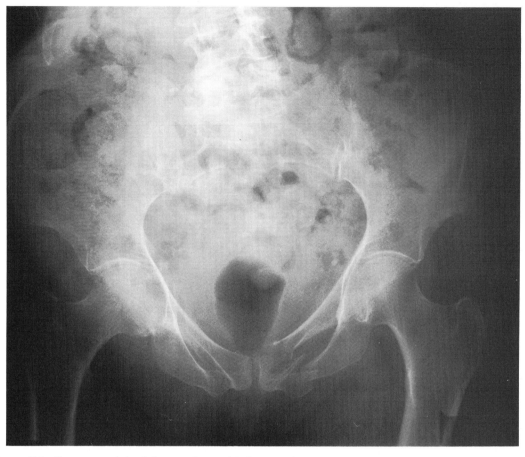

Figure 7.3 Fractures of the left superior and inferior pubic rami in an 86-year-old woman.

NON-OPERATIVE MANAGEMENT OF FRACTURES OF THE EXTREMITIES

Occasionally the situation arises where non-operative treatment is indicated for a fracture that in a younger person would normally require surgery or manipulation. In this circumstance the basic techniques are early mobilization without any form of cast, functional bracing and traction. Whenever one uses this approach in the older patient, there is a tacit acceptance that what might be unacceptable management in a young and fit patient may be perfectly reasonable in a frail elderly person, who may be unable to cope

with more aggressive treatment and whose functional demands are relatively minor in comparison. Occasionally the corollary argument may hold.

The usual reasons for making such a decision are if the bone quality is so poor either due to osteoporosis or comminution that internal fixation is technically impossible, if the patient is mentally or physically unfit for any intervention and if the patient refuses surgery. In such cases it is surprising how often a functionally good result is obtained. Like so many accepted methods of treatment in medicine there are few prospective randomized controlled trials in the litera-

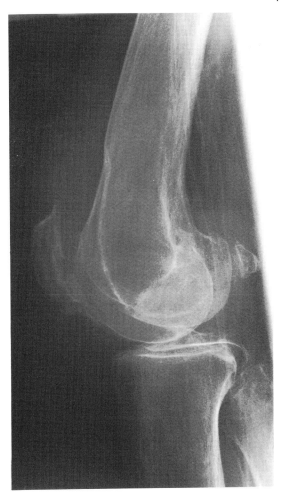

Figure 7.4 A patellar fracture in an 86-year-old woman, treated successfully with full early mobilization.

are often treated with an attempt at open reduction and internal fixation or lengthy cast immobilization. Experience has shown that many of these injuries do well with active mobilization from a very early stage, as soon as the initial discomfort is settling (Rowe, 1965).

The other fracture of the elbow region that may be treated in this way is the very severely comminuted fracture of the distal humerus, colloquially known as the 'bag of bones' technique. In some of these injuries even a limited reconstruction of the articular surface is beyond the most proficient surgeon and the outcome in terms of pain, stiffness and stability is no worse after treatment with a sling and early mobilization than if an operation with its concomitant risks had been performed.

Impacted sub-capital fractures of the femoral neck may also be treated conservatively, and many probably are, albeit unwittingly. Most orthopedic surgeons are familiar with the elderly patient presenting a few weeks after a minor fall with a twinge of hip pain on walking, whose radiographs reveal an impacted fracture of the femoral neck. For conservative therapy to succeed, good quality AP and lateral radiographs are essential to confirm impaction in a slightly valgus position. Partial weight bearing is advisable initially and regular clinical and radiographic review is required until the fracture is considered to have healed.

ture, and inevitably the evidence supporting these protocols is largely anecdotal. We nevertheless believe that such treatment provides a valuable alternative to surgery, particularly in the elderly.

EARLY MOBILIZATION

Undisplaced and minimally displaced fractures of the olecranon and patella (Figure 7.4)

FUNCTIONAL BRACING

The primary site of use of the functional brace in the elderly is the knee. In recent times a number of authors, most notably Sarmiento and Latta (1981) have pioneered the use of this technique in numerous fractures of the upper and lower limbs, and there is considerable published evidence of its effectiveness.

85

The essence of any functional brace is that it permits early joint motion while maintaining stability of the fracture. This has particular attractions in the elderly, in whom prolonged recumbency has a high morbidity and mortality. Braces for the knee are essentially full length casts of the leg, with a carefully sited hinge over the joint. They are constructed from a variety of materials including plaster of Paris, various thermoplastics and fiber glass bandages, such as Scotchcast. The hinges are available ready made, in several sizes.

In the femur it may be used in most distal femoral fractures, in the shaft, the metaphysis and in intra-articular fractures. A particular problem seen more frequently in the older patient is a fracture through the femur adjacent to the tip of the femoral component of a knee or, more commonly, a hip replacement. In all of these injuries a period of two to four weeks of bed rest and traction, which allows the soft tissues to settle and callus to start to form, usually precedes the application of the brace. In the elderly fractures of the tibial condyles are relatively common injuries. These nearly always involve the articular surface to some extent, and tend to be comminuted, with considerable impaction of the cancellous bone and consequent depression of the joint surfaces. Bracing has been shown to be effective as a primary treatment of undisplaced and minimally displaced fractures in all ages (Delamarter and Hohl, 1989), and even if joint surface incongruity is present the clinical outcome is not inevitably bad, provided early joint motion is achieved. Hence bracing is a useful alternative to surgery in patients who are unsuitable for operation for the reasons listed above. Most patients can have the brace applied within a few days of injury, once the initial pain and swelling have begun to subside.

TRACTION

The dangers of using traction as a definitive treatment of lower limb fractures in the elderly are the risks of prolonged bed rest: deep vein thrombosis, pulmonary embolus, pressure sores, urinary tract infection, atelectasis, chest infection and so on, as has already been stressed in this chapter. The advantages are that it may be possible to avoid the hazards of surgery and anesthesia.

In practice traction is now usually employed as an adjunct to other treatments, mostly in fractures of the femur as a preliminary to functional bracing. In addition, 'overnight' skin traction is widely used to relieve the pain from proximal femoral fractures prior to surgery.

When applying any form of traction, great care must be taken to adequately protect the soft tissues. The skin of elderly patients is often fragile, bruising and breaking down with minimal trauma. Adhesive skin traction must therefore only be used when absolutely necessary, and for as short a time as possible. A variety of non-adherent devices are currently available which are suitable for short-term traction, for example prior to fixation of a proximal femoral fracture. If it becomes necessary to use traction for more than a week it is wise to use skeletal traction. A Denman pin is preferred as it has a screw thread in its midshaft which provides good purchase on the bone. This is easily introduced about two-and-a-half centimetres posterior to the tibial tuberosity, using a sterile technique and local anesthetic infiltration. In a patient with porotic bone these pins can cut out of the tibia when subjected to traction forces, and must therefore be inspected daily. All long-term traction set ups should be monitored on a daily basis to check the following:

- fracture alignment, including rotation;
- limb circulation;
- sensory and motor function;

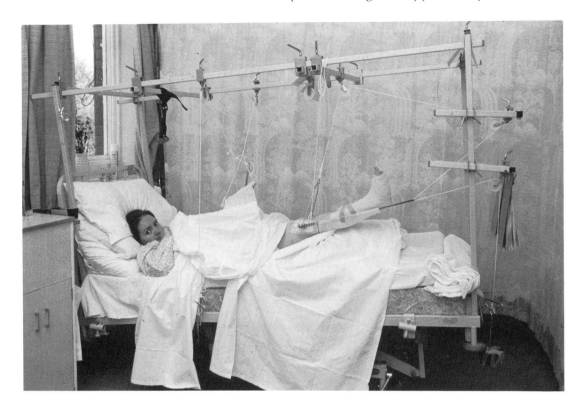

Figure 7.5   The use of sliding traction, allowing active movement of the knee and hip.

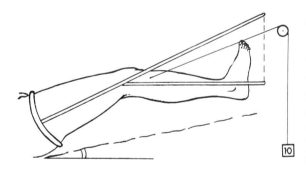

Figure 7.6   A diagram showing the arrangement of traction when using a knee flexion piece with a Thomas splint.

- all pressure areas, particularly in relation to the ring encircling the proximal thigh on a Thomas splint, in the groin and at the ischial tuberosity;

- the pin sites, looking for cutting out or infection.

The commonest use of traction as the definitive treatment in the elderly is probably in managing acetabular fractures, as outline above. If Hamilton Russell sliding traction (Figure 7.5) is used it is possible to begin passive and active joint motion from an early stage.

Occasionally it is still necessary to treat femoral fractures definitely with ten to twelve weeks of traction. In these circumstances a period of four to six weeks of fixed traction in a Thomas splint will let enough callus form to stabilize the fracture sufficiently to apply a knee flexion piece for the remainder of the time (Figure 7.6). Although such treatment is essentially non-operative, it may be necessary to actually apply the splint and reduce the fracture under an anesthetic. The alternative is to perform a femoral nerve block using local anesthetic, often in combination with a mild sedative such as midazolam.

The intricacies of these and other traction techniques are clearly explained in Charnley's classic work (1961), to which the interested reader is referred.

REFERENCES

Armstrong, A.L., Thomas, G., Wallace, W.A. and Green, D. (1992) Letter – vertebral fractures. *Br. Med. J.*, **304**, 1308.

Charnley, J. (1961) *The Closed Treatment of Common fractures*, 3rd edn, Churchill Livingstone, Edinburgh, London, New York.

Cooper, C. and Melton, L.J. (1992) Vertebral fractures. How large is the silent epidemic? *Br. Med. J.*, **304**, 793–4.

Delamarter, R. and Hohl, M. (1989) The cast brace in tibial plateau fractures. *Clin. Orthop.*, **242**, 26–31.

Eastell, R., Ceder, S.R., Wahner, H.W. *et al.* (1991) Classification of vertebral fractures. *J Bone Miner. Res.*, **6**, 207–15.

Helfet, D.L., Borelli, J. DiPasquale, T. and Sanders, R. (1992) Stabilisation of acetabular fractures in elderly patients. *J. Bone Joint Surg*, **74A**, 75–65.

Jensen, G.F., Christiansen, C., Boesen, J. *et al.* (1982) Epidemiology of postmenopausal spinal and long bone fractures. *Clin. Orthop.*, **166**, 75–81.

Melton, L.J., Sampson, J.M., Morrey, B.F. and Ilstrup, D.M. (1981) Epidemiologic features of pelvic fractures. *Clin. Orthopaed.*, **155**, 43–47.

Melton, L.J., Kan, S.H., Frye, M.A., *et al.* (1989) Epidemiology of vertebral fractures in women. *Am. J. Epidemiol.*, **129**, 1000–11.

Romness, D.W. and Lewallen, D.G. (1990) Total hip arthroplasty after fracture of the acetabulum. Long-term results. *J. Bone Joint Surg.*, **72B**, 761–74.

Ross, P.D., Ettinger, B., Danis, J.W. *et al* (1991) Evaluation of adverse health outcomes associated with vertebral fractures. *Osteoporosis Int.*, **1**, 134–140.

Rossvol, I. and Finsen, V. (1989) Mortality after pelvic fractures in the elderly. *J. Orthop. Trauma*, **3**, 115–17.

Rowe, C.R. (1965) The management of fractures in elderly patients is different. *J. Bone Joint Surg.*, **47A**, 1043–59.

Sarmiento, A. and Latta, L. (1981). *Closed Functional Treatment of Fractures*, Springer-Verlag, Berlin, Heidelberg, New York.

Shikata, J., Yamamuro, T., Iida, H. *et al.* (1990) Surgical treatment for paraplegia resulting from vertebral fractures in senile osteoporosis. *Spine*, **15**, 484–9.

Smith, D.P., Enderson, B.L. and Maull, K.L. (1990) Trauma in the elderly: determinants of outcome. *Southern Med. J.*, **83**, 172–7.

Spencer, R.F. (1989) Mortality after pelvic fractures in the elderly. *J. Orthop. Trauma*, **3**, 115–17.

Storm, T. Thamsborg, G., Steiniche, T. *et al.* (1990) Effect of intermittent cyclical etidronate therapy on bone mass and fracture rate in women with postmenopausal osteoporosis. *New Engl. J. Med.*, **322**, 1265–71.

Woolf, A.D. and Dixon, A.St.J. (1988) *Osteoporosis: a Clinical Guide*, Dunitz, London.

8

Shoulder and upper humeral injuries in elderly people

PAUL STABLEFORTH, WILLIAM MACLENNAN
and LOREN LATTA

INTRODUCTION

Shoulder fractures and dislocations form 5–10% of all bone and joint injuries.

In older patients they can cause difficulties with self care, domestic routine or leisure activities; in those with a spinal or lower limb disorder loss of shoulder comfort, strength or stability can lead to loss of independence.

Injury of the acromio-clavicular joint, clavicle or scapula is rare and sub-coracoid dislocation is infrequent in the older patient; proximal humeral fractures are common. A rotator cuff tear may follow a strain or shoulder dislocation.

CAUSES OF DISABILITY

(a) Stiffness

Gleno-humeral movement is usually restricted after shoulder injury but stiffness alone is not usually a cause of major disability if scapulo-thoracic motion is retained. If there is a combined range of 95 degrees of shoulder flexion, and 50 degrees of internal and external rotation then most activities of daily living are possible.

(b) Pain

Pain may follow articular surface damage or disturbance of blood supply with later fibrous ankylosis or post-traumatic arthritis. Pain may also be caused by impingement of displaced bone fragments against the coraco-acromial arch or glenoid, or may result from post-injury algodystrophy.

(c) Instability

Transient inferior gleno-humeral subluxation may result from a large effusion or from short-lived muscle atony after injury. Permanent incongruity or instability may follow nerve or tendon damage, capsular or ligamentous avulsion, or damage to an articular surface.

EIDEMIOLOGY
By W.J. MacLennan

Though fractures involving the upper end of the humerus are very much less common than those of the proximal femur, they show a similar exponential increase in old age

Skeletal Trauma in Old Age
Published in 1994 by Chapman & Hall, London
ISBN 0 412 48750 0

(Bengner, Johnell and Redlund-Johnell, 1988). Their incidence is similar in men and women up to the age of 45 years beyond which there is a preponderance of women, so that after the age of 75 years the condition is 2.5 times as common in this group. There has also been an increase in its incidence over the last thirty years, which has been most dramatic in individuals over the age of 75 years, the magnitudes of change in men and women being 3.4 and 2.4 times respectively.

Relatively few studies have been conducted on factors influencing the incidence of fractures of the upper end of the humerus. It might well be that more extensive investigation would find that these were similar to those associated with fractures of the proximal femur.

BONE DENSITY

In a longitudinal study of women from the USA, fractures of the proximal humerus were 7.5 times as common in women from the lowest quartile of bone density as in that from the highest one (Kelsey *et al.*, 1992).

OTHER FACTORS

The same study identified a decline in health status, insulin dependent diabetes mellitus, poor mobility and neuromuscular weakness as additional risk factors from the fracture. A study from Denmark found that the fracture was usually sustained in the patient's own home, that traffic and work accidents were rarely involved and that the incidence peaked during the months of December and January (Lind, Kroner and Jensen, 1989).

BIOMECHANICS
By Loren L. Latta

Following fractures in the upper humerus there are often only small islands of trabecu-

lar bone left in the osteoporotic head which has a very vulnerable blood supply (Hall and Rasser, 1963). Surgical intervention may therefore not achieve good fracture stability and there is a high risk of causing avascular necrosis (Mouradian, 1986; Hawkins and Kiefer, 1987). Thus, closed methods of treatment which can provide for early motion of the shoulder provide an attractive alternative to internal fixation in many of these fractures (Sarmiento *et al.* 1977; Zagorski *et al.* 1987). One can expect that a certain limitation of shoulder motion will occur in these cases with closed treatment due to the inability to achieve full range of motion in the early phases of healing. However, this is often a small price to pay for achieving good healing in a viable humeral head. A collar and cuff can provide adequate initial immobilization during the acute phases and allows for adequate early motion by pendulum exercises (Sarmiento *et al.*, 1977; Zagorski *et al.*, 1987; Charnley, 1968; Perkins, 1955). A hanging cast also provides for comfortable means of early immobilization but will tend to create internal rotation deformities and limits early gravity alignment in motion of the shoulder (Sarmiento and Latta, 1981; Zagorski *et al.*, 1987). Therefore it is recommended that a hanging cast be removed at a very early stage while the fracture site is still quite mobile and the patient begins functioning in elbow extension with a functional brace. The brace provides comfort through soft tissue compression but will not stabilize the fracture and therefore, early gravity alignment can occur through pendulum exercises and early limited range of motion (Figure 8.1). The most important aspect of either form of closed treatment is the therapy with progressive range of motion beginning passively and progressing to active range of motion of the shoulder during the healing process.

In instances when internal fixation is necessary, the best cancellous bone for screw fixation is located on the postero-medial

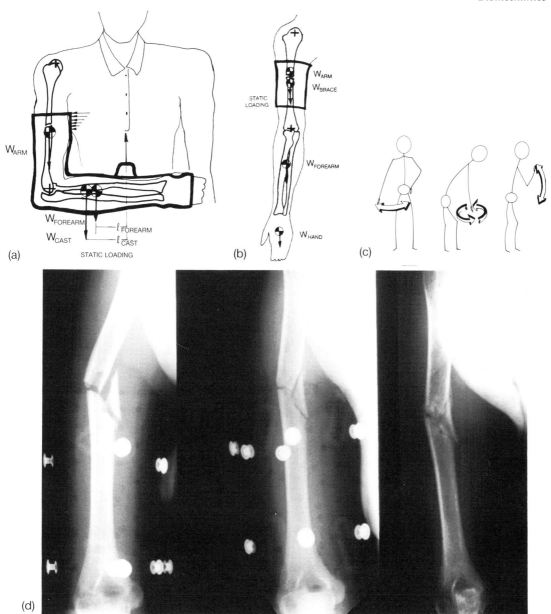

(a)
(b)
(c)
(d)

Figure 8.1 The use of a hanging cast is excellent for providing traction during the early stages of repair of the humerus fracture, (a). However, with the elbow fixed in 90° of flexion, and the forearm internally rotated across the front of the body, there will naturally be a varus angulation and internal rotation deformity of the humerus in this position, (d). In a functional brace which allows for full motion of the shoulder and elbow, (b), it is possible to begin early pendulum exercises, (c), which promotes gravity alignment of the fracture fragments while the fracture is still stable. This realignment is possible, (d), only because the functional brace does not effectively stablize the fracture site but provides comfort which promotes the early functional activity and natural realignment of the limb (Sarmiento and Latta, 1981; Zagorski *et al.*, 1987).

91

portion of the head in the late stages of osteoporosis and may be the only island of bone with adequate strength for screw fixation (Hall and Rosser, 1963; Saitoh, Latta and Milne, 1990), A T-plate can be utilized to achieve distal fixation in the cortical bone but one must be careful in achieving good cancellous fixation in the postero-medial region with a single lag screw on the first attempt of fixation. Even when this is achieved the fixation is much weaker than in normal bone (Figure 8.2), so post-operative rehabilitation must be protected and gradual. Radiographic assessment of the contralateral humerus may be helpful in evaluation of the quality of this bone as well as its location.

For extra-articular fractures, locking intramedullary nails (Henley, Monroe and Tencer, 1991), rush pins with tension bands (Robinson and Christie, 1993) or external fixation (Kristiansen and Koefed, 1987) may be appropriate to achieve adequate fixation for these difficult proximal fractures with minimal surgical intervention. Because of the poor quality of cancellous bone, cortical locking devices provide the best mechanical stability (Henley Monroe and Tencer, 1991). Although anatomical alignment may not be achievable by this technique, it is excellent in providing adequate stability for early range of motion and has been associated with a high percentage of excellent functional results (Zagorski *et al.*, 1987). With both intramedullary rods and plate fixation, supplementary fixation may be achieved with the use of methylmethacrylate bony cement to significantly enhance the mechanics of fixation in osteoporotic bones.

THE INVESTIGATIONS OF HUMERAL FRACTURES

An A-P X-ray of the shoulder and an axial view of the scapula are the essential minimum views needed after injury (Figure 8.3). The Stripp view (Horsfield and Jones, 1987) is helpful if the arm cannot be abducted, or the axial view is not diagnostic and dislocation is suspected.

An axillary projection is often helpful in the non acute situation.

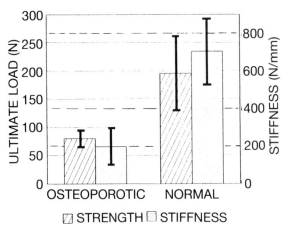

Figure 8.2 A laboratory simulation of fracture fixation with a T-plate for humeral head fractures demonstrated a significant loss of strength and stiffness of fixation in osteoporotic bones even when fixation was optimal under these well-controlled conditions (Saitoh, Latta and Milne, 1990).

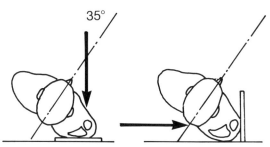

Figure 8.3 These two basic projections; the A-P of the shoulder and the axial of the scapula are the minimum requirements for the management of shoulder injury and can be taken with the patient standing or supine.

Shoulder ultrasonography, arthrography, particularly with CT scanning and MRI scanning are all of proven value for more detailed examination of complex shoulder injuries.

ACROMIO-CLAVICULAR JOINT AND CLAVICLE INJURY

A fracture of the clavicle is uncommon in the elderly. The thin skin may split over the site of injury. There is bruising, soft tissue swelling and some deformity. The diagnosis is confirmed by antero-posterior X-ray. A broad-fold sling and analgesics are prescribed until pain eases. Fractures heal in 6–8 weeks and arm use is restored in 12 to 16 weeks. Late pain, dysfunction or significant deformity are rare.

Acromio-clavicular dislocation is rare; the step at the joint is usually obvious. Treatment is symptomatic with analgesics and an elbow support sling, going on later to range of movement exercises. Final function is usually good though discomfort and a permanent bump at the joint are common.

GLENO-HUMERAL DISLOCATION

ACUTE-SUB-CORACOID DISLOCATION

This usually follows a fall onto the elbow or the outstretched arm. In those over 50 years old the supraspinatus tendon is often stretched or torn; it may heal poorly, causing continuing shoulder stiffness or discomfort (Johnson and Bayley, 1981; Astley, 1986).

In 10–15% of patients there is an avulsion fracture of the greater tuberosity; the fragment usually realigns as the dislocation is reduced, but redisplacement may occur and it is prudent to take a further X-ray 7–10 days after injury. A 'winged' greater tuberosity lying elevated or in the subacromial space needs open reduction and fixation through a superior subacromial or posterior approach (Gschwend, 1984; Bennet, 1941) if cuff function and shoulder motion are to be restored.

The axillary nerve is stretched in 20–30% of anterior dislocations; the deltoid muscle may be weakened or paralysed with inconsistent numbness over its insertion (Brown 1952; Blom Dahback, 1970). Recovery is usual but the 2–3 month delay before muscle function starts to return results in shoulder stiffness.

The elderly do not tolerate the prone lying needed for the 'hanging arm' reduction (Stimson 1900) and the Kocher's or the Hippocratic maneuvers under sedation or general anesthetic is usually required (Beattie *et al.*, 1986).

Rapid or forced manipulation of the arm, or attempted closed reduction of a dislocation more than 7–10 days old may cause a spiral fracture of the humeral shaft.

Following reduction, biplanar X-rays should be taken to confirm congruous and concentric reduction of the humeral head.

RECURRENT SUBCORACOID DISLOCATION

In patients over 50 years old the anterior capsular tear that allows acute dislocation heals and recurrent dislocation is uncommon (Reeves, 1968). Self-care and shoulder movements may be safely started at once. Persistent shoulder stiffness or weakness from a rotator cuff strain may make hand use at or above shoulder height difficult but disabling symptoms are uncommon.

If it does occur the clinical presentation is of an acute traumatic dislocation and later painful instability on unguarded or incautious use, occasionally during self-care or sleep, more often with the arm high or away from the body.

Apprehension when the abducted arm is moved into external rotation or a positive anterior translation test may be the only clinical findings.

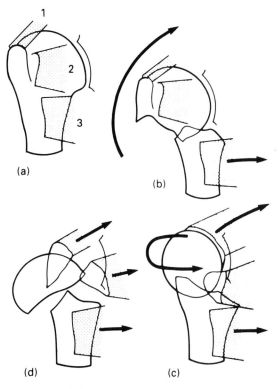

(a) (b) (d) (c)

Figure 8.4 The '4-segment' classification; after fracture the pull of the three major muscle groups determines the direction of movement of the segments.

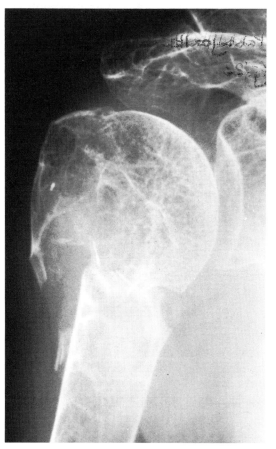

Figure 8.5 A relatively undisplaced fracture of the humerus.

Anterior stabilization with inferior capsular reattachment (Bankart, 1938) or anterior capsular plication and subscapularis reefing (Osmond-Clarke 1948) may be needed. Rarely an anterior glenoid deficiency may require a bone augmentation procedure (Hindmarsh and Lindberg, 1967), and where necessary a large posterior humeral head defect may make a rotation osteotomy more appropriate.

OLD UNREDUCED SUBCRACOID DISLOCATION

Persistent dislocation after an unremembered fall may present as a painful 'frozen shoulder' with little apparent deformity; it is therefore prudent to take X-rays of the elderly patient's shoulder before physiotherapy or other treatment is started.

The painless stiff shoulder is probably best left but a humeral neck rotation osteotomy may improve the arc of movement for low arm use. Intrusive pain may be an indication for open reduction through an anterior approach.

Exploration is difficult as the soft tissue planes are distorted and adherent; the subscapularis tendon is Z lengthened and the capsule widely released. A glenoid rim deficiency may need augmentation by a bone

94

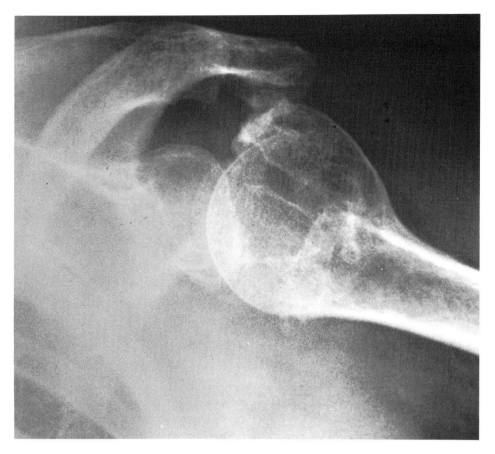

Figure 8.6 The displacement of this 3-segment fracture was accepted; the greater tuberosity has healed high. Subacromial impingement limits elevation.

block and humeral head replacement is sometimes needed.

Pin transfixion of the head and glenoid by a stout pin will compromise shoulder function and is not a good alternative to adequate soft tissue release. Pain is usually eased and low forward and rotation movement are increased, but the overall range of motion is often disappointing.

FRACTURE OF THE PROXIMAL HUMERUS

Most fractures are little displaced and neuro-vascular complications are uncommon. Cir-cumflex humeral or axillary vessel damage is rare, but exceptionally a tensely swollen axilla needs decompression or an arterial tear needs repair to prevent hand or forearm ischemia.

The displaced humeral head may some-times press on the medial cord or the branches of the brachial plexus to produce sensorimotor dysfunction in the hand and forearm. Neurological recovery is usual but is slow and crippling. Hand stiffness is common despite dedicated physiotherapy (Stableforth, 1984).

The fracture type and displacement is established by bi-planar shoulder X-rays

(Codman, 1934). Use of the '4-segment' or the AO classification aids decisions on management (Figure 8.4).

85% of these fractures are little displaced and do not need manipulation or surgery (Figure 8.5).

Fracture union is usual by 6–8 weeks. Pain usually eases after 3–4 days though sleep disturbance may persist; independent self-care is usual by 3–4 weeks; shoulder mobility and strength improve for 3–6 months and sometimes longer.

In 15% of fractures the bone segments are grossly malrotated or displaced and cause gleno-humeral mismatch, subacromial bone impingement or rotator cuff muscle dysfunction and lead to a painful or functionally poor outcome. Manipulation or surgery should be considered.

Those 2-segment fractures more than 40% displaced or malrotated have an improved outcome after manipulation.

If fracture impaction is not possible percu-taneous wire or external skeletal fixation will prevent redisplacement and allow earlier remobilization, though skilled open reduction and internal fixation will give the best result.

Reduction may be easier if the proximal segment is 'captured' with a Schanz screw which is used to pull the fracture into alignment; a second pin can be drilled into the proximal shaft and an external fixation frame constructed to hold an unstable fracture (Kristiansen and Koefed, 1987). In this circumstance the pins are removed after 3–4 weeks.

In 3-segment fractures the articular segment may be grossly malrotated and/or the isolated tuberosity pulled away from its insertion; painful shoulder dysfunction is then common (Figure 8.6). Closed reduction is difficult and the position rarely stable but capture of the articular and tuberosity segments aids reduction and application of a frame will prevent redisplacement.

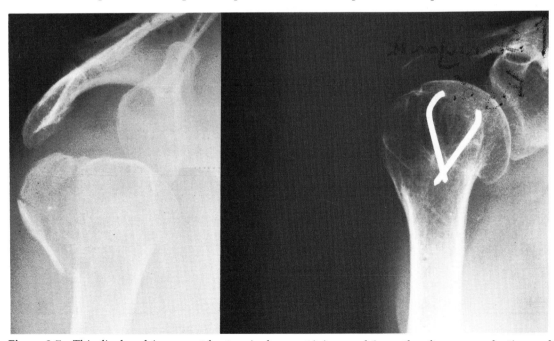

Figure 8.7 This displaced 4-segment fracture is shown at injury and 6 months after open reduction and internal fixation by K wires and *5 Ethibond tension banding.

Open reduction of an irreducible or unstable 3-segment fracture and stabilization by K wires and tension band or by T-plate may be needed but the surgery can be difficult, the post-operative regimen is prolonged, and the final outcome often disappointing (Hawkins, Bell and Gurr, 1986).

In the 4-segment fracture the articular segment may be stripped of its soft tissues and both tuberosities widely displaced; shoulder function is often poor, stiffness usual and pain common after non-operative management.

In these older patients proximal humeral reconstruction around a Neer prosthesis will,

with a compliant patient and skilled after-care, give a comfortable functional shoulder (Stableforth, 1984; Neer 1969). Open reduction and internal fixation may be indicated if the articular segment still has its soft tissue attachments (Figure 8.7).

PATHOLOGICAL FRACTURE OF THE PROXIMAL HUMERUS

Metastases from breast or bronchial carcinoma, less commonly from a thyroid, renal or other primary neoplasm, may erode and destroy the humeral head, neck or proximal

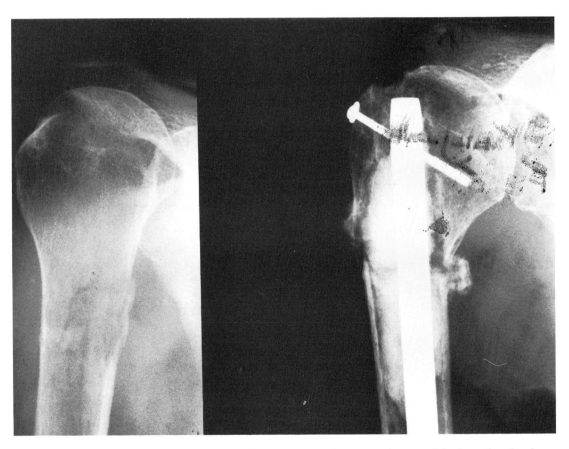

Figure 8.8 This pathological fracture through a metastasis from a carcinoma of the bronchus has been managed by curettage, intermedullary nail and bone cement fixation.

shaft. There may be increasingly severe upper arm pain with sleep disturbance, or sudden onset severe pain from pathological fracture.

X-ray guided fine needle aspiration, large needle, or open biopsy, from the edge of the lesion may provide the diagnosis if no primary tumor is found and a radionuclide bone scan will identify other skeletal metastases.

If more than one third of the humeral cortex has been destroyed, fracture may occur before radiotherapy or chemotherapy causes tumor regression and allows bone healing. 'Bone splintage' using a closed intramedullary nailing technique or two tensioned Rush pins may be adequate before a fracture has occurred.

A pathological fracture can be managed in the same way particularly if stability is increased by fracture impaction before fixation. A better alternative where little proximal cortex remains, is to expose the fracture through the anterior approach, currette the metastasis, stabilize the bone by locked intramedullary fixation and fill any defect with bone cement (Figure 8.8). Rarely tumor curettage, humeral impaction and stabilization with bone cement and T-plate fixation may be possible.

TEARS OF THE ROTATOR CUFF

An acute supraspinatus tear may follow a fall with the arm outstretched or as a consequence of subcoracoid dislocation in the older patient. There is marked local swelling and tenderness, shoulder movements are painfully restricted.

Satisfactory but incomplete recovery with pain relief and a return to self care and domestic routine usually follows non-operative treatment. Self-care is encouraged from the start; active low rotation and flexion exercises follow as pain eases; gentle resistance work starts at 4–6 weeks.

If pain or stiffness persists for 6–8 weeks a subacromial injection of steroid and local anesthetic or shoulder manipulation under anesthetic may speed recovery. If pain, sleep disturbance, or difficulty with arm use persist, further investigation may suggest a supraspinatus rupture or subacromial impingement; repeated steroid injection will not help and surgery should be considered. Anterior acromioplasty (Neer 1972) overcomes the impingement and predictably eases pain. Cuff repair is rarely indicated in these older patients. Recovery may take 5–6 months.

REFERENCES

Astley, T. (1986) Dislocation of the shoulder in the elderly. *J. Bone Joint Surg.*, **68B**, 676.

Bankart, A.S.B. (1938) The pathology and treatment of recurrent dislocation of the shoulder. *Br. J. Surg.*, **26**, 23–39.

Beattie, T.F., Studman, D.J., McGowan, A. and Robertson, C.E. (1986) A comparison of the Milch & Kocher techniques for acute anterior dislocation of the shoulder. *Injury*, **17**, 348–52.

Bengne, U., Johnell, O. and Redlund-Johnell, I. (1988) Changes in the incidence of fracture of the upper end of the humerus during a thirty year period. A study of 2125 fractures. *Clin. Orthop.*, **231**, 179–82.

Bennett, G.E. (1941) The posterior approach to the shoulder joint. *J.A.M.A*, **117**, 510-14.

Blom, S. and Dahback, L.O. (1970) Nerve injuries in dislocation of the shoulder joint and fracture of the neck of the humerus. *A. Chir. Scand.* **136**, 461–6.

Brown, J.T. (1952) Nerve injuries complicating dislocation of the shoulder. *J. Bone Joint Surg.*, **34B**, 526.

Charnley, J. (1968) *The Closed Treatment of Common Fractures.* 3rd. edn, William and Wilkins, Baltimore.

Codman, E.A. (1934) The shoulder, rupture of the supraspinatus tendon and other lesions in or about the subacromial bursa, T Todd, Boston.

Gschwend, N.A. (1984) A surgical approach to rotator cuff tears, in *Surgery of the Shoulder* (J.

Bateman edn and R.P. Walsh), The C.V. Mosby Company, Philadelphia.

Hall, M.C. and Rosser, M (1963) The structure of the upper end of the humerus with reference to osteoporotic changes in senescence leading to fractures. *Can. Med. Ass. J.*, **88**, 290–4.

Hawkins, R., Bell, R. and Gurr, K. (1986) 3 part fractures of the proximal humerus. *J. Bone Joint Surg.*, **68A**, 1410–14.

Hawkins, R. and Kiefer, G.N. (1987). Internal fixation techniques for proximal humerus fractures. *Clin. Orthop.*, **223**, 77–85.

Henley, M.B., Monroe, M. and Tencer, A.F. (1991), Biomechanical comparison of methods of fixation of a midshaft osteotomy of the humerus. *J. Orthop. Trauma*, **5**, 14.

Hindmarsh, J. and Lindberg, A. (1967) Eden Hybbinette's operation for recurrent dislocation of the shoulder. *Acta Ortho. Scand.* **38**, 459–78.

Horsfield, D. and Jones, S.N. (1987) A useful projection in radiography of the shoulder. *J. Bone Joint Sur.*, **69B**, 338.

Johnson, J.R. and Bayley, J.I.L. (1981) Loss of function following acute anterior shoulder dislocation. *J. Bone Joint Sur.*, **63B**, 663.

Kelsey, J.L., Browner, W.S., Seeley, D.G. *et al.* (1992) risk factors for fractures of the distal forearm and proximal humerus. The Study of Osteoporotic Fractures Research Group. *Am. J. Epidemiol.*, **135**, 477–89.

Kristiansen, B. and Koefed, H. (1987) External fixation of displaced fractures of the proximal humerus. Technique and preliminary results. *J. Bone Joint Surg.*, **69B**, 643–6.

Lind, T., Kroner K. and Jensen, J. (1989) The epidemiology of fractures of the proximal humerus. *Arch.Orthop.Trauma Surg.* **108**, 285–7.

Mouradian, W.H. (1986) Displaced proximal humeral fractures. *Clin.Orthop.*, **212**, 209–218.

Neer, C.S. (1969) Prosthetic replacement of the humeral head; indications and operative technique. *Surg.Clin.N.Am.*, **43**, 1581–97.

Neer, C.S. (1972) Anterior acromioplasty for the chronic impingement syndrome. *J. Bone Joint Surg.*, **54A**, 41–50.

Osmond-Clarke, H. (1948) Habitual dislocation of the shoulder. The Putti-Platt operation. *J. Bone Joint Surg.*, **30B**, 19–22.

Perkins, G. (1955) Rest and motion. *J. Bone Joint Surg.*, **37A**, 101.

Reeves, B. (1968) Experiments on the tensile strength of the anterior capsular structures of the shoulder in man. *J. Bone Joint Surg.*, **50B**, 858–65.

Robinson, C.M. and Christie, J. (1993) The two-part proximal humeral fracture: a review of operative treatment using two techniques. *Injury*, **24**, 123–5.

Rockwood, C.A. and Green, D.P. (1975) *Fractures and Dislocations*, J.B. Lippincott, Philadelphia, pp. 589–90.

Saitoh, S., Latta, L.L. and Milne, E.L. (1990) Osteoporosis of the proximal humerus. *Trans 36th Orthop. Res. Soc.*, **15**, 12.

Sarmiento, A. Kinman, P.B., Galvin, E.G. *et al* (1977) Functional bracing of fractures of the shaft of the humerus. *J. Bone Joint Surg.*, **59A**, 596–601.

Sarmiento, A. and Latta, L.L. (1981) *Closed Functional Treatment of Fractures*, Springer Verlag, Berlin.

Stableforth, P.G. (1984) Four part fractures of the neck of the humerus. *J. Bone Joint Surg.*, **66B**, 104–8.

Stimson, L.A. (1900) An easy method of reducing dislocations of the shoulder and hip. *Med. Rec.*, **57**, 256–7.

Zagorski, J.B., Zych, G.A., Latta, L.L. and McCollough, N.C. (1987) Modern concepts in functional fracture bracing – upper limb, in *AAOS Instructional Course Lectures*, Vol XXXVI, Chap. 24, AAOS, Chicago, Illinois.

9

Fractures of the elbow in elderly people

JOHN DENT

INTRODUCTION

Fractures around the elbow are a common occurrence in the elderly. They are caused by minimal trauma, often by a stumble in the home and although they are often uncomplicated, occasionally they may be extremely comminuted and displaced. When assessing the management of any particular fracture the needs of the patient as a whole must be assessed and adequate pain control commenced early. The overriding goal of management is the restoration of a functional pain-free limb. To this end treatment must be directed to finding a method of controlling the fracture while at the same time allowing active mobilization of both the affected joint and the neighbouring joints at the earliest possible opportunity.

Although the literature is replete with papers on the management of elbow fractures in adults in general there are few which discuss the management of these injuries in the elderly in particular.

FRACTURES OF THE RADIAL HEAD

Falls on the outstretched hand which produce a valgus force at the elbow will cause an impaction fracture of the radial head on the capitellum. This injury occurs with various degrees of comminution according to the amount of force sustained and may be associated with an avulsion fracture of the medial epicondyle thus creating an unstable joint.

Classically the fractured radial head is painful when palpated during supination and pronation movements, and the grip is characteristically weak. The radiological appearances of the injury were classified by Mason and Shutkin in 1943. Primary excision of the radial head was once popular for all fracture types but it is now realized that this will produce further disability. In particular the inferior radio-ulnar joint may become symptomatic due to proximal migration of the radius (Taylor and O'Connor, 1964). Mason and Shutkin advocated early mobilization of radial head fractures after an initial period of splinting at 90 degrees to allow pain to settle. Early aspiration of the hemarthrosis may lead to a quicker return of motion and relief of pain. Excision of the radial head is now reserved for cases with severe cases of comminution and displacement (Bakalim, 1970) or as an elective procedure after therapy if loss of motion persists. Prosthetic re-

Skeletal Trauma in Old Age
Published in 1994 by Chapman & Hall, London
ISBN 0 412 48750 0

placement should be carried out at the same time (Benjamin, 1982) using a silastic radial head prosthesis. Fractures of the radial head associated with a fracture of the coronoid process, a Type IV fracture (Johnston, 1962), must be managed by prosthetic replacement if the radial head is to be excised. Recent work suggests that a metal prosthesis may have a significant biomechanical advantage over the traditional silastic spacer (Knight *et al.*, 1993).

FRACTURES OF THE OLECRANON

This injury is the most common one to be seen around the elbow in elderly patients. The mechanism of injury is usually a fall on to the elbow. The X-ray appearances have been classified by Murphy, Greene and Dameron (1987) as being transverse, oblique or comminuted. They describe the percentage of the articular surface involved in the proximal fragment of the olecranon as being the extent of the articular component. Patients with 60% or greater articular involvement tended to have poorer results after fracture fixation. Excellent results can be achieved with internal fixation (Van der Kloot, 1964). The device of choice is a tension band wire loop. This is more suited to the porotic bone of the olecranon in this age group than is lag screw fixation. The technique involves the use of a Rush nail or two parallel Kirschner wires drilled across the fracture into the cortical bone of the proximal ulna. A figure-of-eight wire loop is passed round the ends of the wire across the fracture and through a drill hole in the proximal ulna cortex. Simultaneous twisting of both limbs of the loop gives equal compression to the fracture (Deliyannis, 1974; Figure 9.1). Backing out of the Rush nail or Kirschner wires may however be a problem and the subcutaneous position of the tension band wire may cause symptoms. The twisted ends of the wire loop should be carefully buried in the bone or soft tissue and the proximal ends of the Rush nail or Kirschner wires must be buried deep to the triceps tendon, to avoid these problems. Non-sliding pins have been described by Netz and Stromberg (1982). These pins allow the wire to be threaded through an eye in their head so that compression on the fracture is still exerted when active elbow movement has begun. Pin slippage can therefore be prevented (Larsen and Jenson, 1991).

All types of olecranon fractures involving up to 80% of the articular surface were treated by excision of the fragments and advancement of the triceps to the distal olecranon by McKeever and Buck (1947). This technique was specifically recommended for the elderly patient, and did not lead to instability of the elbow. Satisfactory results with equal elbow strength and fewer complications than tension-band wiring have been reported more recently (Compton and Bucknell, 1989; Gartsman, Sculco and Otis 1981).

FRACTURES OF THE HUMERUS

The most difficult type of fracture of the distal humerus to manage in the elderly patient is the intercondylar T or Y shaped fractures. Fortunately these are rare. The vertical limb of the fracture usually passes through the trochlear sulcus into the humeral fossa. There may be greater or lesser degrees of comminution at the fracture site. This injury is usually caused by simple falls on the elbow causing impaction of the humeral shaft onto the olecranon (Wilson and Cochrane, 1925) or vice versa. In either case the condyles are already prestressed by contraction of the forearm muscles (DeLee, Greene and Wilkins, 1984). Considerable soft tissue injury is associated with these fractures. The importance of good quality radiographs cannot be over-emphasized for accurate classification of the injury. If surgery is being proposed these can be supplemented by computed

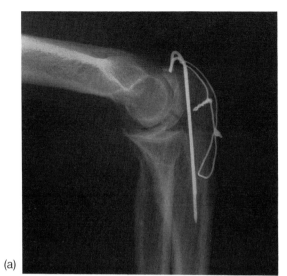

Figure 9.1 A displaced fracture of the olecranon, with tension band wire fixation.

(a)

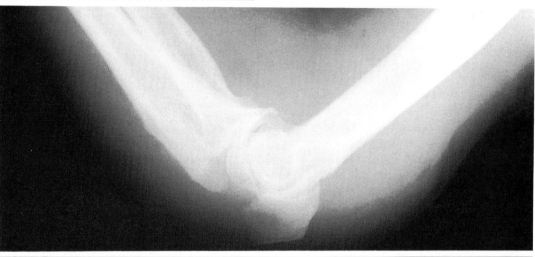

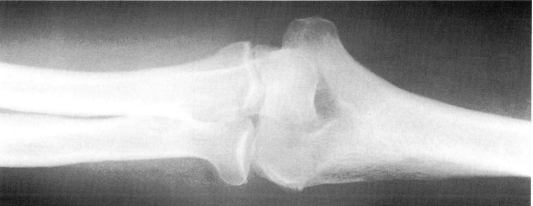

(b)

tomography (CT) to further clarify of the fracture. The fracture can be classified by the AO method (Muller *et al.*, 1979) or by one of the four types described by Riseborough and Radin in 1969. These classifications help to suggest the appropriate treatment and the expected prognosis but really each case must be carefully assessed individually and at all times the patient needs to be made aware of the gravity of this particular injury. Traction may have a role in restoring the alignment of the bony fragments by soft tissue moulding. This can be achieved by skin traction or skeletal traction via an olecranon pin. Some early elbow motion is possible with this technique. It is suitable if the patient is unfit for surgery, in the presence of a contaminated wound or if the surgeon considers that anatomical reduction of a severely comminuted fracture is not possible. However, the treatment may not be tolerated well by elderly patients and requires prolonged in-patient care. The so called 'bag of bones' technique (Eastwood, 1937) involves suspending the arm in a collar and cuff sling and allowing movement of the elbow as soon as it becomes comfortable. This treatment can be carried out as an out-patient. A functional range of motion can be achieved using this technique but usually with some loss of full extension (Brown and Morgan, 1971). Functional bracing of the arm provides a similar form of treatment. It controls angulation at the fracture site but gives insufficient stability to the fracture to allow adequate early mobilization.

The advent of more refined techniques of internal fixation has led to the possibility of rigid fixation of the fracture sufficient to allow early active mobilization (Muller *et al.*, 1979). Either the transolecranon approach (Cassebaum, 1969) or the posterior approach is recommended (Delee, Green and Wilkins, 1984) for good access to the supra-condylar columns and safe utilization of AO/ASIF internal fixation devices which may be required, according to the appearance of the fracture fragments at operation. The techniques used may include malleable reconstruction and third tubular plates, lag screws and tension band wiring. Initial Kirschner wire stabilization of the fragments greatly facilitates the accurate positioning of the definitive fixation devices, and may be used as guides for cannulated drills and screws which are of great value in this technically demanding surgery. (Figure 9.2). Excellent and good results were reported in all the fifteen patients over the age of sixty-five treated in this way by Jupiter and colleagues (1985). Postoperative rehabilitation can be facilitated by the use of a continuous passive motion splint, and pain control during this period can be continued by placing a cannula in the brachial plexus sheath for the administration of local anesthetics (Letsch *et al.*, 1989).

FRACTURES OF THE ARTICULAR SURFACE

The anterior shear fracture of the capitellum is entirely intra-articular and may have no soft tissue attachments whatsoever. The shearing force on the capitellum is sustained by a fall on the outstretched hand. With some degree of flexion at the elbow the radius impinges on the articular surface. Women are particularly affected and there may be an anatomical vulnerability caused by the characteristic cubitus valgus in the female elbow (Grantham, Norris and Bush, 1981). The fracture may involve part of the articular surface of the trochlear (Kocher-Lorenz Type I fracture). Alternatively the fracture may literally be the articular surface of the capitellum with very little subchondral bone attached (Kocher-Lorenz Type II fracture). Satisfactory holding of Type I fractures following closed reduction is difficult and if articular congruity is to be maintained and early mobilization possible then internal fixation with a small fragment screw is indicated.

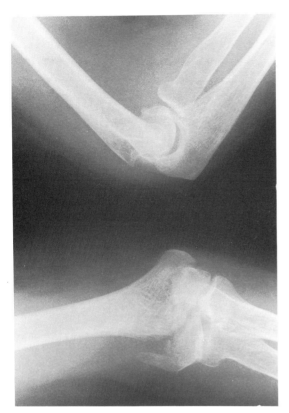
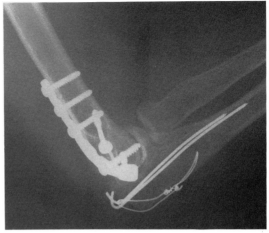
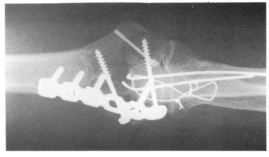

Figure 9.2 A comminuted intra-articular fracture of the distal humerus in a 67-year-old woman. The transolecranon approach was used, and the humeral fracture reconstructed using a plate and screws, with autologous bone graft. Function at six months was excellent.

For Type II fractures, excision of the fragment and irrigation of the joint can be followed by early mobilization.

COMPLICATIONS

Complications of intracondylar fractures of the humerus include post-traumatic arthritis, periarticular fibrosis, avascular necrosis of the bony fragments and non-union at the fracture site which results in a stiff, painful elbow with a poor range of movement. A non-union rate of 2% has been reported by Sim (1985). The presence of periarticular fibrosis and joint stiffness may potentiate the non-union by causing increased stress at the fracture site. Possible treatments include functional bracing, resection arthroplasty, open reduction with internal fixation and bone grafting and total elbow replacement. The use of a functional brace may give some stability to the non-union site but is probably insufficient to allow a significant increase in mobility. Resection arthroplasty will provide pain relief but the joint is unstable and weak. A repeat attempt at open reduction and internal fixation together with allograft bone grafting is recommended by Ackerman and Jupiter (1988). In their series of non-union of intra-articular and extra-articular fractures in patients aged between twenty and seventy years, union was achieved in 95% of cases. However, this procedure does not address the problem of any coexisting joint disease. Total elbow replacement has a higher complication rate when used in the treatment of post-traumatic arthritis than it does in cases of rheumatoid arthritis (Morrey *et al.* 1981) but its use in post-traumatic arthritis is probably more acceptable in the elderly than in young patients who will put greater demands on the prosthesis. Figgie *et al.* (1989) reported the use of a semi-constrained prosthesis for non-union in 14 patients with an average age of 65 years. The procedure was carried out three years after injury and combined with an anterior capsulotomy. The indications for surgery were loss of function in the limb, difficulties with activities of daily living, pain and a flail limb with pain at the non-union site. Other indications included marked intra-articular disease and osteoporosis or inadequate bone stock for satisfactory internal fixation. At follow-up five years later their elbow scores as measured by the Hospital for Special Surgery scoring system (Inglis and Pellicci, 1980) had improved from 17 to 84. Three of their 14 cases failed because of deep infection, dislocation or early loosening.

In the elderly the risk of devitalization of skin flaps must be guarded against. Large flaps should not be dissected as the skin is often very thin and its blood supply may be tenuous. Every attempt must be made to avoid pressure over the point of the elbow from dressings or plaster casts.

CONCLUSIONS

Fractures around the elbow in the elderly patient are often seen but fortunately the more severe comminuted types are rare. It is important to be able to classify the fractures accurately if the correct management is to be given. Although a number of these injuries can be treated conservatively, it must be emphasized that prolonged immobilization is deleterious to both the joint and the patient. Whatever the appointment treatment, it should always be combined with the earliest possible introduction of joint mobilization.

REFERENCES

Ackerman, G. and Jupiter, J.B. (1988) Non-union of the fractures of the distal end of the humerus. *J. Bone Joint Surg.*, **70-A**, 75–83.

Bakalim, G. (1970) Fractures of the radial head and their treatment. *Acta Orthop. Scand.*, **41**, 320.

Benjamin, A. (1982) Injuries of the Forearm, in *Watson-Jones Fractures and Joint Injuries*, 6th edn (ed. J.N. Wilson), Churchill Livingstone, Edinburgh, pp. 655–6.

Brown, R.F. and Morgan, R.G. (1971) Intercondylar T-shaped fractures of the humerus: results of ten cases treated by early mobilisation. *J. Bone Joint Surg.*, **53-B**, 425–8.

Cassebaum, W.H. (1969) Open reduction of T and Y fractures of the lower end of the humerus. *J. Trauma*, **9**, 915–25.

Compton, R. and Bucknell, A. (1989) Resection arthroplasty for comminuted olecranon fractures. *Orthop. Rev.*, **18**, 189–192.

DeLee, J.C., Green, D.P. and Wilkins, K.E. (1984) Fractures and dislocations of the elbow, in *Fractures in Adults*, 2nd edn (eds C.A. Rockwood and D.P. Green), J.P. Lippincott, Philadelphia.

Deliyannis, S.N. (1974) Comminuted fractures of the olecranon treated by Weber–Vasey technique. *Injury*, **5**, 19–24.

Eastwood, W.J. (1937) The T-shaped fracture of the lower end of the humerus. *J. Bone Joint Surg.*, **19**, 364–69.

Figgie, M.P., Inglis, A.E., Mow, C.S. and Figgie, H.E. (1989) Salvage of non-union of supracondylar fractures of the humerus by total elbow arthroplasty. *J. Bone Joint Surg.*, **71-A**, 1058–65.

Gartsman, G.M., Sculpo, T.P. and Otis, J.C. (1981) Operative treatment of olecranon fractures. *J. Bone Joint Surg.*, **63-A**, 718–21.

Grantham, S.A., Norris, T.R. and Bush, D.C. (1981) Isolated fracture of the humeral capitellum. *Clin. Orthop*, **161**, 262–9.

Inglis, A.E. and Pellicci, P.M. (1980) Total elbow replacement. *J. Bone Joint Surg.*, **62-A**, 1252–8.

Johnston, G.W. (1962) A follow-up of one hundred cases of fracture of the head of the radius with a review of the literature. *Ulster Med. J.*, **31**, 51–6.

Jupiter, J.B., Neff, V., Holzach, P. and Allgower, M. (1985) Intercondylar fractures of the humerus. *J. Bone Joint Surg.*, **67-A**, 226–39.

Knight, D.J., Rymaszewski, L.A., Amis, A.A. and Miller, J.H. (1993) Primary replacement of the fractured radial head with a metal prosthesis. *J. Bone Joint Surg.*, **75-B**, 572–6.

Larsen, E. and Jensen, C.M. (1991) Tension-band wiring of olecranon fractures with non-sliding pins: report of twenty cases. *Acta Orthop. Scan*; **62**, 360–2.

Letsch, R., Schmit-Neuerburg, K.P., Sturmer, K.M. and Walz, M. (1989) Intra-articular fractures of the distal humerus. *Clin. Orthop.*, **241**, 238–44.

Mason, J. A. and Shutkin, N.M. (1943) Immediate active motion treatment of fractures of the head and neck of the radius. *Surg. Gynecol. Obstet.*, **76**, 731–7.

McKeever, F.M. and Buck, R.M. (1947) Fracture of the olecranon process of the ulna: treatment by excision of fragment and repair of triceps. *J.A.M.A.*, **135**, 1–5.

Morrey, B.F., Bryan, R.S, Dobyns, J.H. and

Linscheid, R.L. (1981) Total elbow arthroplasty. *J. Bone Joint Surg.*, **63-A**, 1050–63.

Muller, M.E., Allgower, M., Schneider, R. Willenegger, H. (1979) *Manual of Internal Fixation. Technique recommended by the AO-Group*, 2nd Edn, Springer, New York.

Murphy, D.F., Greene, W.N. and Dameron, T.B. (1987) Displaced olecranon fractures in adults: clinical evaluation. *Clin. Orthop.* **224** 215–23.

Netz, P. and Stromberg, L. (1982) Non-sliding pins in traction absorbing wiring of fractures: a modified technique. *Acta Orthop.*, **234**, 215–23.

Riseborough, E.J. and Radin, E.L. (1969) Intercondylar 'T' fractures of the humerus in the adult: a comparison of operation and non-operative treatment in twenty-nine cases. *J. Bone Joint Surg.*, **51A**, 130–41.

Sim, F.H. (1985) Non-union and delayed union of distal humeral fractures in the elbow and its disorders (ed. B.F. Morrey), W.B. Saunders, Philadelphia, pp. 340–54.

Taylor, T.K.F. and O'Connor, B.T. (1964) The effect upon the inferior radio-ulnar joint of excision of the head of the radius in adults. *J. Bone Joint Surg.*, **46-B**, 83–8.

Van der Kloot, J.F.V.R. (1964) Results of treatment of olecranon fractures. *Arch. Chir. Neerlandicum*, **16**, 237–49.

Wilson, P.C. and Cochrane, W.A. (1925) *Fractures and dislocations*, J.P. Lippincott, Philadelphia.

10

Fractures of the distal radius in elderly people

MARGARET McQUEEN, WILLIAM MACLENNAN
and LOREN LATTA

INTRODUCTION

Although 209 years have passed since Pouteau (1783) first described the fracture of the distal end of the radius it still remains one of the commonest and most challenging fractures encountered by the orthopedic surgeon. Considerable controversy continues on the best method of management, ranging from those who believe that no specific treatment is required (Cassebaum, 1950; Benjamin, 1982) to advocates of functional bracing (Sarmiento *et al.*, 1975; Dias *et al.*, 1987b; Ferris *et al.*, 1989), internal (Clancey 1984) and external fixation (Howard *et al.*, 1989; Kongsholm and Olerud, 1989; Edwards, 1991).

EPIDEMIOLOGY
With W.J. MacLennan

Fractures of the distal radius account for 20% of the new Fracture Clinic attendances in the Orthopaedic Trauma Unit of the Royal Infirmary of Edinburgh. Of 2500 fractures occurring in a 4-year period from 1988 to 1992, the mean age of the patients was 57 years and almost half of the patients were over 64 years of age. Studies performed in Scandinavia (Schmalholz 1988; Robertsson,

Jonsson and Sigurjonsson, 1990) revealed marked increases in the age-specific incidence of the injury in women in the 40 to 60-year-old age group. Most fractures occur out of doors, in winter. It would seem therefore that fracture of the distal radius is a fracture of middle-aged to elderly women, three-quarters of whom are likely to be osteoporotic (Dias, Wray and Jones, 1987a).

Figure 10.1, taken from an Icelandic survey, shows that, in women between the ages of 40 and 60 years, there is a sharp increase in the incidence of the fracture to at least five times that of its previous level. The condition remains common in elderly women, but its incidence either plateaus, or shows only a marginal increase with advancing years. Though some surveys have shown an increase in elderly men, this is rarely dramatic. In a Swedish survey, for example, the ratio of men to women over the age of 70 years with the fracture was one to four (Malimin and Ljunghall, 1992).

The severity of the fracture also increased with age in the Scandinavian series. In the Edinburgh series the malunion rate rises from 62% in the seventh decade to 100% in the tenth decade, implying increasing severity with age.

Skeletal Trauma in Old Age
Published in 1994 by Chapman & Hall, London
ISBN 0 412 48750 0

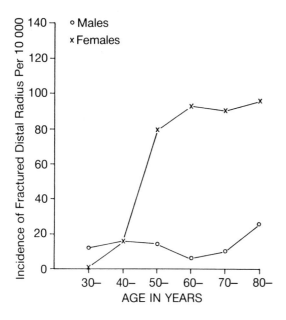

Figure 10.1 Incidence of fracture of the distal end of the radius related to age in men and women from Iceland (Robertsson, Jonsson and Sigurd-jonsson, 1990).

Benner and Johnell (1985) have found an increasing age-specific incidence in Sweden over the last twenty-five years. With the increasing age of the population it is evident that in common with proximal femoral fractures distal radial fractures are likely to increase dramatically as we enter the twenty-first century.

Since the age distribution of fractures to the distal radius is different from that of the proximal femur, it might be expected that there would be some differences in the pattern of risk factors, and, indeed, such is the case.

BONE DENSITY

The association of fractures of the distal radius and bone rarefaction is illustrated by a cohort study from the USA in which women aged 65 years and over from the lower age adjusted quartile for bone mineral density of the proximal radius had 4.1 times the risk of fractures to those from the upper quartile (Kelsey *et al.*, 1992).

FALLS

Most fractures of the distal radius are asso-ciated with a fall (Kelsey *et al.*, 1992). One of the factors contributing to this is an increased level of sway identified by posturography in postmenopausal women, and more marked in those with fractured wrists than age-matched controls (Crilly *et al.*, 1987). Further support for the menopause as a cause for imbalance was a postal survey of women in the Oxford Region of the United Kingdom in which the risk of falling reached a peak in women between the ages of 55 and 59 years, falling off to a trough between 70 and 75 years, and rising thereafter with increasing age (Winner, Morgan and Evans, 1989).

TRAUMA

Table 10.1 presents data from a survey of fractures of the distal radius in which it emerges that, in women, three-quarters of

Table 10.1 Types of trauma responsible for fractures to the distal radius (Robertsson, Jonsson and Sigurjonsson, 1990)

	Percentage with injury	
Type of trauma	Men	Women
Fall on level ground	49.2	73.4
Fall from height	29.2	7.6
Fall on stairs	6.2	13.0
Traffic accident	10.7	1.1
Other	4.7	4.9

fractures resulted from a fall on level ground (Sowers *et al.*, 1991). The injury in men was more likely to be due to a fall from height or a traffic accident, probably reflecting the greater degree of force required to fracture more dense bones.

DIET

In a study from the United States of women from areas with different quantities of calcium and fluoride in the water supply, there was no relationship with the amount of calcium, but an increased incidence of fractures of the distal radius in women from areas where there were increased quantities of fluoride (Sowers *et al.*, 1991).

HORMONAL CHANGES

Evidence from the relationship between sway and the menopause described already suggests that the effect of estrogen deficiency on balance may be at least as important as the change in bone mass as a determinant of fractures of the distal radius (Winner, Morgan and Evans, 1989).

OTHER FACTORS

In a longitudinal study of women over the age of 65 years in the USA it emerged that both poor vision and a high level of mobility were associated with an increased incidence of fractures to the distal radius (Kelsey *et al.*, 1992).

CLASSIFICATION

Many classification systems have been proposed for distal radial fractures from simple to very complex. Several simple classifications are commonly used in clinical practice. Eponymous terms are probably the most familiar – a Colles' fracture being a dorsally displaced fracture (Figure 10.2), a Smith's

fracture being a fracture with volar displacement (Figure 10.3), and a Barton's fracture being a fracture of the dorsal lip of the distal radius. The volar lip fracture is often termed the reverse Barton's fracture. However the eponymous terms can lead to confusion and it is probably better to refer to these fractures in anatomical terms, e.g. the volar displaced fracture of the distal radius.

More complex classification systems include Frykman's system (Frykman, 1967) and the more recent AO system of fracture classification (Muller *et al.*, 1990). The Frykman classification divides distal radial fractures into eight groups depending in joint involvement (including the radio-carpal and distal radio-ulnar joints) and the presence of a fracture in the distal ulna (Table 10.2). The AO system is more complex and requires considerable practice to use with ease in the clinical situation. It comprises three main groups each with nine subdivisions and is based on the complexity of articular involvement, articular comminution and metaphyseal comminution.

In practical terms the most useful simple classification is probably the differentiation between a stable and an unstable distal radial fracture. Stability of a distal radial fracture may be defined as maintenance of an adequate reduction in plaster until healing occurs. The unstable distal radial fracture is one which displaces following adequate reduction and cast application and without further intervention would result in a malunion.

The prediction of instability based on the original X-rays is multifactorial and therefore very difficult to assess with any degree of accuracy. Increasing age, severe initial angulation or shortening, metaphyseal comminution, intra-articular extension and ulnar fracture have all been implicated in the development of instability (Abbaszadegan, Jonsson and von Sivers, 1989; Lafontaine, Hardy and Delince, 1989). Ideally it should be

111

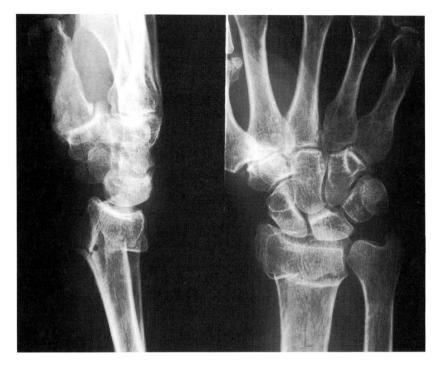

Figure 10.2 A dorsally displaced or Colles' fracture.

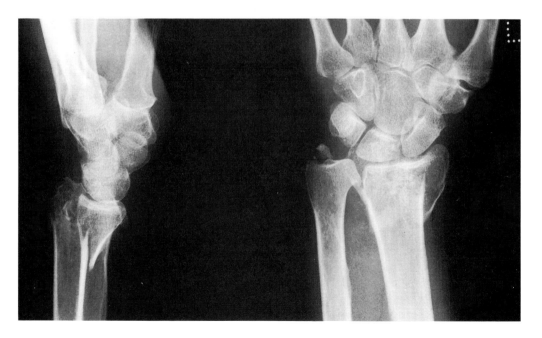

Figure 10.3 A volar displaced or Smith's fracture.

Table 10.2 Frykman's (1967) classification system for distal radial fractures

Joint involvement	No ulnar styloid fracture	Ulnar styloid fracture
Extra-articular	1	2
Radiocarpal	3	4
Distal radio-ulnar	5	6
Both	7	8

possible to make the diagnosis of instability on the day of injury thus reducing delays in definitive management. In practice this is not possible and the diagnosis of instability is made 7 to 10 days after injury based on the behaviour of the fracture in plaster (Figures 10.4 and 10.5).

BIOMECHANICS
By Loren L. Latta

Many authors agree that most distal radial fractures can be treated quite adequately by conservative methods, beginning with reduction and stabilization in plaster or with percutaneous pins while allowing early motion and minimizing the period of immobilization (Dias, Wray and Jones, 1987; Clyburn, 1987; Sarmiento *et al.*, 1975; Zagorski *et al.*, 1986, 1987). Colles' fractures heal quite rapidly and treatment is generally only required for a relatively short time to achieve adequate bony stability. There are two key mechanical factors related to maintenance of good anatomic position in the distal radius fracture: (1) the condition of the volar cortex and relationship of the distal radial fragment to it (Zagorski *et al.*, 1986, 1987); and (2) the condition of the distal radial-ulnar joint and the triangular fibrocartilage complex, or TFCC (Moore, Lester and Sarmiento, 1985).

The volar cortex provides the buttress to resist axial translation or shortening of the distal radius. The hand must be reduced so that the mechanical axis of the wrist lies to the volar half of the radius and the volar cortex must be reduced to assure that the major loading in the forearm will be located on the volar cortex (Figure 10.6). The distal fragment is usually dorsally displaced and the hand becomes dorsally displaced also. In this position, the mechanical axis (or line of loading) through the wrist, falls to the dorsal side of the radius and has no mechanical support to resist shortening of the distal radius. Thus, with the reduction of the distal radius and reapproximation of the dorsal tilt and radial length, the volar cortices must be abutted and the hand must be realigned to the volar side of the radius. A cast which holds the wrist in volar flexion and ulnar deviation can maintain this volar cortical abutment through the method of ligamentotaxis. Ulnar deviation places tension on the ligaments and soft tissues of the radial side of the distal radial fragment to resist radial deviation of this fragment. Volar flexion at the wrist provides tension on the dorsal soft tissue structures which attach to the distal radial fragment and helps to maintain the volar cortical abutment. This position of reduction can be best achieved in a relaxed supination position of the forearm as described by Sarmiento, Zagorski and Sinclair (1980) (Figure 10.7). It is common practice to attempt this in a pronated or 'cotton-loader' position which is adequate but not as effective as supination, probably because of the mechanical role of the brachio-radialis.

The TFCC plays a very important mechanical role in the medial-lateral stability of the wrist and the attachment of the distal radial fragment to the distal ulna. If this complex is dislocated with a Colles' fracture, maintenance of length of the radius without support of internal fixation is very difficult. The ability to use the TFCC for ligamentotaxis on the distal radial fragment is lost, so closed

113

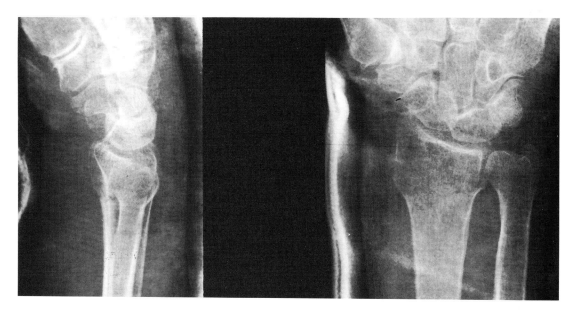

Figure 10.4 The same fracture as in Figure 10.2 after reduction.

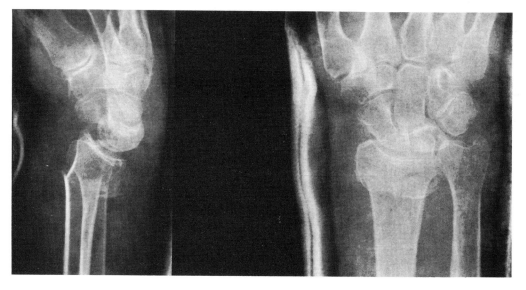

Figure 10.5 The same fracture as Figures 10.2 and 10.4 one week after reduction and cast immobilization. The fracture has redisplaced implying instability.

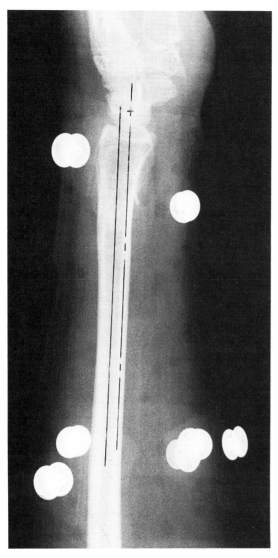

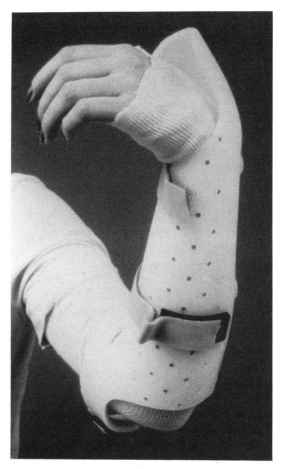

Figure 10.7 One method of maintaining the position of the distal radial fragment is to hold the arm in relaxed supination and block pronation of the forearm by the extensions over the elbow of the cast of fracture brace; maintain the hand in slight ulnar deviation and volar flexion and block radial deviation and dorsiflexion. This can be accomplished in plaster, a custom fracture brace, (Sarmiento *et al.*, 1975) or a prefabricated brace (Zagorski *et al.*, 1986) as shown here.

Figure 10.6 The lateral view of the normal wrist shows that a centre line along the axis of the radius will always fall to the dorsal side of the center rotation of the wrist. And a line parallel to the axis of the radius passing through the center of the wrist will generally fall nearer the volar cortex of the radius. This line through the center of the wrist parallel to the axis of the radius is considered to be the 'mechanical axis' of the wrist and probably best represents the alignment of the average resultant force at the wrist for most functional activities (Zagorski *et al.*, 1987).

treatment with joint positioning for stability is ineffective. The TFCC also provides axial stability by holding the distal radial fragment to the distal ulna. Radial length can only be lost through angulation of the distal radial fragment if the TFCC is intact and the volar cortex is aligned. A cast which holds the wrist in ulnar deviation and blocks dorsiflexion and pronation, has a very good leverage through ligamentotaxis to resist angulation of the distal radial fragment.

In instances where there is volar cortical comminution and/or TFCC dislocation, it may be impossible to maintain length of the radius by non-invasive techniques and the surgeon may choose to provide continued traction across the wrist by use of external fixation or provide volar cortical abutment with ORIF with a volar plate (Clyburn, 1987; Cooney, Linscheid and Dobyns, 1979; Clancey, 1984; Grana and Kopta, 1979; Smith *et al.*, 1988; Vaughan *et al.*, 1985; Husband, 1992). Since the volar abutment is the key to the stability of radial length, in most instances a volar plate need only be fixed on the proximal side of the fracture site to hold the distal fragments from displacing volarly. Another alternative is to allow the distal radius to collapse and heal in a shortened position with the expectation that ulnar shortening or removal of the distal ulna can be performed at a later date (Hartz and Beckenbaugh, 1979; Burkhalter, 1985; Rayhack, Gassa and Latta, 1991). Of these procedures those which leave the distal ulna and TFCC intact are mechanically superior. Wrist stability is compromised by disruption of the TFCC and the radial-ulnar joint (Moore, Lester and Sarmiento, 1985).

MANAGEMENT OF THE DISTAL RADIAL FRACTURE.

INITIAL TREATMENT

Early treatment depends on the degree of initial displacement. If the fracture is undisplaced then it is sufficient to immobilize the wrist for a period of three to four weeks in a forearm cast with the wrist in the neutral position. It is essential to leave the metacarpal phalangeal joints and the thumb free to permit early mobilization of the fingers.

In the displaced fracture a decision must be made about the severity of the displacement and the need for reduction. McQueen and Caspars (1988) found significant functional deficit in patients with dorsal angulation of more than 10 degrees and this would seem a reasonable level over which manipulation should be recommended. In the volar displaced fracture reduction should be performed for those with volar angulation greater than 15 degrees (Keating, Court-Brown and McQueen, 1993).

Manipulation is usually performed under regional anesthesia (Bier's Block) or local anesthesia with infiltration of local anesthetic into the fracture site. Local anesthesia has the advantage of avoiding potential problems with accidental failure of the tourniquet in a Bier's Block but has been demonstrated by Abbaszadegan and Jonsson (1990) to give poorer pain relief and a less satisfactory reduction of the fracture. Regional anesthesia is preferable provided there are sufficient experienced personnel available.

Closed reduction can be achieved in a high proportion of cases by longitudinal manual traction using a 'hand shake' grip with counter-traction applied by an assistant on the forearm or upper arm. This achieves disimpaction of the fracture. Further reduction can be achieved by thumb pressure on the dorsum of the distal radius and slight flexion of the wrist in dorsally displaced fractures and volar pressure and slight extension of the wrist in volar displaced fractures. It may occasionally be necessary to reduce a Colles' fracture in supination, to overcome brachoradialis as outlined above. A forearm cast is applied while traction is maintained. In the Edinburgh series this method resulted in a satisfactory reduction in 95% of fractures.

MANAGEMENT OF THE STABLE DISTAL RADIAL FRACTURE

The stable distal radial fracture will by definition remain in the reduced position in plaster and requires no further operative treatment. Nevertheless there are several areas of contention in the management of the stable fracture. These disputes revolve around the type of casts used, the position of the wrist, the time during which immobilization is required and the value of early mobilization.

A forearm cast with the wrist in slight flexion and ulnar deviation is more commonly used for a distal radial fracture although varying positions of the wrist and forearm or long arm casts have also been advocated. Poole in 1973 was the first to report on a prospective study of various types of plaster and positions of immobilization of the wrist and forearm. He recommended that below elbow casts should be used because he found no advantage in long arm casts in relation to radiological or functional outcome. Some patients whose fractures were immobilized in a long arm cast had permanent loss of supination. Five different types of forearm casts were evaluated by Van der Linden and Ericson (1981). They concluded that the anatomical and functional results were similar regardless of the type of cast or position of the wrist. Adequacy of the initial reduction was a major factor in determining the final outcome.

The second controversy surrounding the management of stable distal fractures is the value of early mobilization. The principle of early movement is achieved by immobilizing the wrist in a brace which allows some controlled movement of the wrist. This was advocated by Sarmiento *et al.* in 1975 who stated that it seemed to reduce swelling, stiffness and incapacity. This was not, however, a comparative study. Stewart Innes and Burke (1984) performed a comparison between forearm casts, above elbow cast braces and below elbow cast braces and found that bracing conferred no functional or anatomical advantage. They concluded that there is no indication to change from using the conventional plaster cast, although functional bracing of Colles' fractures continues to be investigated and is claimed by some to have a clinical role (Ledingham *et al.*, 1991).

Early mobilization may confer a slight advantage in reduction of swelling and recovery of motion in the early weeks after injury (Dias, Wray and Jones, 1987) but this does not persist in the long term. Ferris *et al.* (1989) felt that brace treatment increased hand swelling during the first week after injury and required more frequent review than conventional plaster cast.

The length of time for which these fractures are splinted is usually 5–6 weeks. It is likely that this is unnecessarily long. McAuliffe and his co-authors (1987) found that splintage of reduced fractures for 3 weeks rather than 5 weeks led to significantly less pain and a more rapid recovery without compromising the anatomical results.

In undisplaced or minimally displaced fractures not requiring reduction there seems to be no disadvantage in omitting splintage altogether (Davis and Buchanan, 1987; Abbaszadegan, Conradi and Jonsson, 1989).

Reduction in splintage time is of benefit to the elderly patient in reducing the inconvenience of a plaster cast to a minimum and allowing earlier resumption of domestic skills. Displaced fractures requiring reduction which are then stable in plaster are therefore best treated by a forearm cast with the wrist in neutral or slight flexion for 3–4 weeks. If the fracture is undisplaced or minimally displaced a support bandage will suffice in the majority of cases.

MANAGEMENT OF THE UNSTABLE DISTAL RADIAL FRACTURE

Instability of the distal radial fracture implies that malunion is inevitable unless further intervention is undertaken. Before a decision is made on further treatment the potential consequences of malunion must be considered.

Frykman (1967) stated that the functional end results of distal radial fractures deteriorated with increasing deformities. In common with many authors his functional assessment was based on subjective findings and the range of movement of the wrist. Porter and Stockley (1987) found decreased grip strength in elderly patients with a dorsal angle of more than 20 degrees, while Solgaard (1988) found that the presence of deformity three years after fracture had a strong influence on final function. McQueen and Caspers (1988) reviewed a series of patients more than four years from injury and performed a comprehensive objective assessment of hand and wrist function. There was a statistically significant decrease in mass and specialized grip strength, the ability to perform the normal activities of daily living and the range of movement in those patients with malunion. This is of particular importance to the elderly patient as the difficulties with the activities of daily living include lifting a pan full of water and lifting and holding dinner plates. If an elderly patient is independent and active then achieving an anatomical position after distal radial fracture allows the best chance of a good functional outcome and contributes towards maintenance of their independence.

Although reduction of the unstable distal radial fracture is relatively simple, maintenance of that reduction until union occurs is one of the most challenging aspects of the management of these injuries. Several methods are used to achieve this.

Remanipulation and plaster cast immobilization

Closed remanipulation and cast immobilization in the elderly patient is an illogical and generally unsuccessful method of treatment.

If the fracture has not remained in the reduced position in plaster initially it is unlikely to do so one week later. In 1986 McQueen, MacLaren and Chalmers found that remanipulation resulted in lasting improvement in only one-third of cases over the age of 60 years and even in these the anatomical result was poor. Schmalholz (1989) reported a 62% failure rate of remanipulation. In a prospective study currently being carried out in Edinburgh the malunion rate for remanipulation is 81%. Remanipulation and cast immobilization is not a reliable method of achieving a lasting reduction and should be abandoned.

Closed external fixation

External fixation of the distal radius depends on maintaining continuous traction across the fracture until healing occurs. Provided it is possible to reduce the fracture by closed techniques this method is usually successful in maintaining a near anatomical result (Cooney, Linscheid and Dobyns, 1979; Jonsson, 1983; McQueen, Michie and Court-Brown, 1993). Modern fixators (Figure 10.8) are lightweight and easy to apply. The use of the hand for light tasks is possible during the period the fixator is in place thus making this a suitable method for the independent elderly patient. Complications can occur in 18% (Jonsson, 1983) to 61% of patients (Szabo and Weber, 1988). These include pin track infection, reflex sympathetic dystrophy and carpal tunnel syndrome (McQueen, Michie and Court-Brown, 1993).

One suggested problem of external fixation in the elderly patient is pin loosening or breakage because of osteoporotic bone and this has resulted in several authors avoiding their use in the elderly (Jenkins *et al.*, 1987; Howard *et al.*, 1989). In practice however this complication is rare. In Edinburgh there has been one pin track fracture in 640 fixator pins in the last four years. Advanced age should

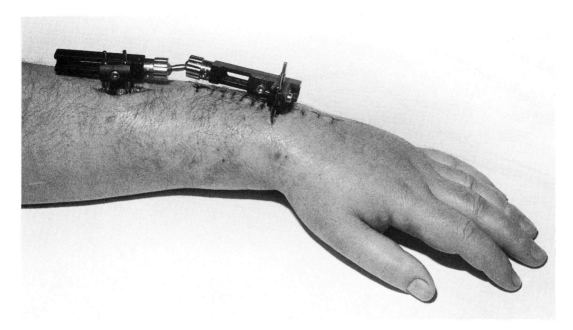

Figure 10.8 A lightweight external fixator.

not be a contra-indication for this technique provided the patient is mentally and physically active. The fixator is removed after 5–6 weeks when physiotherapy is usually started. Hand and wrist function recovers well provided complications can be avoided (McQueen, Michie and Court-Brown, 1993).

Internal fixation

Open reduction and internal fixation is used in the elderly for the volar displaced fracture of the distal radius. A small buttress plate is used (Figure 10.9) which maintains the angulation of the radius although some shortening can occur. The forearm is subsequently protected in a cast. Functional results are satisfactory and dependent on the severity of the initial fracture (Keating, Court-Brown and McQueen, 1993). Open reduction and internal fixation with bone grafting should also be used in cases with severe articular displace-

ment. However these are rare in elderly patients.

Closed reduction and percutaneous pinning have been advocated in the management of the distal radial fracture. This is effective in the stable distal radial fracture particularly in young strong bone but is unlikely to maintain reduction in the truly unstable, comminuted osteoporotic fracture. Clancey (1984) reports 'overall good results' in his series of 30 unselected cases despite loss of position in 10%. This is the rate of instability one might expect in fractures without fixation implying that K wires do not confer sufficient added stability.

COMPLICATIONS

The major complication rate of a series of 565 distal radial fractures is quoted by Cooney, Dobyns and Linscheid (1980) as 31%. Common problems are median neuropathy, malunion, reflex sympathetic dystrophy and tendon ruptures. These may or may not be

119

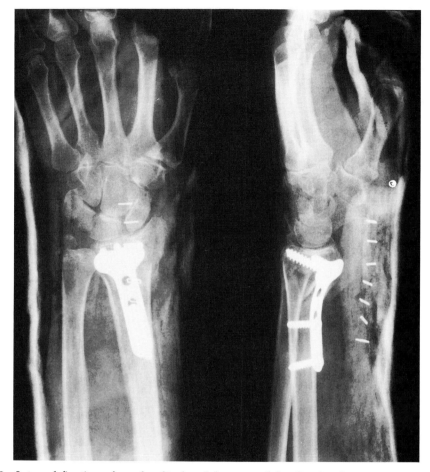

Figure 10.9 Internal fixation of a volar displaced fracture of the distal radius.

treatment related. Prevention if possible is mandatory since complications have a deleterious effect on final function (McQueen and Caspars, 1988; McQueen, Michie and Court-Brown, 1993). Significant carpal tunnel syndrome should be decompressed promptly. Malunion should be prevented by adequate treatment. Physiotherapy should be instituted at the first suspicion of finger stiffness or reflex sympathetic dystrophy.

CONCLUSIONS

A fracture of the distal radius if inadequately treated may lead to significant functional loss in the elderly patient. The suggested treatment for the stable fracture has already been outlined. It is essential however to identify instability at the earliest possible opportunity by serial X-rays over the first ten days after injury. In the mentally and physically active elderly patient with an unstable fracture, closed external fixation is a satisfactory method of maintaining an anatomical reduction and allowing the best chance of a good functional outcome. Serious complications should be promptly and aggressively treated in order to obtain maximal functional recovery.

REFERENCES

Abbaszadegan, H., Conradi, P. and Jonsson, U. (1989a) Fixation not needed for undisplaced Colles' fracture. *Acta Orthop. Scand.*, **60**, 60–2.

Abbaszadegan, H., Jonsson, U. and von Sivers, K. (1989b) Prediction of instability of Colles' fractures. *Acta Orthop. Scand.*, **60**, 646–50.

Abbaszadegan, H. and Jonsson, U. (1990) Regional anaesthesia preferable for Colles' fracture. *Acta Orthop. Scand.*, **61**, 348–9.

Bengner, U. and Johnell, O. (1985) Increasing incidence of forearm fractures. *Acta Orthop. Scand.*, **56**, 158–60.

Benjamin, A. (1982) Injuries of the forearm, in *Watson-Jones Fractures and Joint Injuries*, 6th edn, vol 2 (ed. J.N. Wilson), Churchill Livingstone, Edinburgh, pp. 650–709

Burkhalter, W.E. (1985) Upper extremity fractures in the elderly, in *Orthopaedic Care of the Geriatric Patient*, Ch 10 (ed. T.P. Sculco), C.V. Mosby, St. Louis, Missouri.

Cassebaum, W.H. (1950) Colles' fracture: a study of end results. *J.A.M.A.*, **143**, 963–5.

Clancey, G.J. (1984) Percutaneous Kirschner wire fixation of Colles' fractures. *J. Bone Joint Surg. (Am.).*, **66A**, 1008–14.

Clyburn, T.P. (1987) Dynamic external fixation for comminuted intra-articular fractures of the distal end of the radius. *J. Bone Joint Surg.*, **69A**, 248–54.

Cooney, W.P., Linscheid, R.L. and Dobyns, J.H. (1979) External pin fixation for unstable Colles' fractures. *J. Bone Joint Surg. (Am.)*, **61A**, 840–5.

Cooney, W.P., Dobyns, J.H. and Linscheid, R.L. (1980) Complications of Colles' fractures. *J. Bone Joint Surg. (Am.)*, **62A**, 613–19.

Crilly, R.G., Delaquerrier Richardson L., Roth, J.H. *et al.* (1987) Postural stability and Colles' fracture. *Age Ageing*, **16**, 133–8.

Davis, T.R. and Buchanan, J.M. (1987) A controlled prospective study of early mobilisation of minimally displaced fractures of the distal radial metaphysis. *Injury*, **18**, 283–5.

Dias, J.J., Wray, C.C. and Jones, J.M. (1987a) Osteoporosis and Colles' fracture in the elderly. *J. Hand Surg.*, **12**, 57–9.

Dias, J.J., Wray, C.C., Jones, J.M. *et al* (1987b) The value of early mobilisation in the treatment of

Colles' fractures. *J. Bone Joint Surg. (Br.)*, **69B**, 463–7.

Edwards, G.S. (1991) Intra-articular fractures of the distal part of the radius treated with the small AO external fixator. *J. Bone Joint Surg. (Am.)*, **73A**, 1241–50.

Ferris, B.D., Thomas, N.P., Dewar, M.E. *et al.* (1989) Brace treatment of Colles' fractures. *Acta Orthop. Scand.*, **60**, 63–5.

Frykman, G. (1967) Fracture of the distal radius including sequelae, shoulder-handfinger syndrome, disturbance in the distal radio-ulnar joint and impairment of nerve function. A clinical and experimental study. *Acta Orthop. Scand.* Suppl. 108: 1–153.

Grana, W.A. and Kopta J.P. (1979). The Roger Anderson device in the treatment of fractures of the distal end of the radius. *J. Bone Joint Surg.*, **61A**, 1224–8.

Hartz, G.R. and Beckenbaugh, R.P. (1979) Long term results of resection of the distal ulna for post-traumatic conditions. *J. Trauma*, **19**, 219–26.

Husband, J.B. (1992). Fractures of the distal radius (not just another Colles' fracture). *Trans 4th. Current Concepts in Trauma Care* 11–5.

Howard, P.W., Stewart, H.D., Hind, R.E. *et al.* (1989) External fixation or plaster for severely displaced comminuted Colles' fractures? A prospective study of anatomical and functional results. *J. Bone Joint Surg. (Br.)*, **71B**, 68–73.

Jenkins, N.H., Jones, D.G., Johnson, S.R. *et al.* (1987) External fixation of Colles' fractures. An anatomical study. *J. Bone Joint Surg. (Br.)*, **69B**, 207–11.

Jonsson, U. (1983) External fixation for redislocated Colles' fractures. *Acta Orthop Scand.*, **54**, 878–83.

Keating, J., Court-Brown, C.M. and McQueen, M.M. (1993) Internal fixation of volar distal radial fractures *J. Bone Joint Surg.*

Kelsey, J.L., Browner, W.S., Seeley, D.G. *et al.* (1992) Risk factors for fractures of the distal forearm and proximal humerus. The Study of the Osteoporotic Fractures Research Group. *Am. J. Epidemiol.*, **135**, 477–489.

Kongsholm, J. and Olerud, C. (1989) Plaster cast versus external fixation for unstable intraarticular Colles' fractures. *Clin. Orthop.*, **241**, 57–65.

Lafontaine, M., Hardy, D. and Delince, P. (1989)

Stability assessment of distal radial fractures. *Injury*, **20**, 208–10.

Ledingham, W.M., Wytch, R., Goring, C.C. *et al.* (1991) On immediate functional bracing of Colles' fractures. *Injury*, **22**, 197.

McAuliffe, T.B., Hilliar, K.M., Coates, C.J. *et al.* (1987) Early mobilisation of Colles' fractures: a prospective trial. *J. Bone Joint Surg. (Am.)*, **69A**, 727–9.

McQueen, M.M. MacLaren, A. Chalmers, J. (1986) The value of remanipulating Colles' fractures. *J. Bone Joint Surg. (Br.)* 68B: 232–3.

McQueen, M.M. and Caspers, J. (1988) Colles' fracture: does the anatomical result affect the final function? *J. Bone Joint Surg. (Br.)* **70B**, 649–51.

McQueen, M.M., Michie, M. and Court-Brown, C.M. (1993) Hand and wrist function after external fixation of unstable distal radial fractures. *Clin. Orthop.*, **285**, 200–4.

Mallmin, H. and Ljunghall, S. (1992) Incidence of Colles' fracture in Uppsala. A prospective study of a quarter-million population. *Acta Orthop. Scand.*, **63**, 213–15.

Moore, T.M., Lester, D.K. and Sarmiento A. (1985). The stabilising effect of soft tissue constraints in the artificial Galeazzi fractures. *Clin. Orthop.*, **194**, 189.

Muller, M.E., Nazarian, S., Koch, P. *et al.* (1990) *The Comprehensive Classification of Fractures of Long Bones*, Springer Verlag, Berlin.

Poole, C. (1973) Colles' fracture. A prospective study of treatment. *J. Bone Joint Surg. (Br.)* **55B**, 540–4.

Porter, M. and Stockley, I. (1987) Fractures of the distal radius. Intermediate end results in relation to radiologic parameters. *Clin. Orthop.*, **220**, 241–52.

Pouteau, C. (1783) Oeuveres posthumes de M. Pouteau. Memoire, contenant quelques reflexions sur quelques fractures de l'avant-bras, sur les luxations incomplettes du poignet et sur le diastasis. Paris, PhD, Pierres.

Rayhack, J.M., Gasser, S.L. and Latta, L.L. (1991). Oblique versus transverse ulnar shortening osteotomies: a clinical and biomechanical study. *Orthop. Trans.* **15**, 738.

Robertsson, G.O., Jonsson, G.T. and Sigurjonsson, K. (1990) Epidemiology of distal radius fractures in Iceland in 1985. *Acta Orthop. Scand.*, **61** (5), 457–9.

Sarmiento, A., Pratt, C.W., Berry, N.C. *et al.* (1975) Colles' fractures. Functional bracing in supination. *J. Bone Joint Surg. (Am.)*, **57A**, 311–17.

Sarmiento, A., Zagorski, J.B. and Sinclair, W.F. (1980) Functional bracing and Colles' fractures: A prospective study of immobilisation in supination v pronation. *Clin Orthop.*, **146**, 175.

Schmalholz, A. (1988) Epidemiology of distal radius fracture in Stockholm 1981–82. *Acta Orthop Scand.*, **59** (6), 701–3.

Schmalholz, A. (1989) Closed rereduction of axial compression in Colles' fracture is hardly possible. *Acta Orthop Scand.*, **60**, 57–9.

Smith, R.S., Crick, J.C., Alonso and Horowitz, M. (1988) Open reduction and internal fixation of volar lip fractures of the distal radius. *J. Orthop. Trauma.*, **2**, 181.

Solgaard, S. (1988) Function after distal radius fracture. *Acta Orthop Scand.*, **59**, 39–42.

Sowers, M.F., Clark, M.K., Jannausch, M.L. and Wallace, R.B. (1991) A prospective study of bone mineral content and fractures in communities with differential fluoride exposures. *Am. J. Epidemiol.*, **133**, 649–60.

Stewart, H.D., Innes, A.R. and Burke, F.D. (1984) Functional cast-bracing for Colles' fractures. A comparison between cast-bracing and conventional plaster casts. *J. Bone Joint Surg. (Br.)*, **66B**, 749–53.

Szabo, R.M. and Weber, S.C. (1988) Comminuted intra-articular fractures of the distal radius. *Clin. Orthop.*, **230**, 39–48.

Van der Linden, W. and Ericson, R. (1981) Colles' fracture. How should its displacement be measured and how should it be immobilised? *J. Bone Joint Surg. (Am.)*, **63A**, 1285–8.

Vaughan, P.P., Lui, S.M., Harrington, I.J. and Maistrelli, G.L. (1985) Treatment of unstable fractures of the distal radius by external fixation. *J. Bone Joint Surg.*, **67B**, 385–9.

Winner, S.J., Morgan, C.A. and Evans, J.G. (1989) Perimenopausal risk of falling and incidence of distal forearm fracture. *B.M.J.*, **298**, 1486–8.

Zagorski, J.B., Zych, G.A., Latta, L.L. and Fin-

nieston, A.R. (1986) Management of Colles'
fractures with prefabricated braces. *Ortho
Trans.*, **10**, 471.

Zagorski, J.B., Zych, G.A., Latta, L.L. and McCollough, N.C. (1987) Modern concepts in functional fracture bracing – upper limb, *in AAOS*
Instructional Course Lectures, Vol. **XXXVI**, Chap
24, AAOS, Chicago, Illinois.

FURTHER READING

Jupiter, J.B. (1991) Fractures of the distal end of the
radius. *J. Bone Joint Surg. (Am.)*, **73A**, 461–9.

11

Fractures of the hip in elderly people

SUNE LARSSON, NILE R. LESTRANGE,
WILLIAM MACLENNAN and LOREN LATTA

EPIDEMIOLOGY
By W.J. MacLennan

INCIDENCE

A large number of surveys have confirmed that fractures of the proximal femur are more common in women than in men, and that there is a striking increase in incidence with advancing age. This is illustrated by a review from New England, where in whites the female to male ratio varied from 2.35 for those aged 65 to 69 years to 1.55 for those aged 90 to 94 years (Figure 11.1) (Fisher *et al.*, 1991). There was an exponential increase in the incidence of fractures so that the ratios for change between subjects aged 65 to 69 years and those aged 90 to 94 years were 14.6 and 34.2 for women and men respectively.

In the same paper it emerged that fractures of the proximal femur were more common in whites than in blacks, and age-matched relative risks of white-black being 1.48 for males and 2.41 for females. This confirms the findings of an earlier study on American females in which the age adjusted fracture rates for whites, Asians, blacks and Hispanics were 140.7, 85.4, 57.3 and 49.7 over

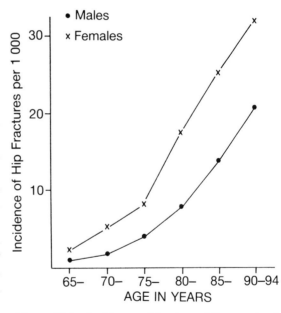

Figure 11.1 Incidence of fracture of the proximal femur in white men and women from new England (Fisher *et al.*, 1991).

100 000 respectively (Silverman and Madison 1988). There is also variation in the ratio of males to females with the injury in different racial groups with the condition being more

Skeletal Trauma in Old Age
Published in 1994 by Chapman & Hall, London
ISBN 0 412 48750 0

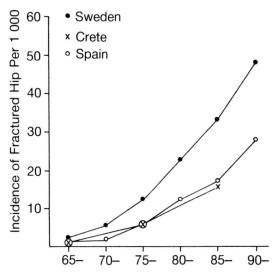

Figure 11.2 Incidence of fracture of the proximal femur in women from Sweden, Crete and Spain (Dretakis, Giarourakis, Steriopoulos, 1992; Nilsson, Lofman, Berglund, Larsson, Toss, 1991; Diez, Puig, Aubia, Vivancos, 1989).

common in male blacks and Asians (Maggi *et al.*, 1991).

Studies from different countries have demonstrated a striking geographical variation in the incidence of fractures of the proximal femur. In general, the fracture is very much more common in Northern Europe and North America than in Southern Europe. Figure 11.2 shows the striking disparity between the age-adjusted incidence for women in Scandinavia and those for women in Spain and Crete (Dretakis, Giaourakis and Steriopoloulos, 1992; Nilsson *et al.*, 1991; Diez *et al.*, 1989). The disparity is even greater in Africa. In a survey of African women between the ages of 75 and 74 years the incidence was one eighty-sixth of that for a comparable group from the United Kingdom (Adebajo, Cooper and Evans, 1991). Even within the United States of America there is considerable regional variation, but the association with latitude is reversed with

age-adjusted rates for women over 65 years with fractures being higher in Southern as opposed to Northern countries (Jacobsen *et al.*, 1990). An observation of particular concern is that there has been a dramatic increase in the age and sex-specific incidence of fractures of the proximal femur over the last 50 years. A review from the county of Ostergotland in Sweden established that there has been a 50% increase in the number of hip fractures (Nilsson *et al.* 1991). This was related in part to the increased number of old and very old people in the population, but shows that, for most five-year age groups over the age of fifty years, there was an increase in the incidence of fractures in both men and women, and that the proportional increase was greater for men than women. Given the age distribution of fractures, the changes in patients over the age of 75 years had the most important effect on overall numbers, and it was predicted that, should current trends continue, there would be a further 70% increase in the absolute number of fractures between 1985 and the year 2000.

Many other countries have had a similar experience with increases in the total number of fractured femurs varying between 50% and in excess of 200% (Della Torre, Petrini and Mancini, 1991; Nydegger *et al.*, 1991; Simoneon, 1991; Boerboom *et al.*, 1991; Martin *et al.*, 1992; Spector, Copper and Lewis, 1990). In all these surveys it has also emerged that a change in the age and sex specific incidence of fractures has been a major factor for the increase in absolute numbers.

Etiology

Bone mass

Although there is a decrease in bone mass and increase in the incidence of hip fractures with increasing age, there is only a modest association between the two variables. One of many papers describes a prospective study in which the density of the distal radius was compared with the incidence of fractured hips in women aged 65 years and over (Cummings *et al.*, 1990). The relative risk of fracture over a mean follow-up period of 1.6 years for subjects with a bone density one standard deviation below the age specific mean was only 1.55, with age itself emerging as a much more important risk factor. When relative risk of fracture in patients with low bone density was related to age, it emerged that this was most important in younger individuals and approached unit, in those over the age of 75 years (Cooper, Wickham and Walsh, 1991).

Falls

There is an association between a history of recurrent falls and fractured hips, and this becomes stronger with increasing age (Gardsell, *et al.*, 1989). Over three-quarters of falls leading to fractures occur in the patient's own home, and often occur when getting up or sitting down (Dias, 1987).

Genetic factors

There is uncertainty as to whether racial differences in the incidence of fractured hips described already relate to genetic or environmental factors. In comparison between Japanese from Okinawa, Japanese from Hawaii and Caucasians from the USA, it was found that the incidences of fractures of the proximal femur were similar in the two Japanese groups and much lower than in the Caucasians, despite the fact that the Hawaiian Japanese had adopted a Western diet and lifestyle (Ross *et al.*, 1991). A retrospective review, from Sweden, of the radiological records from the offspring of patients fracturing their proximal femur, established that the incidence of fractures were no more common in them than in a control group (Gardsell *et al.*, 1989). This suggests that, within racial

groups at least, there is not an important genetic predisposition.

Trauma

Fractures of the proximal femur in young to middle-aged patients are likely to follow severe trauma, whereas, in old age, the trauma is often either moderate or minimal. The severity of trauma also affects the site of the fracture with severe trauma being more usually responsible for fractures of the neck of femur, and moderate trauma leading to pertrochanteric fractures.

Diet

There is considerable debate as to whether the dietary intake of calcium influences the incidence of fractured hips. In a recent case control study from New York on white women there was no difference in recent or teenage intakes of calcium in fracture and control subjects (Nieves, Grisso and Kelsey, 1992). There also was no relationship between calcium intake and fractures in a prospective study of women from the United Kingdom (Wickham *et al.*, 1989). These observations are in contrast to a study on Chinese men and women from Hong Kong where there was a link between intakes of calcium and fractures (Lau *et al.*, 1989). The disparity may be due to the fact that the mean intake of calcium in the Chinese was only a quarter of that in subjects from the United Kingdom or United States.

There is also uncertainty as to the role of Vitamin D deficiency in fractures of the proximal femur. Studies on bone biopsies from fracture patients have placed the prevalence of osteomalacia at between 0 and 2%, suggesting that this is not a major factor in the etiology of fractures (Compston, Vedi and Croucher, 1991; Eventov *et al.*, 1989; Wilton, 1987). Many fracture patients have low plasma calcidiol concentrations, however, and there is evidence that this leads to secondary hyperparathyroidism leading, in turn, to a negative calcium balance and bone rarefaction (Behnamou *et al.*, 1991).

Although there is radiological evidence that there is an increase in the bone density of individuals from areas with high concentrations of fluoride in the drinking water, a number of surveys have suggested that a high concentration of fluoride had either no effect or actually increases the risk of fractured hips (Sowers *et al.*, 1991; Cooper *et al.*, 1990; Sowers, Wallace and Lenike, 1986).

Physical exercise

In a recent survey of men and women living in eight areas within the United Kingdom, it emerged that physical exercise protected against fractures of the proximal femur in that the adjusted odds ratio for the third of the population with a history of the least outdoor activity level against the third with the greatest level was 4.3 (Wickham *et al.*, 1989). This supported the observation from an earlier case control study in the United Kingdom in which patients with fractured hips had had a lower level of physical activity in middle-age than controls. Similar observations also have been made in case control studies from Hong Kong and the USA (Leung *et al.*, 1988; Nieves, Grisso and Kelsey, 1992).

Coffee, alcohol and smoking

Data from the Framingham study suggest that while the consumption of up to two cups of coffee did not increase the risk of hip fractures, there was a marginal increase in risk when the amount taken was in excess of 2.5 cups per day (Kiel *et al.*, 1990). It was thought that the association with coffee consumption might be indirect, and indica-

tive of other behavioral patterns which were more important as causes of the fracture. Evidence for this emerged in a subsequent study from Sweden in which an apparent relationship, in women, between drinking more than three cups of coffee per day disappeared when a stepwise logistic regression model was used to investigate the interrelationship of this to deteriorated dental state, socio-economic status and tobacco consumption (Johansson *et al.*, 1992).

Analysis of data from the Framingham study also revealed an association with alcohol consumption and fractured hips, the relative risk for heavy drinking in men being 1.26 and that in women being 1.54 (Felson *et al.*, 1988). When the relationship was subjected to logistic regression analysis, however, it emerged that there was only a strong association between alcohol consumption and fractures in individuals under the age of 65 years, and that the association did not reach a statistically significant level above this age. It is unclear whether the relationship was due to bone rarefaction, to an increased risk of accidents or to both.

A number of studies have established that there is a relationship between smoking and the risk of hip fractures. One from North Italy established that, in women, the relation for smokers and ex-smokers was 1.7 and 1.5 respectively, and that this increased to 2.5 in individuals smoking more than 25 cigarettes per day (La Vecchia *et al.*, 1991).

Body build

Most reviews have shown a consistent negative relationship between body mass index (weight/height) and the incidence of fractured hips (Grisso *et al.*, 1991; La Vecchia *et al.*, 1991; van Hemert *et al.*, 1990). The association is probably related to the fact that individuals with a low body mass index have a reduced bone mass (Johansson *et al.*, 1992).

Hormonal changes

In view of the accelerated loss of bone in women after the menopause, it is not surprising that there is an association between fractures of the proximal femur and estrogen levels (Riggs and Melton, 1986). In women under the age of 70 years, the risk increases with the number of years since the menopause, but beyond this age the duration of the menopause is of little significance. The risk of fractures is reduced in postmenopausal women on estrogen replacement therapy. This was illustrated by a review of postmenopausal women in the Framingham study in which the relative risk of fractures in those who had ever been on estrogens was 0.65, and that for those who had been on treatment within the previous two years was 0.34 (Kiel *et al.*, 1987).

Although there are no sudden changes in hormone levels in men, those with hypogonadism are at increased risk of fractures. Evidence for this was a case control study of men with hip fractures against controls in which the proportion of fracture cases with low serum free testosterone was 58.8% as against 26.97% of controls (Stanley *et al.*, 1991).

Drugs

A variety of drugs increases the risk of fractured hips in old people, usually by compromising their balance. A case control study revealed that the relative risk of fractures was 1.7 for patients on benzodiazepines with a long half-life (Ray, Griffin and Downey, 1989). This contrasted with one of only 1.1 for those on benzodiazepines with a short half-life. In a similar study, the relative risk of antidepressants being associated with fractures was 1.6 (Ray, Griffin and Malcolm, 1991).

A review of prescriptions in women over the age of 65 years in Canada revealed that analgesics also may predispose to fractures, the relative risk for codeine being 1.6, and that for propozyphene also being 1.6 (Short *et al.*, 1992). This was even higher in patients who had only recently gone on to treatment, possibly because those on long-term therapy had adapted to side-effects.

Several studies have suggested that patients on thiazide diuretics have a reduced risk of fractures. In one of these the risk was reduced with the duration of therapy (Ray, Griffin and Dourney, 1989). There was a much more modest and statistically insignificant effect in another study on thiazide diuretics and fractures (Felson *et al.*, 1991). When, however, patients on thiazides combined with potassium sparing agents were excluded, the odds ratio for patients on thiazides fell to 0.31. The explanation for the protective effect of thiazides is probably that they reduce the excretion of calcium and thus promote a positive calcium balance.

Neuropsychiatric disorders

There is a particularly high risk of fractures of the proximal femur in elderly patients with neuropsychiatric disorders. An example is a follow up of a group with Alzheimer's disease in which there were three times the incidence of falls associated with fractures as in a control group (Buchner and Larson 1987). The risk was particularly great in patients who wandered or who suffered from drug side-effects. In another study, the odds ratios for fractures in patients with a stroke or with Parkinson's disease were 2.0 and 9.4 respectively (Grisso *et al.*, 1991). In stroke patients the fractured hip is more likely to be on the side of a hemiparesis (White, 1988). Prolonged follow-up of patients with Parkinson's disease established that, over ten years, 27% had sustained a fractured hip (Johansson *et al.*, 1992).

Poor vision is also an important determinant of falls (Grisso *et al.*, 1991). In the

Framingham study the relative risk of fractures in patients with vision between 20/30 and 20/80 was 1.54 rising to 2.17 in those with vision of 20/100 or worse (Felson *et al.*, 1989). The risk of falls also was greater in those with a disparity of vision in the two eyes than those with moderate impairment in both.

Environment

The observation that fractures of the proximal femur are more common in patients from institutions is of little relevance in that this is merely a reflection of the high morbidity of this group. A more interesting finding from Sweden is that the age/sex adjusted incidence of fractures was lower in a rural than an urban area, and that, whereas over ten years the incidence increased in the urban area, there was no change in the rural one (Larsson, Eliasson and Hansson, 1989). A feature of the rural area is that it was mountainous suggesting that a high level of physical activity protected the population against hip fractures.

There is also a seasonal variation in the incidence of hip fractures, peak levels occurring during the winter months, but the precise explanation for the association has not been defined (Jacobsen *et al.*, 1991). Presumably it reflects an increased number of falls in the winter, but changes in vitamin D status also might be important.

INTRACAPSULAR HIP FRACTURES
By N. LeStrange

BIOMECHANICS
By Loren L. Latta

One of the most common types of fracture in osteoporotic bones is the subcapital hip fracture, usually associated with minimal energy. Subcapital hip fractures are often associated with avascular necrosis as the blood supply to the femoral head is precarious following fracture. Because the subcapital fracture generally occurs from compressive overloading on the head of the femur, the fractures are often impacted and relatively stable at the time of initial treatment. If the fracture fragments are impacted, it may be difficult or impossible to separate them in order to achieve reduction and manipulation, and can further jeopardize the blood supply to the head. If the impacted position of the femoral head is accepted, the surgical fixation can be a relatively minor procedure and any fixation system which allows for further collapse with weight bearing is generally adequate (Edwards, Lewallen and Hayer, 1985; Elmerson *et al.*, 1987; Stromquist *et al.*, 1987; Swiontkowski *et al.*, 1987; Van Audekercke *et al.*, 1979; Deyerle, 1980).

With any fixation system, one must keep in mind that the best trabecular bone for fixation is in the centre of the femoral head, and in the subchondral region (Crowell, Edwards and Hayer, 1985; Milne *et al.*, 1988; Smith, Cody and Goldstein, 1992). With osteoporosis very few trabeculae of any mechanical significance can be found through most of the neck area and therefore, fixation and support cannot generally be expected through the neck. With multiple pin fixation, pins are placed in a parallel fashion so that sliding and further collapse of the head is possible with weight bearing. It is, however, necessary to assure that at least one pin is as far inferior through the neck as possible so that the pin will rest directly on the cortical bone of the medial neck for support (Van Audekercke *et al.*, 1979; Nakamura *et al.*, 1987) (Figure 11.3). This seems to be necessary because of the lack of trabecular support through the neck area and if the pins achieve fixation only in the head proximally and at the lateral side of the trochanter distally, then a long unsupported region through the neck will allow for bending of the pins during loading and if they bend significantly, they will bind and

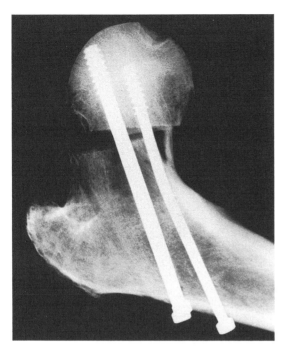

(a)

Figure 11.3 In osteoporotic femora *in vitro*, subcapital osteotomies were created and axial loading applied at a fixed angle to the shaft of the femur to create a simulation of the mechanical behavior of the fracture fixation observed clinically, (a) Two modes of failure were observed in this model based on the location of the sliding screw fixation in the head. When the most distal screw lay close to the medial wall of the neck, impaction of the head of the neck was the typical mode of failure with sliding of the screws and maximum resistance, (b). In instances where the most inferior screw was too central in the head and not supported along the medial neck of the femur in osteoporotic bones, (c), the screw would bend and binding of the screw in the lateral femur prevented sliding and impaction of the femoral head which significantly reduced the resistance to load (Nakamura *et al.*, 1987).

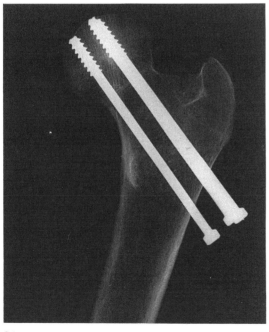

(b)

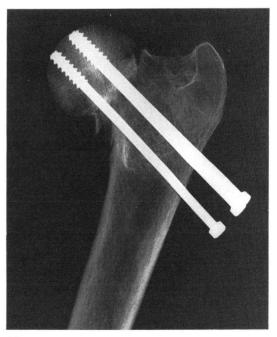

(c)

131

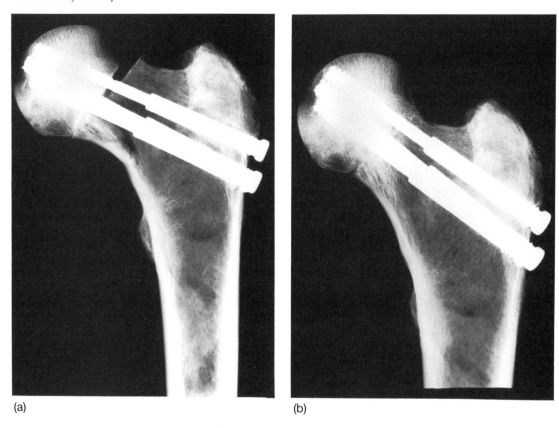

(a)　　　　　　　　　　　　　　　(b)

Figure 11.4　Another alternative for fixation of these fractures is variable length sliding screws (a), (Neustadt *et al*, 1989). Because of the extra support of the telescoping mechanism in the neck, bending was not observed and impaction was much easier to achieve with the initial reduction. Thus, the failure mode generally consisted of fracture of the medial cortex indicating good abutment on the medial side, consistent with the excellent resistance to load measured, (b).

not slide effectively (Figure 11.3). Thus, with multiple pin fixation there is need for some fixation very inferiorly in the neck which will have a corresponding fixation in the inferior portion of the head where trabecular bone is not optimum. Other pins can be placed into the centre of the femoral head and provide the best fixation of the proximal fragment and rotational stability, but those will be the pins which have minimal support throughout their shaft where they traverse the neck.

The quality of fixation in the head is more related to the points of fixation than it is to the type of thread or screw achieving the fixation. In Japan, a popular technique for fixation of subcapital fractures is to use multiple smooth Kirschner pins in a parallel array of 8 to 12 pins through the neck and into the femoral head. Another alternative for maintaining the ability to slide while achieving minimal support through the neck is to utilize a telescoping mechanism in the pin such as that available in the compression hip screw (Neustadt *et al.*, 1989) (Figure 11.4). Another advantage of the telescoping pin is that it is not necessary for the pins to back out

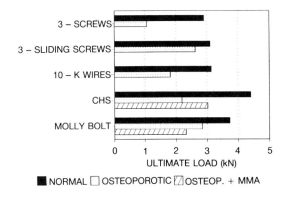

Figure 11.5 A comparison of five different methods of fixation of subcapital fractures demonstrates very little difference in the strength of fixation for any of the devices in normal bone, but major differences in the ability of each device to provide good resistance to loading in osteoporotic bone. Multiple sliding screw fixation was significantly stronger than other methods of multiple pin fixation in osteoporotic bone. In this particular study, the CHS fixation was significantly improved with the addition of methylmethacrylate in the head but there was no significant improvement in the molly bolt fixation with the addition of methylmethacrylate. In all instances, even when optimum fixation was achieved in osteoporotic bone, it was still significantly less than the strength of fixation in normal bone.

laterally in order for impaction of the fragments to occur. When well placed, these achieve comparable stability to the more common multiple pin fixation techniques with screw fixation in the head (Figure 11.5).

Single screw and side plate devices provided the advantage of a much larger diameter of rigid section transversing the unsupported part through the neck and the ability to achieve consistent central fixation of the femoral head where the best trabecular bone is located. The other potential advantage of these devices is the ease of utilizing supplementary methylmethacrylate fixation in the osteopenic areas of the head. Care

must be taken, however, not to allow cement to migrate into the neck and into the area of the fracture, where it may impede fracture healing (Enis, McCollough and Cooper 1974). One must also take care that no pins have penetrated the joint space as it may be possible for the cement to follow. There is clear advantage, however, to the strength of fixation which is achievable with augmentation by methylmethacrylate. Despite all of these 'tricks' for optimizing the strength of fixation in osteoporotic bone, one can never achieve the strength of normal bone fixation (Figure 11.5).

CLINICAL APPROACH

Intracapsular fractures of the hip differ considerably from other proximal femur injuries, even though the clinical symptoms have much in common. This section will deal primarily with fractures of the femoral neck with brief mention of other intracapsular injuries. The history of the treatment of femoral neck fractures parallels the development of orthopedic surgery. Speed, in 1935, referred to femoral neck fractures as 'the unsolved fracture'. This still remains, in many ways, true today.

Classification

Classification of intracapsular hip injuries consists of:

Non-traumatic fractures:
1. stress or fatigue fractures;
2. pathological fractures (tumors, primary or secondary);
3. post-irradiation fractures.

Traumatic fractures:
1. undisplaced femoral neck fractures;
2. impacted femoral neck fractures;
3. displaced and/or comminuted femoral neck fractures.

Complex traumatic intracapsular injuries:
1. dislocation of femoral head;
2. femoral head fractures (with or without posterior hip dislocation);
3. Combined femoral neck fracture and ipsilateral femoral shaft fractures (segmental fractures);
4. fractures of the acetabulum.

Numerous classifications of intracapsular fractures have been proposed throughout the years by Pauwels (1935), Garden (1971), Thompson and Epstein (1951), and the AO classification system (Muller *et al.*, 1991). Such classification systems are generally oriented toward the surgical treatment of fractures and are beneficial in choosing treatment methods and predicting prognosis, as well as outlining programs for surgical aftercare. Perhaps the most commonly used classification of displaced femoral neck fractures is as follows:

1. Subcapital fracture. Occurs immediately beneath the articular surface of the femoral head, along the old epiphyseal plate.
2. Transcervical fracture: The fracture passes across the femoral neck, between the femoral head and the trochanters.
3. Basal cervical fracture: The fracture occurs immediately above the intertrochanteric line at the base of the femoral neck.

In essence, however, many actual fractures do not fall into the above categories because of varying obliquity, comminution, and other geometric combinations which invariably exist.

I. Non-traumatic fractures of the femoral neck

This group of fractures is characterized by the lack of a single traumatic episode in the etiology of the fracture process. Stress fractures of the femoral neck tend to occur, for different reasons, in the young and the elderly. In young vigorous persons they occur with unaccustomed strenuous repetitive activity such as running or marching long distances. In the elderly, stress fractures tend to occur with metabolic disorders of bone. Pathologic fractures occur primarily with metastatic carcinoma and the neck of the femur is a common location. Primary tumors may also occur in the neck of the femur, however these are rare. The first symptoms of malignancy may be local pain, secondary to bone tumor in the hip, or a pathological fracture, secondary to metastatic invasion of the proximal femur. Post-irradiation fractures of the femoral neck were reported by Leabhart and Bonfiglio (1961) to occur in 1.5% of a series of patients who received pelvic radiation. They believed that irradiation affects the metabolism of the bone enough to weaken it and cause pathological fracture, but does not cause overt necrosis with the usual amounts of radiation used. Strangely enough, the post-irradiation fracture progresses slowly, preceded by a prodromal of pain with increasing limp and disability. Successive X-rays may demonstrate a line of increasing density in the femoral neck and coxa vara. Histologically, extensive marrow fibrosis and edema is found with a surprising lack of necrosis. Stephenson and Cohen (1956) noted that the fracture is preceded by the loss of trabecular bulk. Both the cellular elements of bony tissue and the fatty substance within the marrow were destroyed, but the blood supply was not diminished and loss of blood supply was not responsible for bony changes. They believed that the meagre blood supply of the femoral head may even be increased by radiation therapy.

II. Traumatic intracapsular fractures

Traumatic intracapsular fractures are characterized by varying degrees of displacement depending upon the force and type of injury and the strength of the bone, as observed by

Linton (1949, 1944). He believed that the mechanism of injury in femoral neck fractures is primarily external rotation of the femur. The femoral head is fixed in the acetabulum by the iliofemoral ligament anteriorly as the femoral neck rotates externally. The posterior cortex of the femoral neck comes into contact with the posterior acetabular rim, causing fracture and fragmentation of the posterior femoral neck as the rotational force is continued. Then impaction and fragmentation occurs and the femoral neck is driven into the femoral head usually with posterior angulation. In the case of undisplaced fractures, the alignment remains anatomical. With impacted fractures, the femoral neck is driven into the femoral head for varying distances, depending on the force applied and what strength the bone has to resist impaction of the fragments. Commonly, some posterior angulation exists with impacted fractures. It is thus important for the clinician to demand high quality radiographs of all intra-articular fractures, particularly the lateral acetabular view or lateral femoral neck view. Displaced fractures will usually have both angulation and impaction, often with the addition of significant comminution of the posterior cortex. The type and degree of severity of fracture has considerable importance in the surgical management of the fracture.

III. *Complex traumatic intracapsular injuries*

Dislocations of the femoral head are usually posterior. They may occur with or without a posterior acetabular fragment. Dislocation of the hip may also result in a fracture of part of the head of the femur, which is sheared off by the posterior lip of the acetabulum as the femoral head traverses posteriorly over it. The fragments may be small and of little clinical significance, or they may be quite large, necessitating treatment by surgical intervention.

Segmental femoral fractures or intracapsular fractures of the hip combined with ipsilateral femoral fractures are uncommon, but when present, must be correctly diagnosed and both problems treated simultaneously. Henry and Bayumi (1934) reported posterior dislocation of the hip complicated by fracture of the femoral neck or shaft. The incidence of dislocation of the femoral head with fracture of the ipsilateral femur is approximately 1:1 000 000. There is considerable swelling and distortion of the thigh which may mask the hip injury, causing untimely delays of treatment while the femoral fracture alone is treated, potentially resulting in disastrous consequences for the femoral head and sciatic nerve. This underlines the importance of obtaining adequate radiographs of the joints immediately proximal to and distal to all fractures.

History of the management of intracapsular fractures

Before successful surgical treatment of femoral neck fractures, the mortality rate was as high as 85%. These figures have been markedly reduced by internal fixation or prosthetic replacement which makes possible early mobilization. The earliest attempt at internal fixation of a fractured femoral neck was done by driving a metallic nail through the trochanter, across the neck fracture, and into the head of the femur, by Langenbeck and others, in 1878. The procedure of internal fixation was not widely used until perfected by Smith-Petersen, Case and Gordon (1931), however all of these procedures were done as open techniques. Closed reduction or 'blind nailing' was reported by Johansson (1932). Further refinements in the technique of closed reduction with internal fixation followed throughout the years with improvement in anesthetic techniques and the availability of image intensifiers. Results improved, but there were still many failures.

Another step forward in the treatment of intracapsular fractures occurred when Thompson in 1954, and Moore in 1957 devised a replacement arthroplasty for the femoral head to correct the complications of non-union and avascular necrosis. The development of the bipolar prosthesis by Bateman (1974) and cementing techniques for instantly stabilizing the prosthesis in the femoral shaft, further improved the outcome of surgical treatment. Another major advance was the introduction of structured, vigorous post-operative physical therapy and rehabilitation programmes, concentrating on early ambulation with emphasis on muscle strengthening, improved range of joint motion, and early return to activities.

The hip joint is a relatively spherical ball and socket joint which permits a wide range of motion. Its cylindrical capsule is attached proximally to the rim of the acetabulum and extends to attach to the base of the neck of the femur. Synovium lines the inner aspect of the capsule. Therefore, the entire head and a great deal of the neck of the femur is intracapsular. The thick ligamentum teres passes from a recess in the acetabulum to its point of attachment, the fovea centralis, which is in the centre of the femoral head. The ligament contains a small vessel which, it is generally agreed, furnishes a blood supply to only a small area of the femoral head immediately around its attachment, and cannot be depended upon for the healing of fractures of the femoral neck. The arterial supply to the head and neck of the femur is supplied entirely from the extracapsular arterial ring at the base of the femoral neck. This ring gives off branches which penetrate the base of the capsule, and proceed through the base of the neck, up the neck of the femur and into the head. The arterial supply to the neck, and particularly the head of the femur,

is tenuous and a fracture across the neck with any displacement will completely interrupt the blood supply to the femoral head. This is the cause of the frequently seen avascular necrosis phenomenon of the femoral head with transcervical fractures, particularly those which are displaced. Even if a displaced fracture is anatomically replaced, the blood supply to the femoral head and neck, having been completely interrupted at the moment of injury, must completely revascularize the femoral head and must do so before collapse of the femoral head occurs.

Treatment

The primary goal of treatment of any fracture of the hip is to restore painfree function to an injured patient. Mildly or moderately impacted fractures, undisplaced pathological fractures, undisplaced or minimally displaced post-irradiation fractures and stress or fatigue fractures can usually be treated by the technique of closed reduction and internal fixation. If severe damage has been suffered by the head or neck of the femur, the surgeon may elect to remove the head and part or all of the neck and replace it with a prosthesis, usually some form of hemiarthroplasty (Figure 11.6a and b). These two broad categories of surgical procedures available in the treatment of intracapsular fractures will be discussed next, followed by criteria for choosing which procedure would be preferable in specific circumstances.

Prior to surgery all patients should receive a full anesthetic work up. Multiple pathology is rife in the older population, and many of these patients are relatively high risk for anesthesia and surgery. Traditionally, patients presenting with hip fractures are put into skin traction whilst awaiting operation, as this is thought to provide pain relief, although recent work has cast doubt on its value (Anderson *et al.*, 1993).

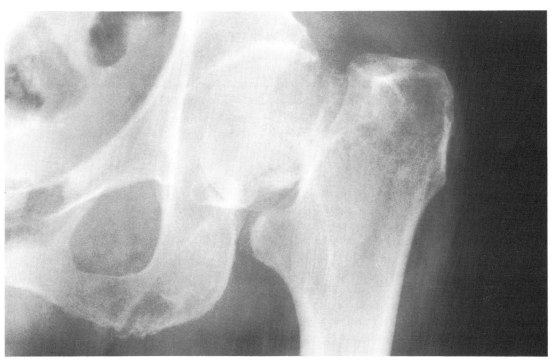

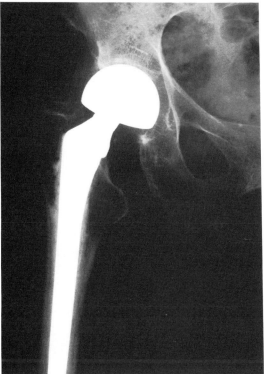

Figure 11.6 A displaced subcapital fracture of the neck of the femur. This has been managed using a bipolar hemiarthroplasty.

Reduction with internal fixation

Preference of surgical techniques and internal fixation devices vary from surgeon to surgeon. In general, the more quickly the procedure is performed, the better overall results can be expected. An adequate general anesthetic or spinal block is required. Spinal anesthesia is attended by less postoperative confusion in geriatric patients, and has other advantages with regard to blood loss and the risk of deep venous thrombosis. The operative fixation is performed on a fracture table which can apply a distracting, rotatory and sometimes flexion force to the involved lower extremity. A fracture table also permits the use of an image intensifier mounted on a C-arm to provide adequate anteroposterior and lateral fluoroscopy. The surgical approach is from the lateral aspect, extending from the greater trochanter, as far distally as necessary, to accommodate whichever internal fixation device is used. Incisions are kept as small as possible and the structures are incised longitudinally, to provide for easy repair after internal fixation is completed. With the use of cannulated screws, usually in undisplaced and minimally displaced fractures, it is often possible to insert the fixation percutaneously through stab incisions.

A variety of internal fixation devices is available and recent improvements have increased their effectiveness. The earliest hip nail only provided fixation across the fracture by securing the femoral head and neck to the remaining base of the neck and the lateral femoral cortex. It was later found that side plate attached to the transfixing nail gave added stability and resisted the varus deforming force. A telescoping capability built into the nail across the fracture site made possible impaction to promote healing. A tensioning screw in the centre of the telescoping device further guaranteed that impaction of the fracture fragments could be accomplished at the time of the surgery. Each

improvement in technique and internal fixation devices produced better clinical results. For a resumé of the various operative techniques the reader is referred to Ganz (1991). Probably the commonest technique for subcapital fracture fixation is the use of two, or preferably three, cannulated screws, placed over parallel guidewires in the femoral neck and head.

Prosthetic replacement of the femoral head

Many intracapsular fractures were not adequately treated by closed reduction and internal fixation. Fractures with marked displacement and considerable comminution frequently could not be reduced. Also, premorbid conditions such as severe osteoporosis, advanced degenerative joint disease, and factors preventing the patient from co-operating with controlled postoperative weight bearing all mitigate for replacing the femoral head and neck with a prosthesis. Opinions vary as to exactly which intracapsular fractures should be treated by internal fixation and which by replacement arthroplasty. In general, when a poor result from internal fixation seems likely, a replacement arthroplasty may be the procedure of choice. Factors favoring prosthetic replacement of the femoral head include the following:

- advanced physiological age;
- severe displacement or comminution of the fracture;
- severe osteoporosis of the femoral head and neck;
- patients who are not expected to resume weight-bearing status;
- fractures that cannot be satisfactorily reduced;
- pathological fractures with extensive tumor replacement of the head and neck;

- severe pre-existent degenerative arthritis of the hip joint;
- patients who are confused or for other reasons are unable to cooperate with a structured postoperative physiotherapy programme, requiring limited weight bearing;
- poor physical condition where there is an absolute contraindication to a second surgical procedure;
- patients in whom immediate full weight bearing is advisable to prevent complications;
- fractures of the femoral head itself, in which the fracture fragment is large or comminuted.

Other intracapsular injuries

Injuries of the hip joint, other than fractures of the femoral neck or head, require varying treatments. Dislocation of the hip must be reduced as quickly as possible to avoid complications, not only of the blood supply to the femoral head, but also to the sciatic nerve. If there is a posterior acetabular rim fracture, where the fragment is of sufficient size to cause the hip to be unstable, the rim fragment must be replaced by open reduction and internal fixation.

In the case of complex fractures involving both the femoral neck and the shaft of the femur, both must be corrected at the same time. A small fracture of the femoral head, if returned to its anatomical position by closed reduction, may heal without intervention. Large fragments may be excised, as long as they do not involve an extensive amount of the weight bearing surface of the femoral head, or internally fixed to the femoral head–neck fragment with small pins recessed beneath the joint surface. The incidence of aseptic necrosis and degenerative arthritis is high and replacement of the entire head and neck with a prosthesis may be preferable.

Surgical procedure of femoral head replacement

The surgical procedure followed for prosthetic replacement of the femoral head varies with the preference and experience of the surgeon. The approach may be anteriorly, posteriorly or laterally (Hastings, Sullivan and Colton, 1991). The operation requires a general anesthetic or, preferably, a spinal block. Antibiotics are given perioperatively, and after the procedure. The author's preferred approach is posterior, and will be outlined here. Those interested in the other approaches are referred to Hastings, Sullivan and Colton (1991). The skin incision is made from just distal to the palpable greater trochanter, coursing proximally and posteriorly along the line of the fibers of the gluteus maximus and in line with the femoral neck. If the incision is in line with the femoral shaft when the hip is flexed, it need not be more than 15–20 cm long. The gluteus maximus is split in its midportion, between the superior and inferior gluteal arteries, where it is least vascular. The hip is then flexed and internally rotated, and the short external rotators are released from their attachment to the posterior intertrochanteric ridge and peeled back off the hip capsule. At this point, the sciatic nerve is identified and demonstrated to the entire operating team to avoid injury. The capsule is opened and the fracture is explored. The femoral head is removed, along with the ligamentum teres, from the acetabulum. A template is used to cut the base of the femoral neck at the proper angle, approximately 1 cm above the lesser trochanter to fit the shoulder of the prosthesis. The acetabulum is inspected and, if not concentric, adequate reaming is done to produce the proper contour. Appropriate reaming and broaching of the femoral canal is done and trial sizings are used with various femoral stems, neck lengths, and prosthetic heads to obtain the ideal fit. Neck length is chosen so that excessive 'pistoning' of the prosthesis in the acetabulum with traction on the femur does not occur. The prosthesis neck length must permit some adduction to occur at the hip. Excessive abductor muscle tension will cause postoperative pain. If the capsule is markedly thickened and synovitis is present, the entire capsule is excised. If the acetabulum is between head sizes, it is advisable to use a smaller rather than a larger prosthesis or to lightly ream the acetabulum to an accurate fit. If a cemented femoral stem is to be used, then pressurized cement techniques are preferred. Some stems, such as the Austin Moore are specifically designed for cementless use. With the posterior approach, it is advisable to impart some anteversion in the placement of the femoral stem in the femoral shaft to avoid posterior dislocation. Above all, it is imperative to avoid retroversion which increases the likelihood of postoperative dislocation. When the surgeon is satisfied with the range of motion of the implanted prosthesis, replacement and repair of the anatomical structures and closure of the wound is carried out.

Surgical aftercare and rehabilitation

A triple assault has occurred on the elderly who have sustained intracapsular fractures, which have been surgically corrected. Firstly, a fall of sufficient severity to produce a major fracture has occurred. Secondly, the surgical procedure and anesthesia is a severe challenge to the body. Thirdly, pre-existing medical conditions frequently found in the elderly must be considered, such as impairment of the cardiovascular, pulmonary, and renal systems. Furthermore, additional factors which caused the fall may be present, such as an unrecognized stroke or fleeting cardiac dysrhythmias. A vigorous effort is necessary to make maximum use of all the faculties remaining in the geriatric patient. This requires a team approach of physicians,

nursing services, physical therapy, and social services.

Rehabilitation is begun the day following surgery, unless medical problems preclude doing so. Treatment must be individualized for each patient, making maximum use of his or her capabilities. In general, range of motion of all extremities, but most particularly the operated extremity, is emphasized actively and passively, twice daily. The patient is encouraged to perform exercises independently, as ability increases. Sitting in a chair, or rarely tilt-table exercises are begun the day following surgery, if possible, and gait training is begun soon after with adequate supervision and with whatever weight bearing is deemed advisable under the close supervision of a trained physical therapist.

Careful regular observation is needed in order to avoid medical problems which may decrease the patient's ability to recover. This includes wound inspection, observation for thrombophlebitis, pulmonary, cardiac, and skin complications and the use of anti-embolism stockings. Emphasis is placed on frequent movement, regular position changes, particularly those which can be instituted by the patients themselves. Small doses of anticoagulants or salicylates may be considered as well.

Hospitalization averages ten days in the United States. Further aspects of postoperative care and rehabilitation are discussed elsewhere in this book.

THE OUTCOME OF INTRACAPSULAR FRACTURES

The outcome is best assessed in two ways, which are to some extent interdependent. Firstly, the results of surgery in relation to the hip joint itself, and secondly, the overall mortality. Using current techniques with cannulated screw fixation, there appears to be virtually no problem with non-union in

Garden grades 1 and 2. Avascular necrosis, in the form of late segmental collapse of the femoral head, occurs in up to 15% of this group of patients, although most series suggest a much lower figure (Barnes *et al.*, 1976; Olerud, Rehnberg and Hellquist 1991). Only a small number of such cases are symptomatic enough to require further surgery. These are undisplaced or minimally displaced fractures with little risk to the blood supply of the femoral head, and one would consequently expect them to do well. The problems lie with the displaced fractures, grades 3 and 4. If they are treated by reduction and internal fixation then the rate of non-union, which usually requires further surgery, is reported as varying between 10 and 40%. Avascular necrosis occurs in 15 to 25% of cases, but generally no more than one-third of these actually require revision surgery (Bray and Templeton, 1993; Christie, Howie and Armour, 1988; Parker, 1992). One of the problems with the current literature is that there are few reports of the results of the most modern fixation techniques, and there is evidence that the use of parallel, as opposed to crossed screws, have significantly reduced the rates of both of these two major complications (Parker *et al.*, 1991). In the United States and Britain, the majority of grade 3 and 4 fractures are treated by hemiarthroplasty. The main disadvantage of this in terms of the hip function is acetabular erosion leading to pain. Unipolar prostheses, such as the Austin Moore and Thompson have a high incidence of this, and there appears to be a direct correlation between the degree of erosion and postoperative longevity and activity levels (Phillips, 1989). It has been proposed that bipolar hemiarthroplasties, in which the hip movement takes place at an inner ball and socket bearing, have a reduced risk of this complication, and medium term studies seem to bear this out (Lestrange, 1990; LaBelle, Colwill and Swanson, 1990). When one compares internal fixation with hemiarthroplasty for these displaced fractures, internal fixation is superior in terms of immediate postoperative complications, duration of stay and cost of primary treatment, but is associated with a three times increased risk of reoperation, mainly due to non-union (Parker, 1992). The issue is as yet unresolved.

There are many important factors influencing the final outcome after surgery. The overall six month mortality for subcapital fractures in a group of 158 patients was 17%. However, only about 10% of the patients who were operated on had died, whereas 60% of those treated conservatively had succumbed (Ions and Stevens, 1987). While this reflects in part the fact that those treated conservatively were unfit for surgery, there is a clear implication that operation and early mobilization will minimize the mortality. Using stringent multivariate analysis, the most significant predictors of mortality at six months were, in order, dementia, postoperative chest infection, malignancy, old age and deep wound infection (Wood *et al.*, 1992). The social and functional outcome of the survivors is most closely related to two factors: the pre-injury mental ability of the patient, and the presence of an integrated multidisciplinary rehabilitation program (Zuckerman *et al.*, 1992).

INTRACAPSULAR FRACTURES – CONCLUSION

Each improvement in anesthetic and surgical technique will hopefully produce a similar improvement in the outcome of intracapsular fractures. Further refinement of postoperative care will maximize the use of the available capabilities in the geriatric patient. Frequently, however, a fall with a resultant fracture is the first symptom of the downward spiral of general health that can only be partially abated by the best of medical care. Early surgical correction and stabilization of the intracapsular injury with early mobilization will minimize morbidity and mortality and maximize the quality and enjoyment of the remaining life of our elderly patients.

EXTRACAPSULAR HIP FRACTURES
By Sune Larsson

BIOMECHANICS
By Loren L. Latta

The most unstable hip fractures which are common in osteoporotic patients are the intertrochanteric fractures. Numerous categories of these fractures have been described in the literature and one clear separation between the groups seems possible by dividing them into the relatively stable versus relatively unstable fractures. The most common fractures by far are the unstable fractures which have three or more pieces with major comminution posteriorly and extensive initial displacement of the fracture fragments (Tronzo, 1984). These fractures are associated with more soft tissue damage and thus, less soft tissue support. It is often difficult or impossible to maintain medial cortical abutment which is critical in maintaining the position of the fragments and resistance to load bearing.

Many of the factors in achieving fixation in these fractures are very similar to the factors of the subcapital hip fracture fixation. The best trabecular bone in the proximal fragment is in the center of the head of the femur and there is minimal trabecular support through the neck of the femur. With intertrochanteric fractures, it is critical to provide plate fixation support to the distal fragment as well as the screw fixation in the head. Most investigators agree that anatomic reduction provides the best resistance to loading and the maintenance of mechanical support from abutment of the medial cortices (Apel *et al.*, 1989; Flores, Harrington and Heller, 1990; Tronzo, 1984; Kaufer, Matthews and Sonstegard, 1974). The compression hip screw (CHS) allows for

controlled impaction of the proximal and distal fragments which helps to achieve and maintain good resistance to loading (Doppelt, 1980; Tronzo, 1984). Because of the fixation strength in the osteoporotic femoral head, the proximal fragment will tend to rotate on the screw into varus under *in vitro* loading and loss of medial cortical abutment occurs at greater frequency than in fixation in normal bones of the same fracture pattern (Latta *et al.*; 1987). Therefore, one technique of supplementing this fixation to the head and helping to maintain resistance to varus angulation is to use methylmethacrylate at the head fixation point (Tronzo, 1983; Latta *et al.* 1987; Bartucci *et al.*, 1985; Harrington, 1975). This can be achieved with CHS or with molly bolt compression hip fixation systems. The result is essentially the same with either type of fixation in that the ability to maintain medial cortical abutment (prevent varus rotation at the head) is significantly improved with the use of supplemental cement fixation in the head.

As long as fixation can be achieved in the center of the femoral head, some advantage can be gained by using the higher nail-plate angle with the CHS to minimize the frictional resistance (Meislin *et al.*, 1990; Yoshimine, Milne and Latta, 1993a,b; Kyle, Wright and Burnstein, 1980). However, the mechanics of loading on the CHS are so variable that the parameters which affect the tendency of the device to slide are far less important than the parameters which affect fracture stability (Yoshimine, Milne and Latta, 1993 a,b). Both in laboratory and clinical evaluations of sliding, the unstable fracture patterns in osteoporotic bones with poor reductions slid the most (Figure 11.7a,b). Maintenance of medial cortical abutment is always associated with greater resistance to load bearing (Apel *et al.* 1989; Flores, Harrington and Heller, 1990; Kaufer *et al.*, 1974; Latta *et al.*, 1987).

Many other methods of achieving stable fixation have been utilized including the

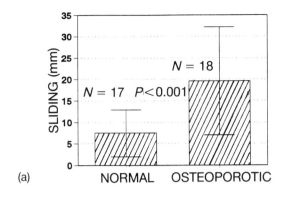

(a)

REDUCTION

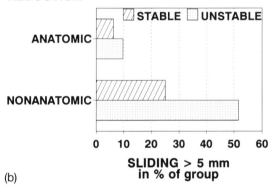

(b)

Figure 11.7 In a similar laboratory study of unstable intertrochanteric fractures comparing 135° to 150° CHS fixation, there was a significant difference in the length of sliding in the osteoporotic bone due primarily to the loss of medial cortical support, (a). In the majority of the osteoporotic bones tested telescoping was the mode of failure which provided a minimal resistance during sliding, which was significantly weaker than in normal bones. A follow-up of clinical cases utilizing the CHS device demonstrated no correlation in those parameters which affect tendency to slide (barrel engagement angle of screw, etc., Kyle, 1980), but significant correlation to the accuracy of the reduction, particularly in unstable fracture patterns, (b). (Yoshimine, 1993b).

valgus osteotomy which attempts to reduce the varus loading on the hip but primarily

provides an accurate, repeatable method of achieving medial cortical abutment (Sarmiento and Williams, 1970; Shannak, Maldawi and Hadidi, 1988). Each of these techniques takes advantage of the fact that it is possible to achieve reasonable fixation in the centre of the head of the proximal fragment and reasonable fixation on the lateral cortex in the distal fragment in order to control the interaction of bone fragments in between. It is those parts between that the surgeon has the least control over during the reduction and fixation process as well as during the impaction of early load bearing, postoperatively.

The most important mechanical goals to achieve are medial cortical abutment, and maintenance of that abutment with good fixation into the femoral head (supplemented by methylmethacrylate if necessary) to maintain controlled impaction on the medial cortex during early load bearing from early function activity. Note again that even if these can all be achieved in osteoporotic bone, the strength of fixation will not be as good as in normal bone. These factors should all be weighted when implementing post operative rehabilitation.

CLINICAL APPROACH

Classification

Extracapsular fractures are usually discussed as one entity although a trochanteric fracture to the surgeon can be anything from a very simple procedure to a highly complex operation. The number and location of fracture fragments, displacement, and bone quality will affect the possibility of obtaining a stable fracture reduction and also the risk of secondary fracture displacement. In order to identify and assess the risk of mechanical complications predictable from radiographs taken prior to surgery, a number of different classification systems have been developed.

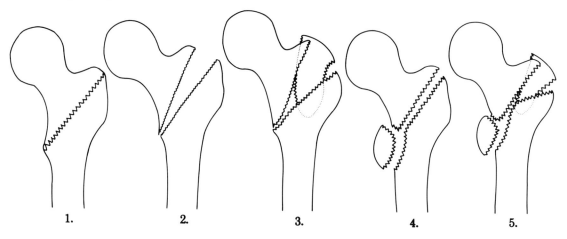

Figure 11.8 Schematic drawings of the Evans–Jensen classification of extracapsular hip fractures.

One most commonly used is the Evans (1949) classification or a modification of it (Jensen, 1980; Figure 11.8). With this classification the integrity of both the medial and posterior aspect of the trochanteric region are considered to determine fracture stability. A successful outcome is highly dependent on the restoration of the medial and posterolateral bone-to-bone support. Two-fragment fractures are defined as stable with type 1 being undisplaced and type 2 displaced. Types 3 and 4 consists of three fracture fragments with either a separate posterolateral fragment from the greater trochanter (type 3) or a medial fragment from the lesser trochanter (type 4). If there are four fragments or more the fracture is defined by a type 5 fracture. Types 3–5 are regarded as unstable due to potential difficulties in achieving a stable reduction and the increased risk of secondary fracture displacement when compared to two-fragment fractures. With this classification approximately two-thirds will be regarded as unstable, while one-third fall into either type 1 or type 2, that is stable fractures.

In Evans' original classification system fractures with a reversed fracture line, where the major fracture line runs through the trochanteric region from medioproximal to distolateral, were distinguished as a separate group due to the inherent instability even in two-fragment fractures of this variation. The instability is due to muscle forces acting to separate the fragments with abductors pulling on the proximal fragment while the adductors are acting on the distal fragment. When using the so-called sliding screw system (see below under Treatment) for internal fixation of such a fracture it is important to realize that this fixation device may not stabilize this fracture type. The basic principle with the sliding screw system is that the implant adjusts by telescoping of the lag screw within the barrel of the sideplate so that the fracture can impact until bone-to-bone contact is obtained. In reversed fractures no such fracture impaction is obtained, instead the device might act as a slide which points the proximal fragment to go laterally thereby causing secondary fracture displacement.

TREATMENT

As most of the patients are elderly with poor bone quality the demands on the operative technique and implant device are very high.

144

Until the late 1950s skeletal traction through the proximal tibia for 12–16 weeks still prevailed as a common treatment. In part, this conservative attitude was supported by the high frequency of technical complications seen in the early series treated surgically. Improvements in surgical techniques and implant design changed this conservative attitude so today surgical treatment with closed and/or open reduction, and internal fixation followed by early mobilization is considered as standard treatment.

Conservative treatment

Traction as the definitive treatment has been almost completely abandoned due to the high complication rate. The most serious complications are related to thromboembolism and superimposed infections causing high morbidity and mortality. These complications are due to the effects of the prolonged bed rest associated with traction in these elderly fragile patients. In very select cases, in whom surgical treatment for any reason is not possible, traction might still be considered an alternative. If the patient can tolerate the prolonged bed rest and general complications can be avoided, fracture healing in an acceptable position can usually be obtained as non-unions and other healing disturbances are uncommon in extracapsular hip fractures.

Surgical treatment

While indications for traction as final treatment are very limited, temporary traction from admission until surgery is very useful, especially if surgery is to be delayed for more than 12 hours, which often is necessary for optimizing the patient's general condition prior to surgery. Temporary skeletal traction of 4–6 kg through the proximal tibia usually affords substantial pain relief and less discomfort. If surgery will be delayed for several days it is sometimes beneficial to increase the

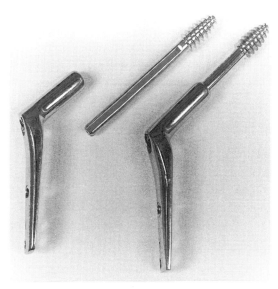

Figure 11.9 Sliding screw implant consists of two parts, a lag screw and a sideplate with a barrel.

load slightly, depending on the weight and muscle function of the patient, in order to avoid soft tissue contraction and fracture shortening especially in comminuted fractures.

A number of different implants have been designed for internal fixation of extracapsular hip fractures. In the early era of internal fixation combinations of a rigid nail and a sideplate as well as rigid one-piece nail-plates were used. These rigid systems were associated with high complication rates especially in unstable fractures, with implant breakage, varus angulation and nail penetration into the acetabular floor. By the introduction of a system that allowed controlled sliding between a screw and a sideplate a new mechanical principle for the treatment of trochanteric fractures was introduced. The sliding screw device is at present probably the most widely used implant for stabilization of extracapsular hip fractures (Figure 11.9).

Recently the conventional sliding screw devices have been challenged by new

145

systems that basically have adopted the sliding screw principle although the sideplate has been replaced by an intramedullary rod. The rod is inserted through the tip of the trochanter and passed down the upper shaft of the femur. A lag screw is introduced through the lateral aspect of the trochanter, passed through a hole in the rod and inserted with the screw tip ending in the femoral head. So far reported results with this type of system are few although theoretically it might be beneficial in certain fractures (Halder, 1992). For example, the so-called reversed trochanteric fracture type, according to Evans' classification system, will probably be better merged with this new type of device compared to the traditional sliding screw system because the intramedullary rod will counteract lateral sliding of the proximal fragment more efficiently (Figure 11.10). Another indication might be combined trochanteric and subtrochanteric spiral fractures. When using traditional sliding screw systems in these fractures the length of the fracture system makes it necessary to use long sideplates. However, fatigue breakage of the sideplate is a known complication due to the inherent fracture instability in combination with a tendency for delayed union. By using an intramedullary rod instead of a sideplate the moment arm acting on the device is reduced and furthermore the rod system will allow some fracture impaction which will further reduce the forces acting on the implant. However, further experience is necessary before these new devices adopting the intramedullary/lag screw principle can find a correct position among the different options available.

Surgical technique

Reduction

The patient is placed on a fracture table. Rotatory or biplane fluoroscopy is used for checking reduction as well as later during surgery to ensure correct positioning of the implant. The most common displacement is external rotation combined with shortening. Reduction can usually be obtained by first applying traction to the leg in the semi-abducted slightly flexed position. Once the shortening through the fracture has been reduced the leg can be internally rotated. Sometimes closed methods will not give an adequate reduced position of the fracture and reduction will then have to be completed by open means following incision. The desired fracture position is anatomical or slightly valgus with reinstitution of the medial bony support and complete reduction of the external rotation and shortening.

Although, as mentioned earlier, several implants have been developed for internal fixation of extracapsular fractures, in this text the sliding screw system will be presented in detail as it has become the most widely used and well documented system.

Internal fixation with the sliding screw system

Approach: Lateral incision through skin and fascia lata over proximal femur, after which the vastus lateralis muscle is elevated slightly anteriorly. This usually provides an adequate view of the lateral part of the proximal femur and the fracture area. By lifting the muscle instead of cutting directly through the muscle compartment the bleeding is greatly reduced.

Procedure: If open reduction is necessary, it can usually be achieved by clamping the fragments into the desired position or by using temporary cerclage wires. In cases where the lesser trochanter is avulsed as a separate fragment there is usually no need to restore its anatomical position if the size of the fragment is less than 4 cm (Figure 11.11). If larger it can usually best be reduced by external rotation of the leg, clamping it to the distal fragment after which it is fixed by a

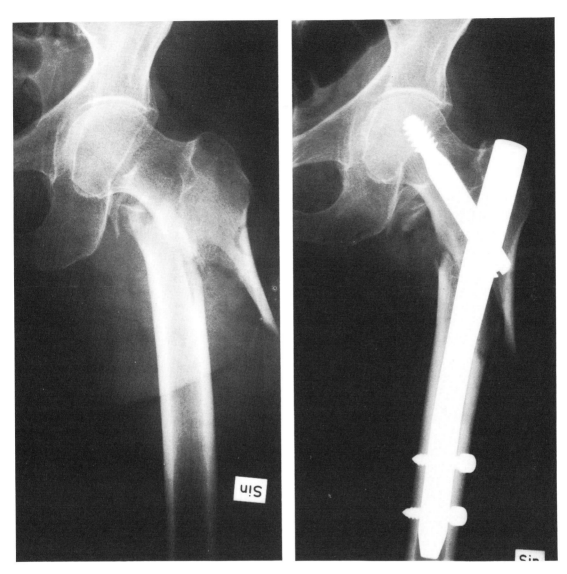

Figure 11.10 Extracapsular fracture with reversed fracture direction. Before surgery (a) and immediately after surgery (b) having been managed with an intramedullary nail incorporating a strong screw.

separate lag screw directed almost in the anterio-posterior direction.

The sliding screw system is produced by several different manufacturers marketing their product under different names although basically they all consists of two major parts,

a plate with a barrel and a screw that can slide within the barrel. The plate is usually available in different angles although in most cases a plate angle between 135 and 150 degrees is sufficient. A larger angle reduces the risk of the screw being jammed in the

147

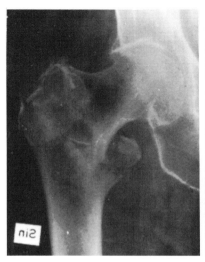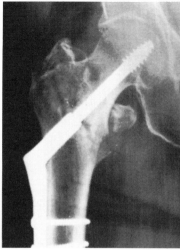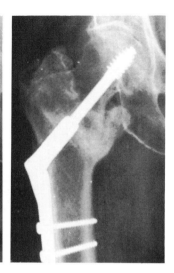

Figure 11.11 Extracapsular fracture type 5 according to the Evans–Jensen classification. Before surgery (left), immediately after stabilization with sliding screw implant (middle) and 3 months after surgery (right).

barrel although on the other hand a large angle increases the risk of cutting out through the superior part of the femoral head. The sliding screw should be placed within the central or inferior part of the femoral neck and head with the tip of the nail within 5–10 mm of the surface of the head. Superior and anterior positions of the screw should be avoided due to subsequent increased risk of cutting out through the femoral head.

The side plate is available in different lengths although in most trochanteric fractures four screws penetrating both lateral and medial cortices is sufficient to stabilize the side plate to the proximal femur (Larsson, Friberg and Hansson, 1990a). Some manufacturers use shorter distances between screw holes making it necessary to use plates with five or more screw holes in order to achieve a secure grip in the distal fragment.

Following surgery the fracture fragments will impact due to physiological loadings until bone-to-bone contact is obtained. The major part of the applied stress will be absorbed by the bone, while only a minor part of the stress will be taken by the implant. Because of the sliding effect of the implant the risk for the tip of the screw cutting out through the surface of the head is significantly reduced compared to when rigid nail/ plate systems are being used. Several sliding screw devices offer the possibility of applying fracture compression during surgery by means of a compression screw between the plate and the sliding screw. This compression can be hazardous especially in osteoporotic bone as too much compression will diminish the holding power of the lag screw within the femoral head and ultimately risk the lag screw being pulled out. After surgery early free weight-bearing can be encouraged provided that stable reduction and accurate implant position have been achieved.

COMPLICATIONS

General complications

Thromboembolic complications including deep vein thrombosis with the potential risk of pulmonary embolus, cerebrovascular accident, and myocardial infarction are the most serious. Together with infectious complications such as pneumonia and septicemia due to upper urinary tract infection, the morbidity and mortality following treatment of trochanteric fractures is considerable. By using prophylaxis with dextran or low-dose heparin the incidence of thromboembolic complications can be reduced, while prophylaxis with antibiotics instituted at the time of surgery and continued for twenty-four hours following the operation reduces the number of postoperative infectious complications substantially (Larsson, Friberg and Hansson, 1990b).

Local fracture complications

The stable fracture types seldom present any problems if the basic guidelines for reduction and internal fixation are followed. Unstable fractures on the other hand, and especially four-part fractures, are accompanied by mechanical complications much more frequently, making reoperation necessary in 4–10% within three months of the primary surgery. The incidence of reoperation is obviously not only dependent on the type of implant but also on the experience of the surgeon and the type of patient in terms of bone quality, weight etc. The secondary procedure is usually caused by technical complications from insertion of the implant or severe secondary fracture displacement. The most frequent complications are cutting out through the superior aspect of the femoral head, penetration of the surface of the femoral head by the screw at surgery or penetration into the acetabulum of the screw tip due to insufficient sliding. Bending or breakage of the implant, so commonly observed when using rigid devices, is a rare complication when using the sliding screw system. Non-unions are seen on 0.5–3%, usually due to inadequate sliding, thereby

counteracting fracture impaction. Most of these mechanical complications can be avoided by simply following the basic guidelines for the device used.

THE OUTCOME OF EXTRACAPSULAR FRACTURES

The overall mortality during the first year following the fracture event is 15–20% which is higher than in age-matched controls. Normal survival rates can be expected after 1–2 years. In a recent study of about 600 patients we found that of those admitted from their own home 60% could be discharged directly back home after on average 18 days in hospital while another 17% could return to their own home after some additional rehabilitation in a geriatric ward. One year following surgery 80% (360/446) of patients who were able to walk without support or with only one cane prior to surgery had regained the prefracture walking ability (Larsson, Friberg and Hansson, 1990b). The surgical procedure, including selection of proper implant, prophylaxis against infection and thromboembolic complications are important cornerstones in the treatment of patients with extracapsular fractures. Comparing the different devices available it seems that for the well documented implants the sliding screw technique today is the best answer for stabilization of trochanteric fractures. However, it must be remembered that the surgical procedure is just the beginning of a long and labour intensive rehabilitation program for the patient. The importance of a complete rehabilitation program, usually including expertise of several disciplines, including home-medical care after the primary rehabilitation, is crucial for a successful outcome when treating the growing number of patients who will sustain an extracapsular hip fracture.

REFERENCES

Adebajo, A.O., Cooper, C. and Evans, J.G. (1991) Fractures of the hip and distal forearm in West Africa and the United Kingdom. *Age Ageing*, **20**, 435–8.

Apel, D.M., Patwardham, A. Pinzur, M.S. and Dobozi, W.R. (1989) Axial loading studies of unstable intertrochanteric fractures of the femur. *Clin. Orthop.*, **246**, 156–64.

Anderson, G.H., Harper, W.M., Connolly, C.D. *et al.* (1993) Preoperative skin traction for fractures of the proximal femur. *J. Bone Joint Surg.*, **75B**, 794–6.

Barnes, R., Brown, J.T., Garden, R.S. and Nicoll, E.A. (1976) Subcapital fractures of the femur. A prospective review. *J. Bone Joint Surg.*, **58B**, 2–4.

Bartucci, E.J., Gonzalez, M.H., Cooperman, B.R. *et al.* (1985) The effect of adjunctive methylmethacrylate on failures and function in patients with intertrochanteric fractures and osteoporosis. *J. Bone Joint Surg.* **67A**, 1094.

Bateman, J.E. (1974) Single-assembly total hip prosthesis: preliminary report. *Orthop. Digest*, **2**, 15.

Behnamou, C.L., Chappard, D., Gauvain, J.B. *et al.* (1991) Hyperparathyroidism in proximal femur fractures: biological and histomorphometric study in 21 patients over 75 years old. *Clin. Rheumatol.*, **10**, 144–50.

Boerboom, F.T., de Groot, R.R., Ratymakers, J.A. and Duursma. (1991) The incidence of hip fractures in the Netherlands. *Neth. J. Med.*, **38**, 51–8.

Bray, T.J. and Templeman, D.C. (1993) Fractures of the femoral neck, in *Operative Orthopaedics*, 2nd edn (ed. M.W. Chapman), J.B. Lippincott Co., Philadelphia, pp. 583–94.

Buchner, D.M. and Larson, E.B. (1987) Falls and fractures in patients with Alzheimer-type dementia. *J.A.M.A.*, **257**, 1492–5.

Christie, J., Howie, C.R. and Armour, P.C. (1988) Fixation of displaced subcapital femoral fractures. Compression screw fixation versus double divergent pins. *J. Bone Joint Surg.*, **70B**, 199–201.

Compston, J.E., Vedi, S. and Croucher, P.I. (1991) Low prevalence of osteomalacia in elderly patients with hip fracture. *Age Ageing*, **20**, 132–4.

Cooper, C., Wickham, C., Lacey, R.F. and Barker, D.J. (1990) Water fluoride concentration and fracture of the proximal femur. *J. Epidemiol. Comm. Health*, **44**, 17–9.

Cooper, C., Wickham, C. and Walsh, K. (1991) Appendicular skeletal status and fracture in the elderly: 14-year prospective data. *Bone*, **12**, 361–4.

Crowell, R.R., Edwards, W.T and Hayes, W.C. (1985) Pullout strength of fixation devices in trabecular bone of the femoral head. *Trans. Orthop. Res. Soc.*, **10**, 189.

Cummings, S.R., Black, D.M., Nevitt, M.C. *et al.* (1990) Appendicular bone density and age predict hip fracture in women. The Study of Osteoporotic Fractures Research Group. *J.A.M.A.*, **263**, 665–8.

Della Torre, P., Petrini, P. and Mancini, G.B. (1991) The epidemiology of fractures of the proximal end of the femur. Change in the incidence among the population at risk in the city of Perugia, Italy between the periods 1975–77 and 1986–88. *Ital. Orthop. Traumatol.*, **17**, 555–62.

Deyerle, W.M. (1980) Impacted fixation over resilient multiple pins. *Clin. Orthop.*, **152**, 102–22.

Dias, J.J. (1987) An analysis of the nature of injury in fractures of the neck of the femur. *Age Ageing*, **16**, 373–7.

Diez, A., Puig, J., Martinez, M.T. *et al.* (1989) Epidemiology of fractures of the proximal femur associated with osteoporosis in Barcelona, Spain. *Calcif. Tissue Int.*, **44**, 382–6.

Doppelt, S.H. (1980) The sliding compression screw – today's best answer for stabilisation of intertrochanteric hip fractures. *Orth. Clin. N. Amer.*, **11**, 507–23.

Dretakis, E.K., Giaourakis, G. and Steriopololoulos, K. (1992) Increasing incidence of hip fracture in Crete. *Acta Orthop. Scand.*, **63**, 150–1.

Edwards, W.T., Lewallen, D.G. and Hayes, W.C. (1985) The effect of pin number and fracture pattern on immediate mechanical fixation of a subcapital hip fracture model. *Trans. Orthop. Res. Soc.*, **10**, 219.

Elmerson, S., Anderson, G.B.J., Pope, M.H. and Zetterberg C. (1987) Stability of fixation in femoral neck fractures. *Acta Orthop. Scand.*, **58**, 109–2.

Enis, J.E., McCollough, N.C. and Cooper, J.S.

(1974) Action of MMA on osteosynthesis. *Clin. Orthop.*, **105**, 283.

Evans, E.M. (1949) The treatment of trochanteric fractures of the femur. *J. Bone Joint Surg. (Br.)*, **31**, 190–203.

Eventov, I., Frisch, B., Alk, D. *et al.* (1989) Bone biopsies and serum vitamin D levels in patients with hip fractures. *Acta Orthop. Scand.*, **60**, 411–3.

Felson, D.T., Anderson, J.J., Hannan, M.T. *et al.* (1989) Impaired vision and hip fracture. The Framingham Study. *J. Am. Geriatr. Soc.*, **37**, 494–500.

Felson, D.T., Kiel, D.P., Anderson, J.J. and Kannel, W.B. (1988) Alcohol consumption and hip fractures: The Framingham Study. *Am. J. Epidemiol.*, **128**, 1102–10.

Felson, D.T., Sloutskis, D., Anderson, J.J. *et al.* (1991) Thiazide diuretics and the risk of hip fracture. Results from The Framingham Study. *J.A.M.A.*, **265**, 370–3.

Fisher, E.S., Baron, J.A., Malenka, D.J. *et al.* (1991) Hip fracture incidence and mortality in New England. *Epidemiol.* **2**, 116–22.

Flores, L.A., Harrington, I.J. and Heller, M. (1990) The stability of intertrochanteric fractures treated with a sliding screw-plate. *J. Bone Joint Surg.*, **72B**, 37–40.

Ganz, R. (1991) Proximal Femur, in *Manual of Internal Fixation* (eds M.E. Muller, M. Allgower, R. Schneider and H. Willenegger), 3rd. ed., Springer Verlag, pp. 522–7.

Garden, R.S. (1991) Malreduction in avascular and necrosis in subcapital fracture of the femur. *J. Bone Joint Surg*, **53b**, 183–97.

Gardsell, P., Johnell, O., Nillson, B.E. and Nillson, J.A. (1989) The predictive value of fracture disease and falling tendency for fragility fractures in women. *Calcif. Tissue Int.*, **45**, 327–30.

Grisso, J., Chiu, G.Y., Mainslin, G. *et al.* (1991) Risk factors for hip fractures in men: a preliminary study. *J. Bone Miner. Res.*, **6**, 865–8.

Grisso, J.A., Kelsey, J.L., Strom, B.L. *et al.* (1991) Risk factors for falls as a cause of hip fracture in women. The Northeast Hip Fracture Study Group. *N. Eng. J. Med*, **324**, 1326–31.

Halder, S.C. (1992) The gamma nail for peritrochanteric fractures. *J. Bone Joint Surg. (Br.)*, **74b**, 340–4.

Harrington, K.D. (1975) The use of methylmeth-acrylate as an adjunct in the internal fixation of unstable comminuted fractures in osteroporotic patients. *J. Bone Joint Surg.*, **57A**, 138.

Hastings, D.E., Sullivan, J.M. and Colton, C.L. (1991) The Hip, in *Atlas of Orthopaedic Surgical Approaches* (eds C.L. Colton and A.J. Hall), Butterworth-Heinemann, Oxford, pp. 1–23.

Henry, A.K. and Bayumi, M. (1934) Fracture of the femur with luxation of the ipsilateral hip. *Br. J. Surg.*, **22**, 204.

Ions, G.K., Stevens, J. (1981) Prediction of survival in patients with femoral neck fractures. *J. Bone Joint Surg.*, **69B**, 384–7.

Jacobsen, S.J., Goldberg, J., Miles, T.P., *et al.* (1990) Regional variation in the incidence of hip fracture. US white women aged 65 years and older. *J.A.M.A.*, **264**, 500–2.

Jacobsen, S.J., Goldberg, J., Miles, T.P. *et al.* (1991) Seasonal variation in the incidence of hip fracture among white persons aged 65 years and older in the United States, 1984–1987. *Am. J. Epidemiol.*, **133**, 996–1004.

Jensen, J.S. (1980) Classification of trochanteric fractures. *Acta Orthop. Scand.* **51**, 803–10.

Johansson, C., Mellstrom, D., Lerner, U. and Ostenberg, T. (1992) Coffee drinking: a minor risk factor for bone loss and fractures. *Age Ageing*, **21**; 20–6.

Johansson, S. (1932) Zur technic der osteosynthese der fraktur colli femoris. *Zentralbl. Chir.* **59**, 2019. (Also, *Acta Orthop. Scand*, **3**, 362, 1932.)

Kaufer, H., Matthews, L.S., Sontsegard, D. *et al.* (1974) Stable fixation of intertrochanteric fractures. *J. Bone Joint Surg.*, **56A**, 899.

Kiel, D.P., Felson, D.T., Anderson, J.J., *et al.* (1987) Hip fracture and the use of oestrogens in postmenopausal women. The Framingham Study. *N. Eng. J. Med*, **317**, 1169–74.

Kiel, D.P., Felson, D.R. Hannan, M.T., *et al.* (1990) Caffeine and the risk of hip fracture: the Framingham Study. *Am. J. Epidemiol*, **132**, 675–84.

Kyle, R.F., Wright, T.M. and Burnstein, A.H. (1980) Biomechanical analysis of the sliding characteristics of compression hip screw. *J. Bone Joint Surg.*, **62A**, 1308–14.

LaBelle, L.W., Colwill, J.C. and Swanson, A.B. (1990) Bateman bipolar hip arthroplasty for femoral neck fractures. A five to ten year follow up study. *Clin. Orthop.*, **251**, 20–25.

Langenbeck, B. (1878) Vorstellung eines falles von veraltaten querbuga der patella, durch analgung von silbernahten geheilt. *Verh. Deutsch. Ges. Chir Kongress VII*, **1**, 92.

Larsson, S., Eliasson, P. and Hansson, L.-I. (1989) Hip fractures in northern Sweden 1973–1984. A comparison of rural and urban populations. *Acta Orthop. Scand.*, **60**, 567–71.

Larsson, S., Friberg, S. and Hansson, L.-I. (1990a) Trochanteric fractures. Influence of reduction and implant position on impaction and complication rate. *Clin. Orthop.*, **259**, 130–9.

Larsson, S. Friberg, S. and Hansson, L.-I. (1990b) Trochanteric fractures. Mobility, complications and mortality in 607 cases treated with the sliding-screw technique. *Clin. Orthop.*, **260**, 232–41.

Latta, L.L., Tronzo, R.G., Amaya, W.P. and Milne, E.L. (1987) Comparative intertrochanteric fracture fixation in osteoporotic and normal femora. *Proc. Internat, Soc. Fracture Repair*, p. 53.

Lau, E., Donnan, S., Barker, D.J. and Cooper, C. (1989) Physical activity and calcium intake in fracture of the proximal femur in Hong Kong. *B.M.J.*, **296**, 1441–3.

La Vecchia, C., Negri, E., Levi, F. and Baron, J.A. (1991) Cigarette smoking, body mass and other risk factors for fractures of the hip in women. *Int. J. Epidemiol.*, **20**, 671–7.

Leabhart, J.W. and Bonfiglio, M. (1961) The treatment of irradiation fracture of the femoral neck. *J. Bone Joint Surg.*, **43A**, 1056–67.

Leung, P.C., Cheng, Y.H., Ho, Y.F. *et al.* (1988) Fractured proximal end of the femur in the elderly – a medico-social study. *Gerontol.*, **34**, 192–8.

Lestrange, N.R. (1990) Bipolar arthroplasty for 496 hip fractures. *Clin. Orthop.*, **251**, 7–19.

Linton, P. (1949) Types of displacement in fractures of the femoral neck and observations on impaction of fractures. *J. Bone Joint Surg.*, **31B**, 184–189.

Linton, P. (1944) Different types of intracapsular fractures of the femoral neck. *Acta. Chir. Scand. Suppl.*, **90**, 1–122.

Maggi, S., Kelsey, J.L., Litvak, J. and Heyse, S.P. (1991) Incidence of hip fractures in the elderly: a cross-national analysis. *Osteoporos. Int.*, **1**, 232–4.

Martin, A.D., Silverthorn, K.G., Houston, C.S. *et al.* (1992) The incidence of fracture of the proximal femur in two million Canadians from 1972 to 1984. Projections for Canada in the year 2006. *Clin. Orthop.*, **266**, 111–8.

Meislin, R.J., Zuckerman, J.D., Kummer, F.J., Frankel, V.H. (1990) A biomechanical analysis of the sliding hip screw. The question of plate angle. *J. Orthop. Trauma*, **4**, 130–6.

Milne, E.L., Latta, L.L., Kimmel, B. and Weiss, C. (1988) Pullout strength of sliding screws in normal and osteopenic femoral heads. *Comtemp. Orthop.*, **17**, 79.

Müller, M.E., Allgöwer, M., Schneider, R. and Willenegger, H. (1991) *Manual of internal fixation*, ed 3, Springer-Verlag, Berlin.

Moore, A.T. (1985) The self-locking metal hip prosthesis. *J. Bone Joint Surg.*, **39A**, 811.

Nakamura, K., Tronzo, R., Wittles, M. *et al.* (1987) Comparative sub-capital fracture fixation in osteoporotic and normal femora. *Orthop. Trans.*, **11**, 117.

Neustadt, J.B., Tronzo, R., Hozack, W.J. and Latta, L.L. (1989) Femoral neck fractures: a biomechanical study of a new form of internal fixation using multiple telescoping variable length compression screws. *Clin. Orthop.*, **248**, 181.

Nicolayesen, J. (1987) Lidt om diagnosen og behandlingen av Fr. colli femoris. *Nord. Med. Arkiv.*, **8**, 1.

Nieves, J.W., Grisso, J.A. and Kelsey, J.L. (1992) A case-control study of hip fracture: evaluation of selected dietary variables and teenage physical activity. *Osteoporos. Int.*, **2**, 122–7.

Nilsson, R., Lofman, O., Berglund, K. *et al.* (1991) Increased hip-fracture incidence in the county of Ostergotland, Sweden, 1940–1986, with forecasts up to the year 2000: an epidemiological study. *Int. J. Epidemiol.* **20**, 1018–24.

Nydegger, V., Rizzoli, R., Rapin, C.H. *et al.* (1991) Epidemiology of fractures of the proximal femur in Geneva: incidence, clinical and social aspects. *Osteoporos. Int.*, **2**, 42–7.

Olerud, C., Rehnberg, L. and Hellquist, E. (1991) Internal fixation of femoral neck fractures. Two methods compared. *J. Bone Joint Surg.*, **73B**, 16–19.

Owens, W.D., Felts, J.A. and Spitznagel, E.L. (1978) A.S.A. physical status classifications:

A study of consistency of ratings. *Anaesthesiol.*, **49**, 239–43.

Parker, M.J. (1992) Internal fixation or arthroplasty for displaced subcapital fractures in the elderly? *Injury*, **23**, 521–4.

Parker, M.J., Porter, K.M., Eastwood, D.M. *et al.* (1991) Intracapsular fractures of the neck of the femur. Parallel or crossed Garden screws? *J. Bone Joint Surg.*, **73B**, 826–827.

Pauwels, F. (1935) Der schenkenhalsbrock, ein mechaniches problem grundlagen des heilungsvorganges pognose und kausale therapie Stuttgart, Beilageheft zur Zettschrift Fur Orthopaedische Chrirgie, Ferdinand Enke.

Phillips, T.W. (1989) Thompson hemiarthroplasty and acetabular erosion. *J. Bone Joint Surg.*, **71A**, 913–17.

Ray, W.A., Griffin, M.R. and Downey, W. (1989) Long-term use of thiazide diuretics and risk of hip fractures. *Lancet*, **1**, 687–90.

Ray, W.A., Griffin, M.R. and Malcolm, E. (1991) Cyclic antidepressants and the risk of hip fracture. *Arch. Intern. Med.*, **151**, 754–6.

Riggs, B.L. and Melton, L.J. (1986) Involutional osteoporosis. *N. Eng. J. Med.*, **314**, 1676–86.

Ross, P.D., Norimatsu, H., Davis, J.Y., *et al.* (1991) A comparison of hip fracture incidence among native Japanese Americans and American Caucasians. *Am. J. Epidemiol.*, **133**, 801–9.

Sarmiento, A. and Williams, E.M. (1970) The unstable intertrochanteric fracture: treatment with a valgus osteotomy and I-beam nail-plate. A preliminary report of one-hundred cases. *J. Bone Joint Surg.*, **52A**, 1309–18.

Shannak, A.O., Maldawi, H.D. and Hadidi, S.T. (1988) The Debrunner–Cech valgus osteotomy in osteoporotic four-part intertrochanteric fractures. *Internat. Orthop.*, **12**, 143.

Shorr, R.I., Griffin, M.R., Daugherty, J.R. and Ray, W.A. (1992) Opioid analgesics and the risk of hip fracture in the elderly: codeine and propoxyphene. *J. Gerontol.*, **47**, M111–5.

Silverman, S.L. and Madison, R.E. (1988) Decreased incidence of hip fracture in Hispanics, Asians and blacks: California Hospital Discharge Data. *Am. J. Public Health*, **78**, 1482–3.

Simoneon, O. (1991) Incidence of femoral neck fractures: senile osteoporosis in Finland in the years 1970–85. *Calcif. Tissue Int.*, **49**, Suppl: S8–10.

Smith, N.D., Cody, D.D., Goldstein, S.A. *et al.* (1992) Proximal femoral bone density and its correlation to fracture load and hip-screw penetration. *Clin. Orthop.*, **283**, 244.

Smith-Peterson, M.N., Case, E.F., Gorder, G.W. (1931) Intracapsular fractures of the neck of the femur, treatment by internal fixation. *Arch. Surg.*, **23**, 715

Sowers, M.F., Clark, M.K., Jannausch, M.L. and Wallace, R.B. (1991) A prospective study of bone mineral content and fracture in communities with differential fluoride exposure. *Am. J. Epidemiol.*, **133**, 649–60.

Sowers, M.F., Wallace, R.B. and Lemke, J.H. (1986) The relationship of bone mass and fracture history to fluoride and calcium intake: a study of three communities. *Am. J. Clin. Nutr.*, **44**, 89–98.

Spector, T.D., Cooper, C. and Lewis, A.F. Trends in admissions for hip fracture in England and Wales, 1968–85. *BMJ*, **300**, 1173–4.

Speed, K. The unsolved fracture. *Surg. Gynaecol. Obste.*, **60**, 341–51, 1935.

Stanley, H.L., Schmitt, B.P., Poses, R.M. and Deiss, W.P. (1991) Does hypogonadism contribute to the occurrence of a minor trauma hip fracture in elderly men? *J. Am. Geriatr. Soc.*, **39**, 766–71.

Stephenson, W.H. and Cohen, B. (1956) Post-irradiation fractures of the neck of the femur. *J. Bone Joint Surg.*, **38B**, 830.

Stromqvist, B., Hansson, L.I., Nilsson, L. and Thorngren, K.-G. (1987) Hook-pin fixation in femoral neck fractures. *Clin. Orthop.*, **218**, 58–62.

Swiontkowski, M.F., Harrington, R.M., Keller, T.S. and Van Patten P.K. (1987) Torsion and bending analysis of internal fixation techniques for femoral neck fractures: the role of implant design and bone density. *J. Orthop. Res.*, **5**, 433–44.

Thompson, F.R. (1954) Two-and-one-half years experience with a vitallium intramedullary hip prosthesis. *J. Bone Joint Surg*, **36A**, 489–500.

Thompson, V.P. and Epstein, H.C. (1951) Traumatic dislocation of the hip: a survey of 204 cases covering a period of twenty-one years. *J. Bone Joint Surg.*, **33A**, 746–78.

Tronzo, R.G. (1983) Augment internal fixation

with fenestrated hip screw and cement. *Orthop. Review*, **12**, 59–64.

Tronzo, R.G. (1984) Fractures of the hip in adults, in *Surgery of the Hip Joint*, 2nd edn (ed. R.G. Tronzo), Springer-Verlag, New York, 264–311.

Van Audekercke, R., Martens, M., Mulier, J.C. and Stuyck, J. (1979) Experimental study on internal fixation of femoral neck fractures. *Clin. Orthop. Rel. Res.*, **141**, 203–12.

Van Hemert, A.M., Vandenbroucke, J.P., Birkenhager, J.C. and Valkenburg, H.A. (1990) Prediction of osteoporotic fractures in the general population by a fracture risk score. A 9-year follow-up among middle-aged women. *Am. J. Epidemiol.*, **132**, 123–35.

Westcott, H.H. (1932) Preliminary report of a method of internal fixation of transcervical fractures of the neck of the femur in the aged. *Va. Med.*, **59**, 197.

White, B.L., Fisher, W.D. and Laurin, C.A. (1987) Rate of mortality for elderly patients after fracture of the hip in the 1980s. *J. Bone Joint Surg.*, **69A**, 1335–40.

White, H.C. (1988) Post-shock hip fractures. *Arch. Orthop. Trauma Surg.*, **107**, 345–7.

Wickham, C.A., Walsh, K., Cooper, C. *et al.* (1989) Dietary calcium, physical activity and risk of hip fracture: a prospective study. *B.M.J.*, **299**, 889–92.

Wilton, T.J., Hosking, D.J., Pawley, E. *et al.* (1987) Osteomalacia and femoral neck fractures in the elderly patient. *J. Bone Joint Surg. (Br.)*, **69**, 388–90.

Wood, D.J., Ions, G.K., Quinby, J. *et al.* (1992) Factors which influence mortality after subcapital hip fracture. *J. Bone Joint Surg.* **74B**, 199–202.

Yoshimine, F., Milne, E.L. and Latta, L.L. (1993a) Sliding characteristics of compression hip screw in the intertrochanteric fracture: A laboratory study. *J. Orthop Trauma* (in press).

Yoshimine, F., Milne, E.L. and Latta, L.L. (1993b) Sliding characteristics of compression hip screw in the intertrochanteric fracture: A clinical study. *J. Orthop. Trauma* (in press).

Zuckerman, J.D., Sakales, S.R., Fabian, D.R. and Frankel, V.H. (1992) Hip fractures in geriatric patients. Results of an interdisciplinary hospital care program. *Clin. Orthop.*, **274**, 213–225.

12

Fractures around the knee in elderly people

RAYMOND ROSS, WILLIAM MACLENNAN and
LOREN LATTA

GENERAL CONSIDERATIONS

The ideal goal of fracture management, despite age, is restoration of normal function (Scalea *et al.*, 1990; van Aalst *et al.*, 1991). Consider pre-injury function before embarking on heroic measures with unrealistic functional aims, particularly as surgery may carry significantly higher risks. We base management of fractures around the hip on the knowledge that non-operative treatment may result in high rates of non-union, and that prolonged bed rest has high attendant risks. The same philosophy applies around the knee but aggressive operative management may not have the same happy outcomes as in the hip, or as in much younger patients with healthy skin and adequate circulation.

EPIDEMIOLOGY
By W.J. MacLennan

Fractures of the shaft of the femur are even less common than those involving the upper end of the humerus (Bengner, Johnell and Redlund-Johnell, 1990). In women, there is an increase in incidence after the age of 60 years, whereas in men there is only a marginal increase with age. Supracondylar fractures are particularly rare, but there is a modest increase in their incidence in both men and women. The numbers of these fractures are so small that it is difficult to be certain that there has been a change in their pattern over time. There is limited evidence, however, that fractures of the shaft of the femur have become more common in elderly women, and that an age trend associated with supracondylar fractures has become apparent over the last thirty years.

The increasing prevalence of fractures of the shaft and supracondylar femur in elderly women over the last thirty years suggests that, whereas these fractures previously were almost entirely the result of severe trauma, an increasing proportion now are the result of bone rarefaction associated with aging (Benger, Johnell and Redlund-Johnell, 1990).

The age-specific incidence of fractures of the shaft of the tibia in women remains steady at between 1 to 4 per 10 000 throughout adult life (Bengner, Johnell and Redlund-Johnell, 1990). In men, it declines from around 5 per 10 000 in the twenties to around 2 per 10 000 over the age of 70 years. There

Skeletal Trauma in Old Age
Published in 1994 by Chapman & Hall, London
ISBN 0 412 48750 0

has been little change in its incidence or age distribution over the last thirty years.

BIOMECHANICS
By Loren L. Latta

The most common distal femoral fracture in osteoporotic bone results from very low energy trauma, is extra-articular and involves the distal junction of the diaphysis and metaphysis (Hubbart, 1974; Hutson and Zych, 1993). Although these fractures will heal adequately in traction, early function can be achieved with functional bracing for distal diaphyseal fractures because they can be adequately stabilized with soft tissue compression (Brown and Preston, 1975; Connolly, Dehne and La Follette, 1978; Daniel and Rice 1979; Hardy, 1983; Mooney *et al.,* 1970; Neufeld, 1972; Wardlaw *et al.,* 1981; Wardlaw, Scott and McLaughlan, 1984) (Figure 12.1).

The stability which can be achieved with plate and screw fixation (particularly the blade-plate or plate with cancellous lag screws) is adequate for early mobilization and early return to function. However, the amount of soft tissue stripping and severity of the surgical procedure coupled with the poor mechanics of the bone, makes this procedure potentially very risky for this group of patients. Also, these screw-plate combination devices generally are applied to the lateral side of the femur requiring that the cancellous fixation be achieved on the medial column of trabeculae of the distal femur. However, it is the medial column of trabeculae which is the first to weaken and disappear in the development of osteoporosis. Thus, the fixation of the distal fragment is precarious by this method (Giles *et al.,* 1982; Thomas and Meggit, 1981; Hubbart, 1974; Hutson and Zych, 1993). Methylmethacrylate augmentation to this fixation of the cancellous bone has been successful (Struhl *et al.,*

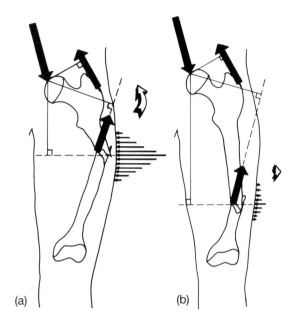

(a) (b)

Figure 12.1 With closed functional treatment of femoral fractures, there is a significant improvement in stability provided by external support through soft tissue compression in fractures which are located in the distal half of the femur, compared to the proximal half. Because of the strong varus angulatory moments in the proximal femur, (a), the leverage that a fracture brace or cast can provide through the soft tissue is very poor and because of the bulk of soft tissue in the proximal thigh it is very difficult to prevent varus angulation. However, the distal thigh is much leaner and the added leverage of the long proximal fragment allows for much smaller pressures in the soft tissue to provide comfortable resistance to varus angulation of the proximal fragment, (b). This is probably why patients treated in fracture braces with distal femoral fractures begin weight bearing earlier (Wardlaw *et al.,* 1981) and angulate less (Sarmiento and Latta, 1981) than proximal fractures.

1990), but still requires an extensive surgical procedure.

With the advent of closed, locked intramedullary nailing of the femur another alternative is available for this group of patients.

This method seems promising because it provides the possibility of minimal surgical risk and the necessary stability for early functional return. Two types of locking intramedullary fixation devices are generally available for fixation of distal fractures: ones with cortical fixation and others with cancellous fixation. Due to the markedly decreased strength of the cancellous bone in these osteoporotic patients, the consistency as well as the mechanical strength of fixation which can be achieved with transcortical locking mechanisms is far superior to cancellous locking mechanisms (Latta *et al.*, 1988). Cancellous fixation can be improved with adjunctive MMA and intramedullary fixation devices also (Stubbs *et al.*, 1975), but is probably not as practical as cortical locking. Although transcortical locking is more difficult, it is certainly far less risky in terms of the biological insult than open reduction and internal fixation.

All these factors should be weighed when choosing the best potential compromise between mechanical strength of fixation and biologic morbidity, and the extent and timing of postoperative rehabilitation.

Another common type of fracture in osteopenic bone is the tibial plateau or proximal tibial fracture (Foltin, 1988). In the elderly, these fractures are generally closed, low-energy injuries, with minimal soft tissue damage, but are often intraarticular. Fractures of the proximal tibia in normal bone tend to involve larger fragments of the proximal tibia and are often extra-articular. With greater degrees of osteoporosis, the fragments of the plateau tend to be narrower and shorter reflecting the minimal amount of load causing the fracture and the lack of shear resistance in the osteoporotic metaphyseal bone (Foltin, 1988).

Incongruity of the joint is critical to the long-term functional result. However, even though most of these fractures are intra-articular, they lend themselves well to a closed functional treatment which can provide for early functional activity before the fracture has united, because the soft tissue damage is usually minimal and they are relatively stable fractures (Apley, 1956, 1979; Beard *et al.*, 1985; Brown and Sprague, 1976; Delamarter and Hohl, 1989; Sarmiento Kinman and Latta, 1979). Isolated fractures of the lateral plateau have the benefit of some support from the fibula and generally tend to be stable enough to maintain adequate position with early weight bearing in a functional brace that has medial and lateral supports across the knee (Sarmiento, Kiman and Latta, 1979). The medial and lateral supports in the functional brace provide the adequate resistance to varus and valgus moments similar to the long leg cast, but allow the benefit of early flexion and extension of the knee (Sarmiento and Latta, 1981; Daniel and Rice, 1979). Bicondylar fractures of the proximal tibia with an associated fracture of the fibula are far less stable than the isolated condylar fracture. However, because of the lack of support from the fibula and the control of varus–valgus angulation by either a long leg cast or a functional brace, they do allow for controlled collapse and impaction of the fragments, with spread of the condyles, but minimal varus–valgus angulation. When early motion can be introduced in these fractures, minor incongruities will often correct themselves with early functional activity. Also, with early motion and functional activity such incongruities are well tolerated and compatible with good functional results. (This is contrary to similar degrees of incongruity in a joint which has been immobilized.) Patients that have been immobilized will usually be symptomatic in the end result (Sarmiento and Latta, 1981; Apley, 1979).

OVERVIEW OF MANAGEMENT STRATEGIES

These are broadly non-operative and operative.

NON-OPERATIVE

The elderly do not tolerate traction well, other than as a temporary measure for early stabilization. Atrophic skin breaks down rapidly if shearing forces are applied through adhesive tapes used for applying traction forces. Pins placed through the bone, to apply skeletal traction, rapidly loosen in osteoporotic bone and infection around such pins inevitably ensues. Pins that have a central thread, such as the Denham may appear to gain better purchase on the cortex but they will ultimately fail through loosening. Low friction couplings, which allow the connecting stirrup to rotate freely while the pin remains virtually static will reduce this problem significantly, as will the use of two parallel adjacent pins to disperse the traction forces in the tibia more evenly. Nevertheless, in carefully selected cases of distal femoral shaft fractures or upper tibial fractures this may be a perfectly satisfactory method of treatment. Early motion of the knee joint can be achieved. Perkins devised a bed which could be split (Figure 12.2). This allows the

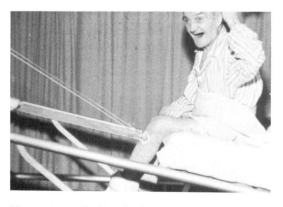

Figure 12.2 Perkins bed.

patient to begin knee flexion while still on traction. The concept of continuous passive motion was not quite achieved but the idea was clearly thought of many years ago. This method was practiced at the Rowley Bristow Hospital by Perkins' successor, Mr. Alan Apley.

Functional bracing (Figure 12.3) has a definite part to play in these fractures. Most modern units construct functional braces from lightweight materials. The short, stumpy, fat lower limb is, however, ill-suited to this technique. The short tubes of material cannot exert anti-buckling forces like longer tubes, and the fat makes close fitting a problem. Excoriation by the brace is avoided by meticulous care of the skin, which is straightforward in younger people but unless there is good social backup from relatives or social services this may prove a problem and contraindication in the elderly. Fiberglass materials are lightweight but extreme care should be taken when using them in this situation. Pay meticulous attention to the edges of this type of casting, where underlying skin necrosis can occur very rapidly. The author has gone back to using thin plaster of Paris cylinders as initial management before bracing, since fewer skin problems occur. A well-padded plaster of Paris cylinder may provide early support that is kind to the skin, whereas fiberglass materials, though light, have to be used with utmost care if skin problems are to be avoided.

OPERATIVE

Onlay devices such as plates with screws tend to fail at the device/bone interface (Figures 12.4, 12.5). This is simply bone failure in another form, but the extra stripping of what may already be a precarious blood supply also contributes to failure. Whether devices like the limited contact dynamic compression plate, developed by the AO group, will help in this respect

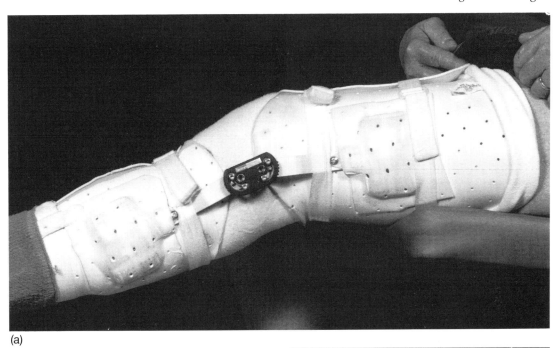

(a)

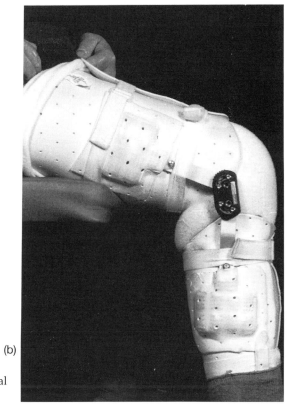

(b)

Figure 12.3 Functional bracing of a distal femoral fracture.

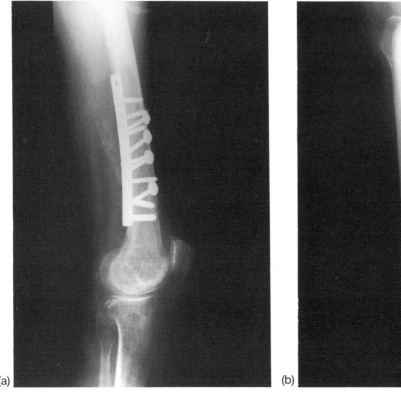
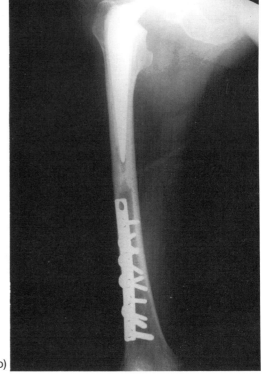

(a)   (b)

Figure 12.4 A femoral fracture below a hip replacment treated by plating and lag screw fixation. This technique has a high risk of failure in the elderly.

remains to be seen. As outlined above, there are advocates of the addition of methylmethacrylate cement in fractures in osteoporotic bones as a means of gaining better screw purchase. In the author's experience this is probably best reserved for fractures secondary to tumor infiltration. While fractures in osteoporotic bone are also pathological, the lifespan of the individual with this type of fracture may be very different to that of the patient with secondary tumor. Failure of healing of a fracture where bone cement has been used may leave a bigger problem to solve. Intramedullary devices are undoubtedly useful but very wide canals make locked or stacked nails essential (Moran, Gibson and

Cross, 1990). A closed technique makes for low infection rates. Very low supracondylar fractures can sometimes be nailed, but modification of certain intramedullary devices may be necessary, usually by removing the distal tip so that the locking screws can have an adequate purchase.

LOWER FEMUR

CLASSIFICATION

The system proposed by the AO group should be adopted (Figure 12.6). The three broad groups are extra-articular, partial-

160

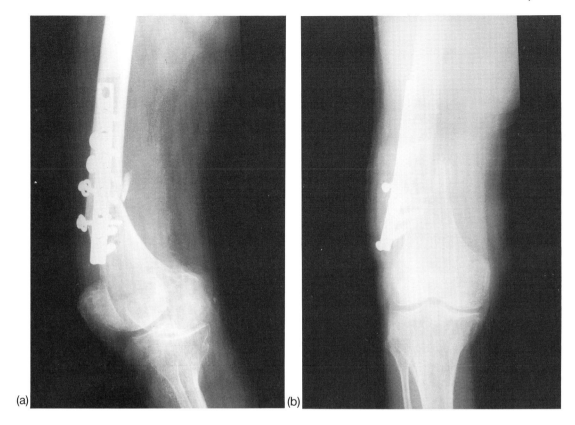

(a)　　　　　　　　　　　　　　(b)

Figure 12.5 The plate and screw fixation have failed. This is a predictable complication.

articular and intra-articular fractures (Muller *et al.*, 1990).

Extra-articular

These may be managed non-operatively. This is not an easy route for the surgeon and requires a lot of attention to care of traction pins and the position of the fracture, as well as the intensive nursing care that a bedbound elderly person must have.

The gastrocnemius muscle crosses the knee and ankle joints, with a flexing action on the knee joint. A supracondylar fracture has a short distal fragment with the gastrocnemius attached. This will produce flexion of the fragment and difficulty in control, unless traction with the knee in 90 degrees of flexion is used. This is not an easy method in this age group, although union is not usually a problem. Conversion to a functional brace by as early as four weeks is the aim.

The trumpet shape of the distal femur makes intra-medullary nailing of these fractures difficult. Locking nails may be adapted as described previously. In general, other devices are better at this level. The AO angle blade plate will stabilize these fractures well, but is technically a difficult device to use, particularly if the surgeon is not using it regularly as part of his armamentarium. The dynamic condylar screw is undoubtedly easier to use. Some degree of latitude is built in as far as placing the plate up the lateral

161

FEMUR DISTAL

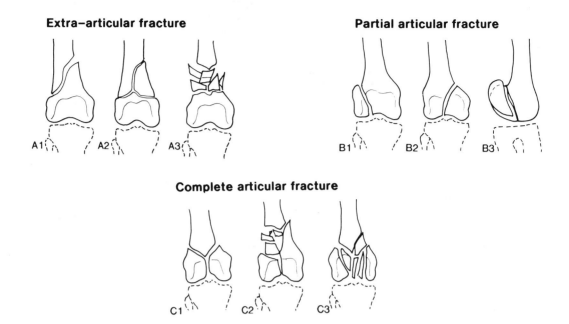

Figure 12.6 Classification of lower femur fractures – system proposed by the AO group.

aspect of the femur, unlike the blade plate, where, once the blade is inserted the position of the plate is decided. If that is incorrect then displacement of the fracture will occur as the plate is forced into alignment with the shaft, or the blade has to be resited – a difficult task! If the condyles are split the condylar screw allows easier insertion of the cross member. Note that rotational problems around the screw can occur. Other devices such as the supracondylar Zickel device or simple Rush rods have advocates. Perhaps this serves to indicate that no device is universally successful in this group. The ideal implant would provide fracture stability, with early knee motion and patient mobility with full weight bearing. So far such a device has eluded production.

Where medial comminution of the shaft is present Mast has described indirect reduction techniques that reduce periosteal stripping (Mast, Jakob and Ganz, 1989). It is essential to avoid wide stripping of the periosteum in bone with an already poor or compromised blood supply. Bone grafting in this group can be a problem since marrow cavities frequently widen and fill with fatty tissue. Poor cancellous bone harvests are therefore likely. There may be an increasing role for bone substitutes in this age group.

Partial-articular fractures

These are only a problem from the point of gaining purchase on bone. Where possible closed reduction and percutaneous screwing are advised. Cannulated screws are valuable in this situation. Screws alone should be supplemented with functional braces postoperatively to permit weight bearing. The elderly cannot be expected to partially weight bear to protect a fixation, since unsteadiness of gait may already be present.

Intra-articular fractures

Fractures of this type in the third or fourth decades are probably best managed by internal fixation. However, there is evidence that restoration of the anatomy may not prevent the onset of osteoarthritis in the over-forties. Since the onset may be quite rapid, even within the first five years, we can no longer say that the elderly will not live long enough to develop osteoarthritis.

There are some very important issues which will apply equally to the section on fractures of the upper tibia, which need to be carefully weighed in the management of an individual case. Knee replacement is now a reasonable option in this age group. If perfect joint congruity is not achieved by a non-operative approach in the first instance, the subsequent development of osteoarthritis can be easily overcome by joint replacement. If on the other hand the degree of deformity of the joint surface, if left, would make the subsequent arthroplasty technically impossible there is a very reasonable argument for open reduction and internal fixation of the fracture. This will at least restore reasonable joint congruity making it suitable for a joint replacement should this become necessary. Restoration of the joint surface may have this limited purpose. Clearly care and judgment must be exercised before embarking on internal fixation. A poor outcome because of skin compromise or infection following internal fixation may prevent a subsequent joint replacement.

The tangential posterior fracture of a single condyle (the Hoffa fracture) is particularly difficult to treat in this age group. The fracture is caused by a shearing of the posterior half or third of one of the condyles and thus total instability of the joint will occur if it is not accurately restored. It must be restored anatomically yet gaining purchase in osteoporotic bone is not easy. In younger patients screws of the Herbert type can be sunk into the articular cartilage since this is usually the only way to insert a lag screw which holds the fractured fragment, under compression, onto the main condylar mass. In this age group using an ordinary screw and burying the head in the articular cartilage is quite acceptable.

In the elderly minimal fixation is preferred in all intra-articular fractures but the use of dynamic condylar screws or t-plates used in buttress fashion may be necessary. The heavy duty condylar buttress plate of the AO system should be used with great care in this age group.

Total knee replacement is now a common operation performed considerably more often in the over-sixty age group than under-sixties. Fracture above a femoral component is a particular problem but may be treated by a dynamic condylar screw (Figures 12.7a, 12.8b). Non-operative treatment using traction and functional bracing is a further possibility.

FRACTURES OF THE UPPER TIBIA

The principles of management of tibial plateau fractures are:

1. reconstruction of joint congruity;
2. re-establishment of tibial alignment;
3. an adequate buttress, with internal fixation and usually bone graft, to maintain these two;
4. repair of meniscus and ligaments.

Consider again the AO classification. In the older age group the aggressive surgeon should remember the complications of internal fixation very seriously. Failure of fixation, infection and wound breakdown with skin loss are not uncommon in fit young adults and in this age group much commoner in the author's experience.

163

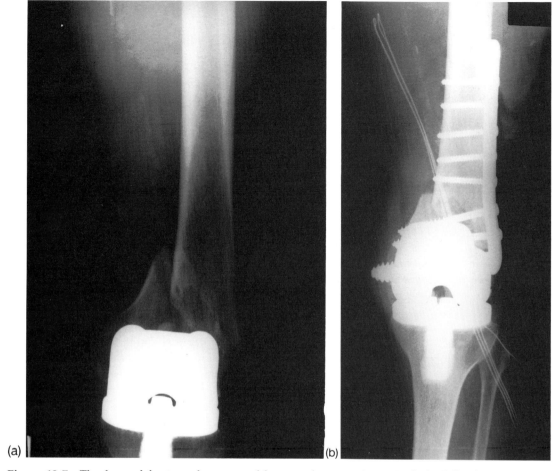

(a)   (b)

Figure 12.7 The femoral fracture above a total knee replacement is particularly difficult to treat. The dynamic condylar screw can be of great value.

Non-operative management may not produce a perfect functional result but it is a safe technique with an adequate outcome for ambulation and transfer. Traction using the split bed Perkin's technique is applicable here. Functional bracing can allow earlier ambulation reducing the period of bedfastness. Sometimes the most comminuted plateau fractures are minimally displaced and where functional bracing is practiced properly, the patient can be assured a reasonable functional outcome with little risk. At worst, if pain persists, or deformity ensues, salvage by a knee replacement is possible – less inviting if sepsis has been present or skin necrosis has already compromised the outcome!

Ligamentotaxis is not a new technique. Every closed reduction of a fracture relies to some extent on the soft tissue envelope for success, as pointed out by Sir John Charnley many years ago. The application of powerful distraction across a joint using external fixators is only an extension of this principle. Ilizarov frames, with thin wires, can be used to advantage in this age group provided

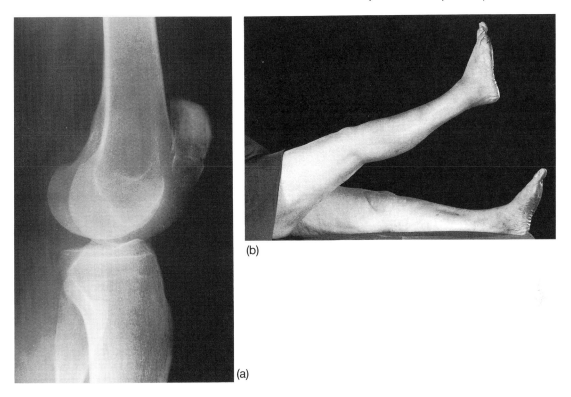

(b)

(a)

Figure 12.8 (a) A displacement fracture of the patella requiring surgery. (b) Following conservative management active extension has been restored.

adequate knowledge and application of the technique has been gained elsewhere (Maiocchi and Aronso, 1991). This will allow early mobilization of both knee joint and patient. Again the result may not be anatomical perfection but functionally adequate.

INJURIES TO THE QUADRICEPS MECHANISM

The quadriceps mechanism is an important group of muscles and tendon producing extension of the knee joint. A large sesamoid bone, the patella, lies in the substance of the tendon. It articulates with the lower end of the femur forming the patello-femoral joint. Since its posterior surface is covered with

articular cartilage nearly all fractures are intra-articular fractures, with all that it implies. Loss of continuity in any part of the mechanism leads to loss of extension of the knee. Thus an important part of the clinical examination when we suspect an injury to the quadriceps mechanism is simply to ask the patient to straight leg raise. Pain may inhibit the ability to do this but if the leg is passively raised and the patient asked to keep the knee straight it will usually be obvious immediately when the mechanism is ruptured. Alternatively, the patient can be asked to extend the knee while lying on their side, which neutralizes the effect of gravity, and may confirm that the mechanism is functioning. Some direct injuries to the patella may fracture it but leave the mechanism intact thus no operative intervention will be required to repair it.

Rectus femoris, vastus lateralis, intermedius and medialis comprise the muscle mass which converges distally to form the quadriceps expansion. This strong coalescence of the four muscles sweeps in from above and both sides of the patella, becoming inseparable from the capsule of the joint. It is unusual for rupture to occur in the expansion proximal to the patella in the elderly, but operative repair is indicated. Repair is done through a straight longitudinal midline incision, the discontinuity is located and repaired with a non-absorbable suture. Plaster of Paris or other lightweight material cylinder is applied and retained for six weeks. In this age group this usually results in considerable stiffness. Quadriceps exercises will be required and in the elderly physiotherapy may be better carried out on an in-patient basis.

The patella may be fractured directly. A fall which results in direct force to the patella will produce a stellate fracture which leaves the quadriceps mechanism intact. A temporary backslab or extension splint for a week to a fortnight with an analgesic may be sufficient to allow pain control before starting full weight bearing and controlled flexion. If facilities exist for continuous passive motion this may be started very early. This contrasts with the fractured patella that has been pulled apart. Usually these fractures are transverse fractures although secondary comminution may occur. The quadriceps expansion is always torn and not infrequently an extension of the tear runs into the capsule on either side. These fractures should be repaired to re-create the articular surface, to restore the quadriceps function and to allow repair of the torn expansion and capsule. Occasionally where there is minimal displacement, or when a medical contraindication to anesthesia exists (Figure 12.8a, b), a plaster cylinder for six weeks may suffice, although tension-band wiring is the treat-

ment of choice in these fractures. The fracture is approached through a midline incision. Some surgeons advocate a transverse incision since this is the direction of Langer's lines and these incisions do heal well, however a longitudinal incision is extensile and if future surgery is required it will not be compromised. Having exposed the fracture any tiny fragments are cleared away, the fracture is reduced and held with appropriate clamps; towel clips can be useful for this. Two 2 mm K wires are driven from proximal to distal across the fracture as far apart from each other as possible. A wire is fed through the expansion just proximally to the upper pole of the patella behind the proximal protruding ends of the K wires, then brought over the front of the patella, crossed so as to form a figure-of-eight and one end is fed through the patellar tendon close to or even through the distal pole. It is then twisted and tightened. This creates a tension band system. When the knee is flexed tensile forces are converted to compressive forces across the fracture. This allows early motion of the knee, reducing recovery time and maintains articular cartilage nutrition. Where comminution occurs screws can be used to bring together major fragments, before tension band wiring. If the fracture is badly comminuted immediate patellectomy is recommended. Unlike younger patients, there is nothing to gain by a 'wait and see' policy in this age group.

A problem the author has noted when using wire across the front of the patella is that it frequently causes discomfort and particularly in this age group where the subcutaneous tissues are often atrophic. It is as well to plan to remove the tension band at the earliest convenient time and to warn the patient this may be necessary.

Patellar tendon injuries rarely occur in this age group. The principles of repair are no different to other age groups. The tendon is exposed and directly repaired with a nonabsorbable suture, then protected by a figure-of-eight wire or artificial ligament.

The principles of managing injuries around the knee joint are similar from skeletal maturity to old age. Hopefully, what this chapter has brought to your attention is how and where these principles need to be modified in dealing with aging tissues.

REFERENCES

Apley, A.G. (1956) Fractures of the lateral tibial condyle treated by skeletal traction and early mobilisation. *J. Bone Joint Surg.*, **38A**, 699.

Apley, A.G. (1979) Fractures of the tibial plateau. *Orthop. Clin. N. Am.*, **10**, 61.

Beard, D.J. *et al.* (1985) Functional bracing: an alternative treatment for peri-articular fractures of the proximal tibia. *J. Bone Joint Surg.*, **67B**, 145.

Bengner, U., Johnell, O. and Redlund-Johnell, I. (1988) Changes in the incidence of fracture of the upper end of the humerus during a 300-year period. A study of 2125 fractures. *Clin. Orthop. A*, **231**, 179–82.

Bengner, V., Ekbom, T., Johnell, O. and Nilsson, B.E. (1990) Incidence of femoral and tibial shaft fractures. Epidemiology 1950–1983 in Malmö, Sweden. *Acta Orthopaed. Scand.*, **61**, 251–4.

Brown, G.A. and Sprague, B.L. (1976) Cast brace treatment of plateau and bycondylar fractures of the proximal tibia. *Clin. Orthop.*, **119**, 184.

Brown, P.E. and Preston, E.T. (1975) Ambulatory treatment of femoral shaft fractures with cast brace. *J. Trauma*, **15**, 860.

Connolly, J.F., Dehne, E. and LaFollette, B. (1978) Closed reduction and early cast brace ambulation in the treatment of femoral fractures. *J. Bone Joint Surg.*, **60A**, 112.

Daniel, E. and Rice, T. (1979) Valgus-varus stability in the hinged cast used for controlled mobilization of the knee. *J. Bone Joint Surg.* **61A**, 135.

Delamarter, R. and Hohl, M. (1989) The cast brace and tibial plateau fractures. *Clin. Orthop.*, **242**, 26.

Foltin, E. (1988) Osteoporosis and fracture patterns. A study of split-compression fractures of the lateral tibial condyle. *Internat. Orthop.*, **12**, 299.

Giles, J.B., DeLee, J.C., Heckman, J.D. *et al.* (1982) Supracondylar-intracondylar fractures of the femur treated with a supracondylar plate and lag screw. *J. Bone Joint Surg.*, **64A**, 864.

Hardy, A.E. (1983) The treatment of femoral fractures by cast-brace application and early ambulation – A prospective review of one-hundred and six patients. *J. Bone Joint Surg.*, **65A**, 56.

Hubbart, M.J.S. (1974) The treatment of femoral shaft fractures in the elderly. *J. Bone Joint Surg.*, **56B**, 96.

Hutson, J.J. and Zych, G.A. (1993) Fractures of the shaft of the distal femur in the elderly. Submitted to *Clin. Orthop.*

Latta, L.L., Zych, G.A. and Greenbarg, P. (1988) Mechanics of distal locking in I.M. Rods – comparison in osteoporotic and normal femurs, in *Femoral Intramedullary Rods: Clinical Performance and Related Laboratory Testing*, ASTM, Philadelphia, PA.

Maiocchi, A.B. and Aronson, J. (eds) (1991) *Operative Principles of Ilizarov*, Williams and Wilkins, Baltimore.

Mast, J., Jakob, R. and Ganz, R. (1989) *Planning and Reduction Technique in Fracture Surgery*, Springer-Verlag, Berlin.

Mooney, V., Nickel, V.L., Harvey, J.P. and Snelson, R. (1970) Cast-brace treatment for fractures of the distal part of the femur. *J. Bone Joint Surg.*, **52A**, 1563.

Moran, C.G., Gibson, M.J. and Cross, A.T. (1990) Intramedullary locking nails for femoral shaft fractures in elderly patients. *J. Bone Joint Surg.*, **72B**(1), 19–22.

Muller, M.E., Allgower, M., Schneider, R. and Willenegger, H. (1990) *Manual of Internal Fixation*, Springer-Verlag, Berlin.

Neufeld, A.J. (1972) A dynamic method for treating femoral shaft fractures. *Orthop. Rev.*, P. 19.

Sarmiento, A., Kinman, P.B. and Latta, L.L. (1979) Fractures of the proximal tibia and tibial condyles: A clinical and laboratory comparative study. *Clin. Orthop.*, **145**, 136.

Sarmiento, A. and Latta, L.L. (1981) *Closed Functional Treatment of Fractures*, Springer-Verlag, Berlin, GFR.

Scalea, T.M., Simon, H.M., Duncan, A.O. *et al.* (1990) Geriatric blunt multiple trauma: Improved survival with early invasive monitoring. *J. Trauma*, **30**(2), 129–36.

Struhl, S., Szporn, M.N., Cobelli, N.J. and Sadler, A.H. (1990) Cemented internal fixation for supracondylar femur fractures in osteoporotic patients. *J. Orthop. Trauma*, **4**, 151.

Stubbs, B.E., Matthews, L.S. and Sonstegard, D.A. (1975) Experimental fixation of the femur with methylmethacrylate. *J. Bone Joint Surg.*, **57A**, 317.

Thomas, T.L. and Meggitt, B.F. (1981) A comparative study of methods for treating fractures of the distal half of the femur. *J. Bone Joint Surg.*, **63B**, 3.

van Aalst, J.A., Morris, J.A., Yates, H.K. *et al.* (1991) Severely injured geriatric patients return to independent living: a study of factors influencing function and independence. *J. Trauma*, **31**(8), 1096–102.

Wardlaw, D., McLaughlan, J., Pratt, D.J. and Bowker, P. (1981) A biomechanical study of cast-brace treatment of femoral shaft fractures. *J. Bone Joint Surg.*, **63B**, 7.

Wardlaw, D., Scott, J.M. and McLaughlan, J. (1984) The recovery of quadriceps function in patients treated by cast bracing. *Injury*, **1594**, 245.

13

Fractures of the ankle in elderly people

P.L.O. BROOS

INTRODUCTION

Ankle fractures are now widely treated by elective internal fixation, based on the philosophy that only accurate restoration of anatomy can result in perfect return of function. Nevertheless rigid internal fixation of complex unstable fractures in old osteoporotic patients is often very difficult to achieve and associated with a high risk of postoperative complications (Lindsjo, 1985; Litchfield, 1987; Fernandez, 1988). Only by good knowledge of the anatomy and indications or limitations of surgical as well as conservative treatment, can good functional results be obtained.

ANATOMY: A FULLY CONGRUOUS AND STABLE MORTISE

The ankle consists of bony and ligamentous structures. The ankle joint includes the talus which articulates with the ankle mortise formed between the fibula and tibia. The ankle joint is fully congruous in all positions of the talus, from full plantar flexion to full dorsiflexion (Inman, 1976; Tile, 1987). The normal ankle has no talar tilt either in valgus or varus in the stance phase of gait and is fully congruous in that position (Gollish, Tile and Begg, 1977; Tile, 1987).

The surrounding ligaments allow normal motion of the joint but prevent excessive movements. There are two groups of ligaments: the inferior tibiofibular ligamentous complex and the collateral ligaments. The inferior tibiofibular ligamentous complex guarantees a tight elastic ankle mortise and consists of the anterior syndesmotic ligament that joints the anterior tibial tubercle of Tillaux-Chaput to the lateral malleolus; the stronger posterior syndesmotic ligament, which joins the lateral malleolus to the posterior tibial tubercle, being the lateral extension of Volkmann's triangle and the interosseous membrane which joins the fibula to the tibia proximal to the syndesmosis.

The collateral ligaments prevent tilting movements. These structures include the lateral collateral ligament with three divisions (the anterior talofibular ligament, the calcaneofibular ligament and the posterior talofibular ligament) and the medial collateral or deltoid ligament which has a tibiotalar and tibiocalcaneal part (Weber and Colton, 1990). Exact anatomic reconstruction of the ankle mortise is necessary for perfect congruity with the talus.

Skeletal Trauma in Old Age
Published in 1994 by Chapman & Hall, London
ISBN 0 412 48750 0

EPIDEMIOLOGY

INCIDENCE

Ankle fractures are common injuries. The incidence of ankle fractures differs from country to country, but has probably risen during the last decade especially in elderly women (Bauer *et al.*, 1985; Lindsjo, 1985; Bengner, Johnell and Redlund-Johnell, 1986; Daly *et al.*, 1987).

About 12% of all patients are aged 65 years or over. These fractures threaten an elderly patient's social and functional independence (Nankhonya, Turnbull and Newton, 1991). The incidence of fractures in a study from the United States was 18.7 per 10 000 (Daly *et al.*, 1987). In youth, the condition is more common in males, whereas, in middle-age, it is more common in females. An apparent increase in elderly males probably was related to the very small number in this group.

In Leuven (Belgium) we treated 915 ankle fractures between 1978 and 1990; 11% were seen in patients of 65 years or older (13% for the women, 7% for the men). In Rochester between 1979 and 1981, ankle fractures occurred with an overall age and sex-adjusted incidence rate of 187 per 100 000 person years; this is over one and a half times the adjusted rate for proximal femur fractures. The ankle fracture rates reported here were higher than those from a study conducted 10 years earlier in the same community (Garraway *et al.*, 1979; Daly *et al.*, 1987). In the Rochester study, 12.5% of the ankle fracture patients were aged 65 years or over. They occurred more frequently in elderly women (18%) compared to elderly men (7%) (Daly *et al.*, 1987). In Uppsala between 1972 and 1975, the number of ankle fractures corresponded to an incidence rate of 114 per 100 000 person years (Lindsjo, 1985). The rising incidence of ankle fractures has also been suggested by the studies of Bengner, Johnell and Redlund-Johnell (1986) and Bauer *et al.* (1987) from Malmö. They noted an incidence rate of 130 per 100 000 persons years between 1980 and 1982, compared with an incidence rate of 70 between 1950 and 1952. This was due to an increase in the proportion of elderly in the population. Elderly women now have an increased age-specific incidence of ankle joint fractures compared to 30 years ago.

Ankle fractures account for approximately 25% of the fractures of the lower extremity in geriatric patients (Miller, 1990). There is also a correlation between age and type of fracture. Bengner, Johnell and Redlund-Johnell (1986) have proved that for unstable bi- and trimalleolar fragility fractures, there is a pronounced increase in women over the age of 65. The increasing number of these complex fractures constitutes a therapeutic problem. These patients may be unsuitable for surgery because of their general health condition and the osteoporotic bone may cause difficulties in achieving stable fixation (Bauer *et al.*, 1987).

ETIOLOGY

The main causes of ankle fractures in the whole population are: traffic accident or fall from a height ('severe trauma', 12%–45%), a fall on level ground due to slipping or stumbling ('moderate trauma', 25%–55%) and sports-related trauma (5%–35%) (Daly *et al.*, 1987; Bisschop, 1989). If the causes of trauma associated with fractures of the ankle are categorized as benign, moderate or severe, it emerges that there is a peak proportion of fractures associated with severe trauma in young men (Daly *et al.*, 1987), and there is a peak proportion of fractures associated with moderate trauma in middle-aged women. An apparent rise in the proportion of fractures associated with moderate trauma in elderly men may well be an artefact

Table 13.1a Causes of ankle fractures (all ages) (N = 915)

	N	%
Traffic accident	242	26
Sports-related trauma	161	18
Fall on ground level	303	33
Fall from a height	172	19
Others	37	4

Table 13.1b Causes of ankle fractures in patients of 65 years or over (N = 103)

	N	%
Traffic accident	10	10
Sports-related trauma	2	2
Fall on ground level	62	60
Fall from a height	24	23
Others	5	5

associated with the very small number in this group.

In elderly people however, the incidence of fractures associated with moderate trauma is increasing, especially in women (Table 13.1a,b). In Leuven a simple fall on level ground was the cause of a fracture in more than 60% of the cases, followed by a fall from a height (23%) (Table 13.1b). As elderly people are less frequently car drivers or motorbikers compared to young adults, the incidence of a traffic accident is rather low (10%). Also sports-related trauma is only a rare cause of an ankle fracture in the elderly population (less than 2%).

Fractures due to moderate trauma showed some of the epidemiologic fractures of osteoporosis-related fractures, such as a greater incidence among women and a rising incidence after midlife. Nevertheless, Seeley and co-workers (1991) have recently proved that in contrast with hip fractures and fractures of the wrist or the humerus, fractures of the ankle, although usually preceded by minimal trauma, are not associated with low

bone mass, so they cannot be considered as typical osteoporotic fractures.

CLASSIFICATION OF ANKLE FRACTURES: THE SIMPLER THE SYSTEM, THE BETTER

There are several classifications of ankle fractures, varying from pure descriptive to a more causative or pathologic-anatomic display. The most common systems are those of Lauge-Hansen that mainly rely on the injury mechanism and the anatomic classification of Danis–Weber (Lindsjo, 1985; Weber and Colton, 1990).

During the 1980s, we also developed our own classification system, based purely on X-ray appearance (Bisschop, 1989; Broos and Bisschop, 1991).

THE LAUGE-HANSEN SYSTEM

In 1942, Lauge-Hansen published his pioneering work on the causative mechanisms of ankle fractures and his 'genetic' classification has gained wide application (Lindsjo, 1985). The fractures were divided into supination-adduction (SA), supination-eversion (SE), pronation-abduction (PA) and pronation-eversion (PE) types, each with a number of sub groups (Figure 13.1) (Bauer *et al.*, 1987). This system has been of historical importance and, when correctly employed, has improved the results of conservative treatment (Lindsjo, 1985).

THE DANIS–WEBER SYSTEM

In 1949 Danis introduced a pathologico-anatomical classification designed for application to operative treatment (Lindsjo, 1985). This has since then been modified by Weber and taken into use by the AO (ASIF) group (Figure 13.2).

According to this system, fracture dislocations at the ankle are divided into three

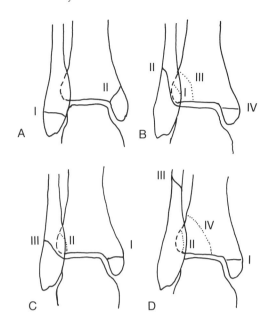

Figure 13.1 Lauge-Hansen classification of ankle fractures.
A: supination – adduction (SA);
B: supination – eversion (SE);
C: Pronation – abduction (PA);
D: Pronation – eversion (PE).

classes, A, B and C according to the height of the fibular fracture in relation to the syndesmosis and to the horizontal tibio-talar joint space. Classified as type A fractures are lateral malleolar fractures below the level of this joint space. In these cases the syndesmosis and deltoid ligament are undamaged. A medial malleolus fracture if present, is often a high, almost vertical fracture. A medial posterior fracture of the tibial margin may occur. Type B fractures are injuries of the lateral malleolus at the syndesmotic level, involving a 75% risk of syndesmotic lesions. On the medial aspect, dislocation may be associated with an injury to the deltoid ligament or a malleolar fracture. A lateral posterior fragment may be present. Type C fractures are fibular fractures above the syndesmotic level,

invariably involving a risk of injury to the syndesmosis. Medially there is an avulsion fracture through the malleolus or damage to the deltoid ligament. A lateral posterior fracture may occur.

THE BROOS–BISSCHOP (B–B) SYSTEM

In this very simple system, ankle fractures were divided into uni- (U), bi- (B) and trimalleolar (T) fractures involving the medial malleolus (M), lateral malleolus (L) posterior (P) and/or anterior tibial margin (A).

Weber's A, B, C classification of fractures of the lateral malleolus was also used. Associated fibular shaft fractures without rupture of the anterior tibiofibular ligament were noted as type F; very high proximal fibular fractures as type P. In this way every single injury can be classified; e.g. a trimalleolar fracture with fibular damage type C was noted as TMLcP (Table 13.2).

IS THERE AN IDEAL CLASSIFICATION SYSTEM?

A good classification system can be defined as a system that is accessible to repetition, that allows for comparison between the different subjects, that is simple and easy to use in daily practice and that gives information that is important for treatment and scientific research (Lindsjo, 1985; Broos and Bisschop, 1991). The Lauge-Hansen system with its 15 subgroups is difficult to use because of the complexity. It is impossible to decide on radiographic ground alone the difference between some types of fractures. Knowledge about the accident is also required.

The Danis–Weber classification is easy, but it does not include fractures in which the lateral malleolus has been spared. The prognostic value of the system is dubious (Heim, 1982; Bauer *et al.*, 1985; Broos and Bisschop,

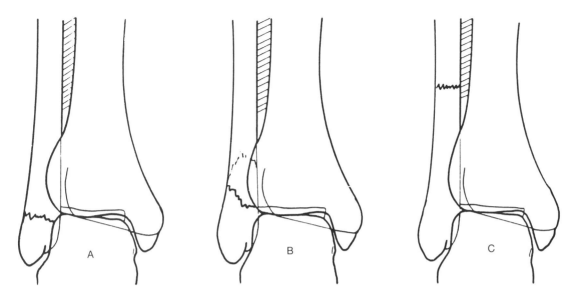

Figure 13.2 Danis–Weber classification of ankle fractures.

Table 13.2 Classification of ankle fractures (N = 915)

		N	%
Unimalleolar	U	467	51
Bimalleolar	B	293	32
Trimalleolar	T	155	17
Lateral malleolus	L		
Weber a	a	119	13
Weber b	b	567	62
Weber c	c	192	21
Fibular shaft	f	18	2
Proximal fibula	p	19	2
Medial malleolus	M	448	49
Posterior margin	P	201	22
Anterior margin	A	20	2

1991). The Broos-Bisschop system has proved to be very easy to use even for young residents and physiotherapists. All ankle fractures without exception can be classified. The prognostic value of the system has been proven (Broos and Bisschop, 1991; Broos in press).

TREATMENT: INTERNAL FIXATION IF POSSIBLE AND IF NECESSARY

There are few problems in traumatology which have been discussed so thoroughly as the treatment of malleolar fractures (Bauer *et al.*, 1985). The most important aim however, in treating elderly people with fractures of the lower limb is to restore their locomotor function as soon as possible. To obtain this goal, unnecessary damage of the soft tissues, prolonged immobilization in non-weight bearing plaster casts, and post-traumatic arthritis have to be avoided. With the methods of internal fixation, according to the AO principles, a stable fixation and anatomical reduction is possible in the younger patient, a plaster of Paris may not be required and unprotected walking can be permitted once the ankle can be extended to a right angle, which may be as soon as 3 or 4 days after the operation (Hooper, 1983). Experiences of older patients, however, indicates that the results of internal fixation are less satisfactory. In 1983 Beauchamp, Clay and Thexton

173

showed that adequate fixation, particularly in women, may be difficult to achieve and that a high risk of postoperative complications was to be expected (Litchfield, 1987).

Therefore the treatment will depend on:

- the general condition of health of the elderly patient and his or her previous ambulatory capacities;
- the type of fracture;
- the bone quality and the condition of the surrounding soft tissues.

THE GENERAL HEALTH AND THE PREVIOUS AMBULATORY CAPACITY

Experience has shown that modern techniques of spinal and even general anesthesia are well tolerated in the elderly patient. A poor general condition is rarely a true contraindication to lower limb surgery. On the other hand, when dealing with patients already definitively bed-ridden and demented at the moment of the ankle fracture, a simple realignment of the bony fragments and immobilization in a well padded plaster of Paris is sufficient.

THE TYPE OF FRACTURE

There is a clear correlation between the final functional result and post-traumatic osteoarthritis. An excellent to good result is noted in 80–90% of the patients without arthritis and in only 0–5% of the patients with completely eliminated joint spaces (Lindsjo, 1985; Bisschop, 1989; Broos and Bisschop, 1991). The development of arthritis in the ankle joint is nearly always due to failure to restore the anatomy and function of the joint (Lindsjo, 1985; Ouzounian and Shereff 1988). Willenegger (1961) found the frequency of arthritis to be 97% among fractures with persistent displacement and 8% among those that were accurately reduced. The criteria of a good reduction were defined as the correc-

tion of talar shift on the antero-posterior radiograph and of posterior talar subluxation on the lateral film. The fibular length has to be restored and maintained (Charnley, 1961; Rowley, Norris and Duckworth 1986). The studies of Bauer *et al.* (1985) and Rowley, Norris and Duckworth (1986) have proved that if a good reduction can be achieved and held then closed treatment is as good as operative treatment. On the other hand, it is generally known that unstable (bi- and tri-malleolar) fractures frequently displace following closed reduction and therefore they are usually treated by open reduction and fixation (de Souza, Gustilo and Meyer, 1985). Also in displaced uni-malleolar fractures reduction can be impossible because of soft tissues incarcerated between the bone fragments making operative treatment mandatory. So for these displaced and unstable fractures operation is indicated and planned as a primary measure without preceding attempts at closed reduction and non-operative treatment. The ideal time for the procedure is within the first 6–8 hours following injury, before any true swelling or fracture blisters develop. The AO technique has to be used. Malleolar fractures are fixed with screws, figure-of-eight tension band wiring, plates and screws or cerclage wires. For the distal fibular fractures screws or a one-third tubular plate are used. If the posterior fragment involves more than 25% of the articular surface, then it is fixed with one to three screws from the front (Figure 13.3). If the play of the distal fibula after reduction, fixation and suturing of the ligaments is more than 2 mm a supra-syndesmotic screw is applied (Muller *et al.* 1977; Heim and Pfeiffer, 1982) (Figure 13.4). There is no need to repair the ruptured deltoid ligament as long as the lateral malleolar fracture is anatomically rigidly fixed and an intra-operative radiograph reveals a normal medial joint space (de Souza, Gustilo and Meyer, 1985). Postoperatively the ankle is elevated and immobilized

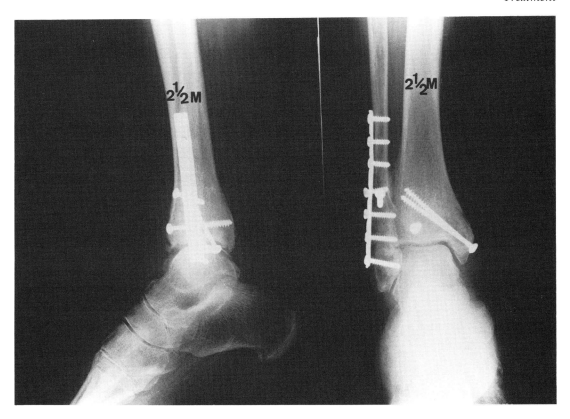

Figure 13.3 Trimalleolar fracture in a 73-year-old woman. Fixation of the posterior margin with a screw from the front.

in a plaster back slab, but joint exercises are allowed. After 5 days, the patients start to walk with floor contact and free ankle movement is encouraged. The importance of early postoperative exercises has been stressed by several authors (Burwell, 1965; Lindsjo, 1985). Early postoperative exercises permit healing of cartilage defects in the joint surfaces, full weight bearing being 6 weeks postoperatively.

Where the fracture fixation is considered to be unstable because of osteoporosis, or when the elderly patient is not able to walk toe touching with crutches the ankle is immobilized in a below-knee walking cast for about six weeks.

THE QUALITY OF THE BONE AND THE CONDITION OF THE SURROUNDING SOFT TISSUES

The cancellous bone of the metaphysis in elderly people is often osteoporotic making an accurate reduction and completely stable fixation more difficult (Lindsjo, 1985; Tile 1987). Because of the compact area of the ankle, swelling may be intense and fracture blisters can occur. These blisters make it very difficult to perform surgery, increasing the risk of infection to 50% (Miller, 1990). In these circumstances, when dealing with patients in good functional condition before injury, anatomical reduction is vital to a

175

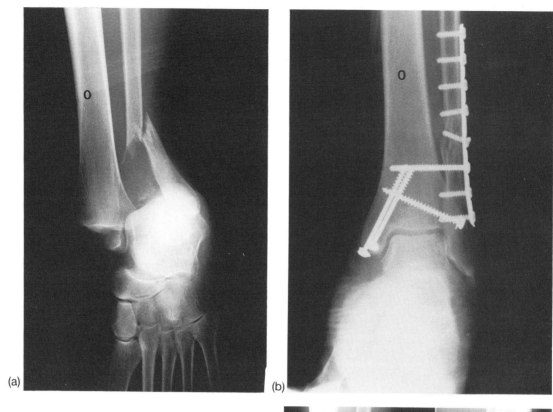

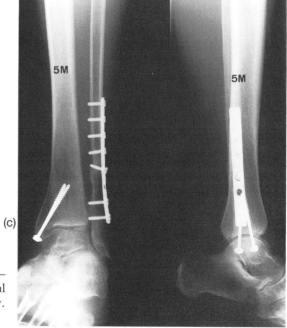

Figure 13.4 (a) Bimalleolar fracture dislocation – Weber$_c$ in a 71-year-old woman. (b) Internal fixation, – presence of a supra-syndesmotic screw. (c) Result after five months.

satisfactory final result (Tile, 1987). In these cases, the operative treatment can be extremely difficult and delicate, and has to be performed by experienced surgeons. In the presence of severe edema and blisters the open reduction must be delayed by at least four days when the soft tissues have settled. Breederveld and co-workers (1988) have shown that a delayed open reduction still gives similarly good functional results. Sometimes the skin vitality can be better evaluated by not using a tourniquet. The soft tissues have to be handled with extreme care, diathermy has to be avoided. If vascularity to the limb is diminished, percutaneous techniques through small stab wounds instead of the standard AO methods, may be sufficient to restore some stability to the ankle without compromising the skin. Since screws do not provide good fixation in osteoporotic bone, Kirschner wire techniques supplemented by tension band wires are preferable. If rotatory stability cannot be obtained the addition of a cast or an external fixator is usually sufficient to prevent displacement of the mortise. In such cases, the maintenance of anatomic reduction must not be sacrificed to early motion. It has been shown that, in these difficult cases, careful operative planning can avoid major complications, and satisfactory results can be obtained (Ali *et al.*, 1987; Litchfield, 1987; Tile, 1987; Ngcelwane, 1990). It is well known that ankle fractures treated in plaster can displace and allow pressure sores to develop, especially if the skin is of poor quality.

PERSONAL EXPERIENCES

From 1978 to 1990, 103 patients (38 men, 65 women) aged 65 years or over were treated in the Department of Traumatology and Emergency Surgery of the University Hospital Gasthuisberg of Leuven, Belgium. Twenty-three patients were treated with a plaster cast only. The indications for this conservative

Table 13.3 Ankle fractures in elderly people (*N* = 73) – postoperative complications

	N	%
Inplant loosening	3	4
Minor wound problems	10	14
Osteïtis	1	0.8
Algoneurodystrophy	3	2
Phlebothrombosis	2	1.5
Pulmonary infection	3	2
Bed sores	1	0.8

treatment were: bed-ridden status before injury (12 times), undisplaced stable unimalleolar fracture (8 times), compromised vascularity of the lower extremely (3 times). The other 80 patients (28 men, 52 women) were operated on following the principles outlined above. Two patients died and five patients were lost for follow-up. For the other 73 patients, a final examination was carried out one year after the accident. This evaluation was done by means of a personal score system based on subjective data and on clinical and radiographic results (de Souza Gustilo and Meyer, 1985; Olerud *et al.*, 1986; Bisschop, 1989). The postoperative complications are listed in Table 13.3. An excellent or good result was obtained in 55 cases (75%), the result was fair in 10 cases (15%) and bad in 8 cases (11%).

All the four cases of implant loosening had a bad result. They were all women with extreme osteoporosis. This confirms Litchfield's findings (1987). There was also a clear relationship between the type of fracture and the final result. As has already been mentioned by other authors, trimalleolar fractures and fractures with a long posterior fragment especially had a bad prognosis (Bauer *et al.*, 1985; Lindsjo, 1985; Tile, 1987). Nevertheless, our results are comparable with those of Ali *et al.* (1987) and of Fernandez (1988). They proved that in elderly patients also, the surgical treatment of ankle fractures gives good and excellent results in the majority of cases.

CONCLUSIONS

The incidence of ankle fractures differs from country to country but is probably rising during the last decades especially in elderly women. About 12% of the patients are 65 years or over.

Despite the fact that an ankle fracture is not associated with a low bone mass, it is caused by a simple fall on ground level in 60% of the cases in elderly people. The most frequently used classification methods are those of Lauge-Hansen and of Danis–Weber. During the 1980s we also developed a simple, purely anatomical system. This system is very easy to use and has a prognostic value.

In treating old people with an ankle fracture, unnecessary damage to the soft tissues, prolonged immobilization and post-traumatic arthritis have to be avoided. So treatment will depend on the general health condition, the ambulatory capacities before the injury, the type of the fracture, the quality of the bone and the conditions of the surrounding soft tissues. Our personal experiences have shown that after surgical treatment, excellent and good results can be obtained in about 75% of the cases.

REFERENCES

Ali, M.S., McLaren, C.A., Rouholamin, E. *et al.* (1987) Ankle fractures in the elderly: nonoperative or operative treatment. *J. Orthop. Trauma*, **1**(4), 275–80.

Bauer, M., Bengner, U., Johnell, O. *et al.* (1987) Supination-eversion fractures of the ankle joint: changes in incidence over 30 years. *Foot and Ankle*, **8**(1), 26–8.

Bauer, M., Bergstrom, B., Hemborg, A. *et al.* (1985) Malleolar fractures: nonoperative versus operative treatment. A controlled study. *Clin. Orthop.*, **199**, 17–27.

Beauchamp, C.G., Clay, N.R. and Thexton, P.W.

(1983) Displaced ankle fractures in patients over 50 years of age. *J. Bone Joint Surg.*, **6**, 329–32.

Bengner, U., Johnell, O. and Redlund-Johnell, I. (1986) Epidemiology of ankle fractures between 1950 and 1980. Increasing incidence in elderly women. *Acta Orthop. Scand.*, **57**(1), 37–7.

Bisschop, A.P.G. (1989) De operative behandeling van enkelfracturen bij volwassenen. Licentiaatsverhandeling motorische revalidatie en kinesitherapie, Leuven, I.L.O.

Breederveld, R.S., van Straaten, J., Patka, P. *et al.* (1988) Immediate or delayed operative treatment of fractures of the ankle. *Injury*, **19**, 436–8.

Broos, P.L.O. and Bisschop, A.P.G. (1991) Operative treatment of ankle fractures in adults: correlation between types of fractures and final results. *Injury*, **22**(5), 403–6.

Broos, P.L.O. (accepted June 1992) A new and easy classification system for ankle fractures. *Int. Surg.* (in press).

Burwell, H.N. and Charnley, D.A. (1965) The treatment of displaced fractures at the ankle by rigid internal fixation and early joint movement. *J. Bone Joint Surg*, **47B**, 634–60.

Charnley, J. (1961) *The Closed Treatment of Common Fractures*, 3rd edn, Churchill Livingstone, Edinburgh and London.

Daly, P.J., Fitzgerald, R.H., Melton, L.J. *et al.* (1987) Epidemiology of ankle fractures in Rochester, Minnesota. *Acta Orthop. Scand.*, **58**, 539–44.

Danis, R. (1949) Les fractures malleolaires, in *Theorie et Pratique de l'Osteosynthese* (R. Danis), Masson et Cie, Paris, pp. 135–60.

de Souza, L.J., Gustilo, R.B. and Meyer, T.J. (1985) Results of operative treatment of displaced external rotation-abduction fractures of the ankle. *J. Bone Joint Surg.*, **67A**, 1066–73.

Fernandez, G.B. (1988) Internal fixation of the oblique, osteoporotic fracture of the lateral malleolus. *Injury*, **19**(4), 257–8.

Garraway, W.M., Stauffer, R.N., Kurland, L.T. *et al.* (1979) Limb fractures in a defined population. Frequency and distribution. *Mayo Clin. Proc.*, **54** (11) 701–7.

Gollish, J.D., Tile, M. and Begg, R. (1977) Fractures of the ankle. *J. Bone Joint Surg.*, **59B**, 510.

Heim, U. and Pfeiffer, K.M. (1982) The ankle joint, in: *Small Fragment Set Manual*, 2nd edn (eds

U. Heim and K.M. Pfeiffer), Springer Verlag, Berlin, pp. 252–331.

Hooper, J. (1983) Movement of the ankle joint after driving a screw across the inferior tibio-fibular joint. *Injury*, **14**, 493.

Inman, V.T. (1976) *The Joints of the Ankle*, Williams and Wilkins, Baltimore.

Lindsjo, U. (1985) Classification of ankle fractures: The Lauge-Hansen or AO System? *Clin. Orthop.*, **199**, 12–6.

Litchfield, J.C. (1987) The treatment of unstable fractures of the ankle in the elderly. *Injury*, **18** (2), 128–32.

Miller, M.D. (1990) Orthopaedic trauma in the elderly. *Emerg. Med. Clin. Am.* **38** (2), 325–9.

Muller, M.E., Allgower, M., Schneider, R. *et al.* (1977) *Manual der osteosynthese*, AO Technik ed 2, Spring Verlag, Berlin, pp. 278–299.

Nankhonya, J.M., Turnbull, C.J. and Newton, J.T. (1991) Social and functional impart of minor fractures in elderly people. *B.M.J.*, **303**, 1514–15.

Ngcelwane, M.W. (1990) Management of open fractures of the ankle joint. *Injury*, **21** (2), 93–6.

Olerud, C., Molander, H., Olssen, T. *et al.* (1986) Ankle fractures treated with non-rigid internal fixation. *Injury*, **17**, 23.

Ouzounian, T.J. and Shereff, M.J. (1988) Common ankle disorders of the elderly: diagnosis and management. *Geriatric*, **43** (12), 73–80.

Rowley, D.I., Norris, S.H. and Duckworth, T. (1986) A prospective trial comparing operative and manipulative treatment of ankle fractures. *J. Bone Joint Surg*, **68B** (4), 610–3.

Seeley, D.G., Browner, W.S., Nevitt, P.C. *et al.* (1991) Which fractures are associated with low appendicular bone mass in elderly women? *Ann. Int. Med.*, **115**, 837–42.

Tile, M. (1987) Fractures of the ankle, in *The Rationale of Operative Fracture Care* (eds J. Schatzker and M. Tile), Spring Verlag, Berlin, pp. 371–405.

Weber, B.G. (1972) *Die Verletzungen des oberen Sprunggelenkes*, 2nd edn, Bern, Stuttgart, Wien, Verlag Hans Huber.

Weber, B.G. and Colton, C.H. (1990) Malleolar fractures, in *Manual of Internal Fixation*, 3rd edn (eds M.A. Muller and M. Allgower), Springer Verlag, Berlin. pp. 595–612.

Willenegger, H. (1961) Die behandlung der luxationskfrakturen des oberen sprunggelenkes nach biomechanischen gesichtspunken. *Helv. Chir. Acta*, **28**, 225.

14

Management and results of bone metastases in the elderly patient

WILHELM FRIEDL

INTRODUCTION

Bone metastases are a sign of tumor dissemination and generally associated with a poor prognosis. The prognosis is not determined by the bone metastases themselves, but they are a sign of dissemination of the tumor to other organs (Manegold *et al.*, 1988; Krempien and Manegold (1992). The life expectancy of patients with bone metastases varies in different studies to between 5 and 15 months following diagnosis (Dittel and Marklin, 1985; Friedl, 1990; Friedl, Ruf and Krebs, 1986; Lies and Rhen, 1984). Therefore, in patients with pathological or impending pathological fractures caused by bone metastases, it is always necessary to achieve an immediate restoration of function if at all possible. In patients with metastases of the lower extremities and the trunk skeleton the weight bearing capacity must be restored. Appropriate management allows rapid mobilization and reintegration with the family. Therefore, in both established and impending pathological limb fractures radiotherapy prior to surgical fixation is rarely indicated.

Table 14.1 Incidence of bone metastases in different carcinomas

Breast cancer	50–85%
Prostate cancer	40–84%
Renal adenocarcinoma	27%
Thyroid cancer	31–50%
Bronchial carcinoma	29–30%

INCIDENCE OF BONE METASTASES

The number of patients requiring surgical therapy for established or impending pathological fractures demonstrates a steep increase in numbers from under 10 in our institute in 1972, to over 50 in 1991. The rate of bone metastases is highest in breast, prostate, bronchial, thyroid carcinoma and renal adenocarcinoma (Table 14.1). Even in tumors with similar bone metastasis rates there are large differences in the incidence of pathological fractures. Only those tumors with osteolytic metastases have a high risk of pathological fracture (Table 14.2).

The increased incidence of pathological fractures has been associated with a change in the primary tumor spectrum. In the review

Skeletal Trauma in Old Age
Published in 1994 by Chapman & Hall, London
ISBN 0 412 48750 0

Table 14.2 Type of metastases and risk of pathological fracture

Osteolytic	76.6%
Mixed	11.1%
Osteoplastic	12.3%

period 1972–1982 breast cancer metastases were the most frequent cause for surgery. In the last 10 years, the incidence of renal adenocarcinoma and bronchial carcinoma have increased significantly (Friedl, 1990; Friedl, 1992). These changes reflect improved techniques in diagnosis of bone metastases, the improvement in operative techniques and stabilization devices for various parts of the skeleton, and the introduction of new anti-osteoclastic drugs such as the bisphosphonates. The use of bisphosphonates is responsible for the falling incidence of pathological fractures in patients with breast cancer (Krempien and Manegold, 1992).

BIOLOGICAL CHARACTERISTICS WITH RELEVANCE FOR SURGICAL MANAGEMENT

The incidence of bone metastases correlates with the blood flow in different parts of the skeleton. Accordingly bone metastases generally occur in cancellous bone or in the medullary space. The incidence of bone metastases is highest in the spine and in 80–90% of patients with bone metastases, the spine is involved (Everbeck, 1992). Cortical bone destruction is generally secondary to the medullary metastatic deposit. Primary cortical bone metastases do occur but these are rare (Fidler, 1981; Galasko, 1974; McBroom *et al.*, 1988; Menck *et al.*, 1988; Mirels, 1989). Distal sites of metastases in the limbs are rare and even lower than may be accounted for by the difference in the blood flow rates in proximal and distal parts of limbs (Krempien and Manegold, 1992).

The distribution of pathological fractures is very different from that of bone metastases. Pathological fractures occur mainly in the heavily loaded parts of the skeleton. Therefore, the incidence is highest in long bones and especially in the femur (Figure 14.1).

The distribution of bone metastases in the skeleton also differs very much with different primary tumors. While in prostate carcinoma multiple bone metastases are nearly always present, in renal adenocarcinoma and thyroid cancer, single metastases are common. Peripheral sites of limb metastases are found predominantly with bronchial carcinoma.

DIAGNOSIS OF BONE METASTASES

Bone scintigraphy is used to screen for bone metastases. Bone scintigraphy is positive only in osteoblastic and mixed bone metastases but not in pure osteolytic metastases. Bone scintigraphy is also positive in all reactive bone remodeling in degenerative and inflammatory diseases. Therefore, bone scintigraphy should be used for screening only in symptomatic cancer patients (Gulenchyn and Papoff, 1987; Monnypenny *et al.*, 1984; Peiss and Bohndor, 1992; Rieden, 1988).

Positive scintigraphy findings must be evaluated alongside plain X-ray examination. Radiographic examination is not reliable as a screening technique because diagnosis of metastasis is possible with plain X-ray films only after a 50% reduction of the bone mass. Classical tomography improves the sensitivity of the X-ray examination considerably.

A less well known method for diagnosis where cortical destruction is present, especially in limb localization, is ultrasonography. Ultra-sonography with a 5–7.5 MHz transducer allows recognition of bone destruction, soft tissue infiltration and also blood flow patterns. (Mende *et al.*, 1992).

If metastases cannot be identified by these methods an axial CT scan or MRI examin-

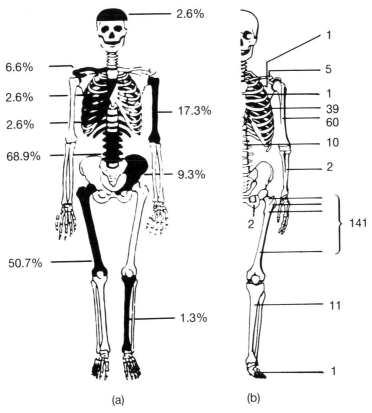

Figure 14.1 Distribution of bone metastases (a) and of pathological fractures (b) in the skeleton. (a) Hecht, Beck and Hecht-Zilch (1979); (b) Our patients treated from 1972–1991.

ation must be performed before planning an operation. The CT scan is superior in the diagnosis of bone destruction whereas the MRI allows one to identify bony marrow and soft tissue infiltration (Peiss and Bohndorf, 1992).

The definitive diagnosis of bone metastases must be performed by biopsy but this is not recommended in all patients with suspected metastases before resection of the tumor. Biopsy before metastasis resection is not necessary in patients with known disseminated carcinoma, primary carcinoma with a high bone metastases rate and existing or impending pathological fracture. Only in a relatively small number of patients is biopsy indicated to exclude benign lesions or second

primary tumors. The presence of single tumor cells in the bone marrow is of questionable biological relevance and no surgical significance (Krempien and Manegold, 1992; Herrmann, 1992). In some cases they can disappear after removal of the primary carcinoma (Manegold *et al.*, 1988; Krempien and Manegold, 1992).

DECISION-MAKING IN PATIENTS WITH BONE METASTASES

There are three questions to be answered when surgery is considered in patients with bone metastases.

1. Which patients should receive surgery?

183

2. When is the right time for operation?
3. How radical should the operation be and which device should be used for stabilization?

The criteria for answering these questions are as follows.

Patient-related characteristics:
1. age;
2. life expectancy;
3. general condition of the patient;
4. morbidity of the surgical management.

Metastasis-related characteristics:
1. type of primary tumor;
2. time interval between primary tumour diagnosis and metastasis occurrence. Growth characteristics of the bone metastases and interval to appearance of second metastases;
3. localization, diameter, number and distribution of metastases in the skeleton;
4. osteolysis;
5. vascularity;
6. impending or existing pathological fracture;
7. efficacy of nonoperative management.

PATIENT-RELATED CHARACTERISTICS

Age

There is no age limit for operative therapy in patients with bone metastases. The biological, rather than the chronological, age should be considered in the type of operation to be performed.

Life expectancy

The mean survival rate in a group of 76 patients with 135 bone metastases which were treated in our hospital between 1972–1982 was 10.8 months (Friedl, 1990; Friedl, Ruf and Krebs, 1986). In a second period from 1982–1989 the mean survival time of 136 patients with 169 pathological fractures (Friedl, 1992), was only 7.5 months (Figure 14.2). This is due mainly to the change in the primary tumor spectrum. The life expectancy in patients with bronchial carcinoma is 3.6–4 months and the life expectancy in patients with breast and prostate cancer 20–29.3 months (Harrington, 1981; Wannenmacher,

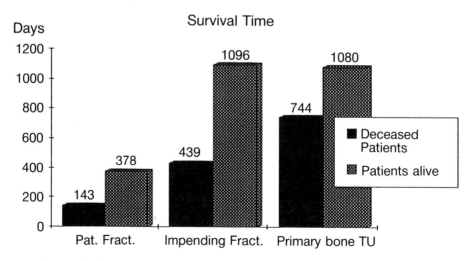

Figure 14.2 Survival of patients with pathological fractures treated between 1982–1989 in our department.

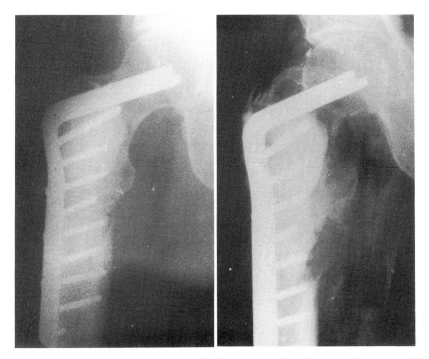

Figure 14.3 Local tumor recurrence in nonradical resection of a femur neck metastasis. Secondary operation and tumor hip prosthesis was necessary.

Rieder and Eble, 1992). Longer survival periods of more than 3–5 years can be observed especially in breast and prostate, but also renal adenocarcinoma and thyroid carcinoma. The life expectancy is much higher in patients with impending fractures (14.9 months) as compared with patients with existing fractures (5 months).

Because of the short life expectancy of these patients an immediate restoration of function and weight bearing capacity is necessary to avoid prolonged immobilization and hospitalization. It is probably not possible to influence the overall survival time with surgery for bone metastases, but the operation should be performed so that two major problems are avoided:

1. Local tumor progression (Figure 14.3).
2. The biomechanical problems of the individual site must be considered so that a

fatigue fracture of the implant or implant dislocation is prevented (Figure 14.4).

METASTASIS RELATED CHARACTERISTICS

Type of primary tumor

Primary breast, thyroid, prostate and renal adenocarcinoma have a favorable prognosis (Becker, 1992; Everbeck, 1992; Friedl, 1990; Friedl, Ruf and Krebs, 1986; Wannenmacher, Rieden and Eble, 1992).

Interval between primary tumor diagnosis and metastasis occurrence

Long intervals between diagnosis of the primary carcinoma and bone metastases and long intervals between the occurrence of

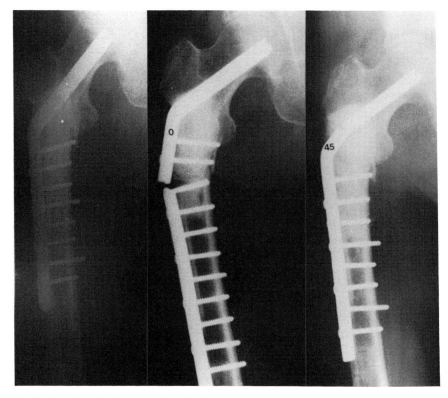

Figure 14.4 Fatigue break of an angle nail plate in a compund osteosynthesis of the proximal femur without medial cortical or implant support.

different metastases are associated with a better prognosis.

Localization, diameter, number and distribution of metastases in the skeleton

Surgical management is ideally indicated in single metastases in loaded parts of the skeleton. Metastases of the lower extremity have the highest risk of pathological fracture. Metastases of the upper and lower extremities can be stabilized with relatively small operations with low morbidity and very low mortality (Friedl, 1992; Heisel, Schmitt and Mittelmeier, 1983; Mutschler, Sabo and Schulte, 1992; Sim, 1990). Since 1972 we

surgically treated all patients with bone metastases and impending or existing pathological fractures of the lower extremity. In the first examination period (1972–1982) some of the metastases of the upper extremity were treated nonoperatively. The functional results were significantly superior following surgery.

In pelvic and spinal metastases radiotherapy is used initially if no neurological symptoms occur and mobilization of the patient is still possible. If neurological symptoms occur the indication to operate is urgent and the operation should be performed within the first 6 hours and not later than 24 hours. After this time, an improvement in the neurological deficit is improbable (Everbeck,

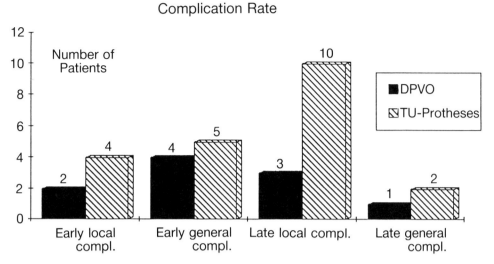

Figure 14.5 Complication rates after DPCO and tumor prosthesis replacement of the proximal femur.

1992). As with other sites, metastatic resection is performed if the life expectancy is over 3–6 months and dorsal stabilization alone is performed only in patients in a poor general condition with a short life expectancy.

The localization and number of metastases is also important in determining the type of operation. Where the metastases are localized close to the bone ends, only tumor prostheses can be used. In other metastases of the long bones, joint preserving techniques such as double plate compound osteosynthesis (DPCO) are used.

Generally therefore metastases should be totally resected and stabilization should be performed with consideration of the biomechanical load of the affected part of the skeleton. According to Windhager *et al.* (1989) the local recurrence rate after intralesional resection of bone metastases is 50%, as compared with extra-lesional resection with a recurrence rate of 15%.

The actual operative technique selected depends on where the tumor is in relation to the joint. A compound osteosythesis can and should be used when the distance from the

resection to the joint is sufficient for stable implant fixation. Due to the high loading in the lower extremity lateral and medial plates – DPCO – may be needed to avoid stress fracture of the implant. We have demonstrated experimentally that the loading capacity of this device, after subtrochanteric resection, is identical to that of control femora (Friedl, 1990; Friedl, Ruf and Mischkowsky, 1986). We compared the results and complication rates of patients treated with a DPCO or a proximal femur tumor prosthesis between 1985 and 1989. Thirty patients were evaluated in each group. Whereas in all patients, in both groups a full weight bearing capacity could be restored, the rate of early and late local complications was significantly higher in the tumor prosthesis group (Figure 14.5). This was due to the high dislocation rate of the hip tumor prostheses. This is caused by the unphysiological fixation of the abductor muscles to the shaft of the prosthesis. Seven of the 30 patients showed a total of 11 hip luxations. There was no case of local recurrence, with the need for a second operation, or instability in either group.

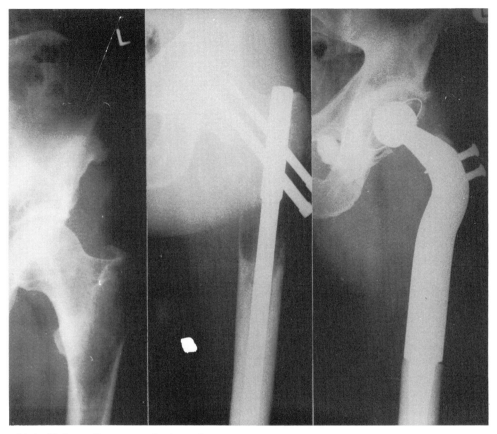

Figure 14.6 Delta nail osteosynthesis without metastasis resection in a patient with renal adenocarcinoma. Local tumor progression with severe instability and pain occured. Therefore secondary proximal femur resection and tumor prosthesis insertion was necessary.

Stabilization, without metastasis resection, should be performed only in patients in a poor general condition and a very advanced stage of carcinoma with a life expectancy of under 3 months. In patients with a life expectancy of under 1 month, surgical management of bone metastases is generally not indicated. If intramedullary stabilization without metastasis resection is performed, in patients with survival time over 6 months, tumor progression with instability, pain, loss or primary lack of function and the need for reoperation should be expected. This problem is illustrated in Figure 14.6.

Localization of metastases is also important in those cases without risk of fracture. A poor response to conservative therapy may lead to the involvement of other parts of the skeleton and necessitate a more extensive operation in the future. This can be the case with metastases close to the acetabulum or major limb joints.

Osteolysis

Osteolytic metastases have a much higher risk of pathological fracture and therefore, are an indication for surgical management.

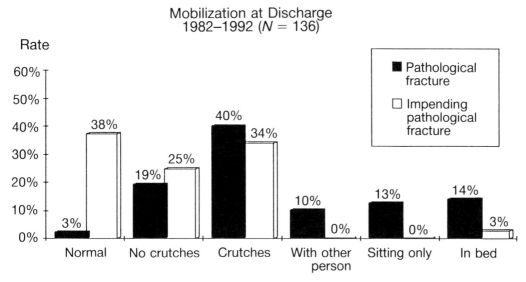

Figure 14.7   Mobilization in patients with pathological fractures in the examination period 1982–1989.

Recalcification of osteolytic metastases after radiotherapy is rare due to the virtually complete destruction of the osteoblasts. Also, in the mixed type metastases, the time to recalcification is 6 to 12 months and therefore is unlikely to occur before the patients die from their disease.

Vascularity

In highly vascular bone metastases, found mainly with renal adenocarcinoma, preoperative selective angiographic embolization may be performed, especially so with difficult operative sites like the spine and pelvis. This helps to reduce blood loss. In spinal metastases the risk of paraplegia, which is approximately 5% (Richter *et al.*, 1992) must be considered, and can occur where emboli affect the spinal cord circulation. Therefore, we do not perform preoperative embolization routinely in spinal metastases, nor in most of the renal adenocarcinoma patients. We recommend the use of preoperative emboli-

zation only in very large highly vascular metastases localized in the lumbar spine.

Impending and existent pathological fractures

There is no doubt today that pathological fractures of the extremities are an indication for surgical management. The special criteria for pelvic and spinal fractures were discussed above.

Surgery on impending pathological fractures shows the best overall functional results and the longest survival time. This is not due only to earlier detection of the bone metastases but also because the rehabilitation is easier and so morbidity lower. In our study 61% of patients with impending pathological fractures were restored to full or nearly full function. In patients with existing fractures the rate was only 8%. 96% of the patients with impending and 62% of patients with existent fractures were able to walk without aids at discharge (Figure 14.7).

There have been many attempts to define

189

Table 14.3 Mirels score for determination of the fracture risk in patients with bone metastases

Number of points	1	2	3
Localization	Arm	Leg	Proximal femur
Pain	Low	Middle	Function dependent
Structure	Osteoblastic mixed	Osteolytic	
Size	< 1/3	1/3–2/3	> 2/3

impending pathological fractures. From the clinical point of view, the appearance of function or load dependent pain at the site of metastasis, is the most important feature. The use of radiological characteristics alone does not correlate very well with fracture risk (Chao *et al.*, 1988; Fidler, 1981; Menck, Schulze and Larser, 1988; McBroom, Cheal and Haynes, 1988).

Mirels (1989) developed a combined score which considers the diameter of the metastasis, localization, primary tumor and the occurrence of pain. At a score of less than 7 the fracture risk is 5% and nonoperative management can be used primarily. With a score of 9 the risk of fracture is 33% and, therefore, early surgery is indicated (Table 14.3).

Effectiveness of nonoperative management

Radiotherapy can be used as another modality in local therapy. Because of the advantages of surgical management, with fast stabilization and short hospital stay, radiotherapy is only performed in metastases of the extremity without fracture risk or when surgery is not indicated because of other reasons.

In spinal and pelvic metastases, radiotherapy is the primary modality if there are no neurological symptoms and there is no risk of deterioration during therapy.

Postoperative radiotherapy is not affected by the implants (Wannenmacher, Rieder and Eble, 1992). Radiotherapy should be used if the metastasis resection was incomplete. However, evidence of tumor cells beyond resection in the bone marrow, is no indication for postoperative radiotherapy in compound osteosynthesis as well as in tumor prosthesis operations.

In spinal metastases where local radical resection cannot be performed as in the extremities, postoperative radiotherapy is not indicated if the stabilization was performed from a ventral or combined ventral and dorsal approach and the preoperative MRI examination proved tumor-free segments at the implant fixation sites. For these reasons the rate of postoperative radiotherapy decreased from 50% in our first review, to 5% in the years 1982–1989. The same change is seen in other studies (Mutschler, Sabo and Schulte, 1992). In contrast to radiotherapy, systemic approaches such as postoperative chemotherapy, hormone therapy, immunotherapy and in recent years, antiosteoclastic therapy with bisphosphonates, are used with increasing frequency. The rate of use of these adjuvant techniques increased from 42% in the first study to 75% in the second.

OVERVIEW OF THE SURGICAL TECHNIQUES IN THE DIFFERENT PARTS OF THE SKELETON

Whereas, in the decade 1972–1982, simple compound osteosyntheses were the most frequent techniques (47%) used in the surgical management of pathological fractures, in the second review period from 1982–1989 the use of devices with a full weight bearing capacity such as DPCO and tumor prostheses increased to about 60% of cases. The use of intramedullary implants, without resection as recommended in older and some more recent American papers (Becker, 1992; Fasno, Olysav and Stauffer, 1988; Manegold *et al.*, 1988), should be restricted to patients with a very short life expectancy.

EXTREMITIES

The devices used today allow reconstruction and restoration of function and weight-bearing capacity at all sites. The operations performed can be divided into three groups:

1. Resection of all the metastasis and stabilization:
   (a) tumor prosthesis;
   (b) compound osteosynthesis.
2. Stabilization only: intramedullary locking nail systems.
   This is indicated in patients with a survival time of under 3 months if the metastases are localized in the upper or lower extremity and in patients with a survival time under 4–6 months with spine and pelvis metastases.
3. Resection of the metastasis only:
   (a) resection of parts of the skeleton without replacement (mainly in the hand and foot).
   (b) amputations are rarely performed today. In the whole period 1972–1989 only one patient had a primary amputation. Amputation is indicated only in patients in a very bad general condition with multiple unstable sites in whom pain relief and nursing facilitation must be achieved.

Lower extremity

Proximal femur

The use of a simple total hip joint prosthesis is possible where the metastasis only affects the femoral head and neck. If used in larger metastases there is a high risk of local recurrence. In patients with trochanteric extension of the metastasis, only a resection of the proximal femur, including the trochanters, can be performed and a tumor prosthesis implanted (Figure 14.6). If the metastasis is localized below the distal end of the lesser trochanter, the DPCO as a joint and muscle insertion preserving device, should be used (Figure 14.8). The use of only one angle nail plate compound osteosynthesis is not possible where the medial cortical support is affected. Owing to the differences of rigidity between bone cement and the metal implant (1 to 100) a fatigue break of the plate will occur when the leg is loaded over a period of time (Figure 14.4). In patients with a very poor prognosis, an intramedullary nail osteosynthesis without metastasis resection can be performed. In cases with pathological fracture the proximal screw of an intramedullary nail should be used statically and not as a sliding device because healing of the fracture cannot be expected and sliding of the proximal femur is associated with pain. Intramedullary nail osteosynthesis gives the patient pain relief and allows partial mobilization and facilitates nursing (Figure 14.9). The use of Ender nails should no longer be recommended because there is no real stabilization of the fracture and no pain relief. Also, other distal unlocked nail systems have no rotational stability and if used in patients with a longer survival period, without metastasis resection, tumor progression and instability will be observed as in the case of Figure 14.6.

Femoral shaft and supracondylar region

A DPCO should be used at these sites. In more distal localized metastases, an inverted insertion of the device in the femoral condyles is necessary. With this device long resections, of up to 20 cm, can be performed. An alternative in metastases of the middle

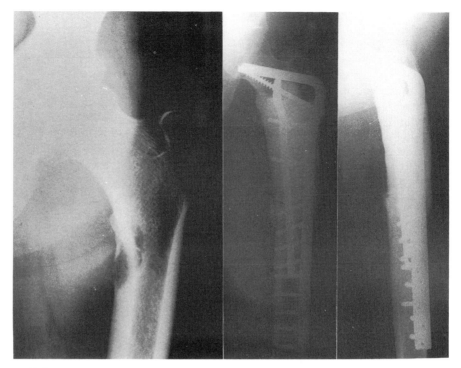

Figure 14.8 If the metastasis is localized below the lesser trochanter a joint preserving resection and DPCO can be performed.

third of the shaft, are custom-made segmental shaft prostheses. A long DPCO without the use of a lateral condylar plate as a tension-belt plate cannot neutralize the tension forces.

Distal femur

If the femoral condyles are affected, a resection of the distal femur end and the implantation of a tumor prosthesis is necessary. Individual prostheses (Figure 14.10) or the Kotz modular system prosthesis can be used.

Tibia

Proximal tibial metastases usually require resection and tumor prosthesis implantation.

If the distance to the joint is sufficient, a joint preserving resection and DPCO should be performed. In proximal metaphyseal metastases, two T-plates (Figure 14.11) and two straight DC plates in the shaft are used.

Distal tibia metastases are very uncommon. If a pathological fracture occurs resection and DPCO with an ankle arthrodesis should be performed.

Foot

Metastases of the foot skeleton are rare and, if surgery is needed, should only be resected. The use of an implant is not recommended because stable fixation in these bones subject to high bending loads, is not possible. On the

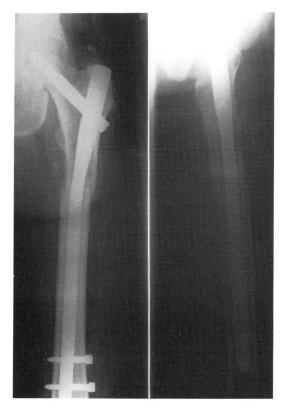

Figure 14.9 In a patient with poor general condition and pathological pertrochanteric fracture stabilization is performed with a locked gamma nail without metastasis resection.

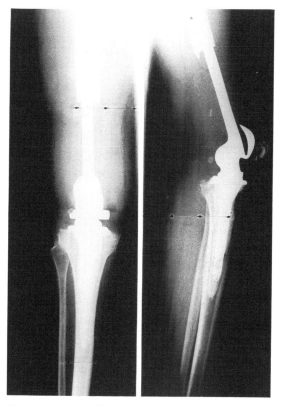

Figure 14.10 When the femoral condyles are involved only resection and knee tumor prosthesis can be performed.

other hand walking can be preserved after simple resection of the metastases.

Upper extremity

Humerus

The arm carries a much lower load than the leg. Therefore, in proximal humeral head and neck metastases, resection of the proximal humerus and prosthetic replacements are performed, without replacement of the glenoid. The prosthesis is generally used without cement and rotatory stability can be ensured with two transfixing screws (Figure 14.12). The rotator cuff, and in larger resections the deltoid, pectoralis and latissimus dorsi muscles are reinserted on to the prosthesis.

In humeral shaft metastases, segmental resection and single femoral dynamic compression plate compound osteosynthesis, performed from a dorsal approach is appropriate (Figure 14.13). If, in more distal metastases, it is not possible to place at least three screws distal to the resection, two tibia DC plates can be used instead.

The use of multiple intramedullary rods may not provide adequate stability for pain

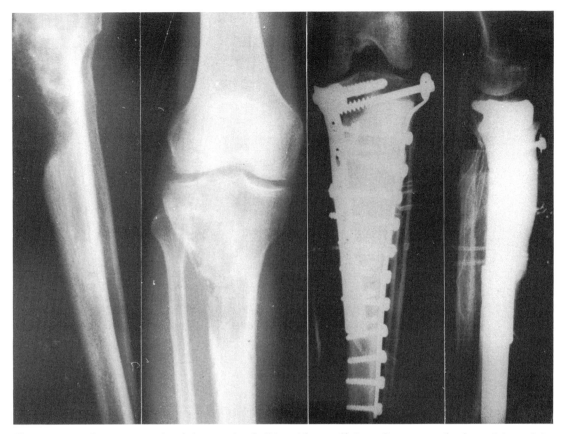

Figure 14.11 In a metastasis of the proximal tibia with a sufficient distance to the knee joint a joint preserving resection and a compound osteosynthesis with two T-plates can be performed.

relief, so that secondary resection and compound plate osteosynthesis may become necessary. Occasionally tumor contamination of the proximal humerus follows surgery to the shaft, and prosthetic replacement should be performed.

In rare cases, where the distal humerus or proximal ulna are affected, elbow joint prostheses can be used. In patients with a poor prognosis in whom resection is not indicated, a locked intramedullary nail should be used. (Figure 14.14).

Forearm

Metastases of the forearm are rare and typical of bronchial carcinoma. The therapy is similar to that of humerus shaft metastases. We recommend the small AO DC plate for this.

Hand

As in the foot, when surgery is needed, only the affected part of the skeleton is resected.

PELVIS

The most frequent indication for surgery in pelvic metastases are acetabulum metastases. Usually, intralesional metastasis resection and reconstruction with special cup plates and bone cement can be performed. A

194

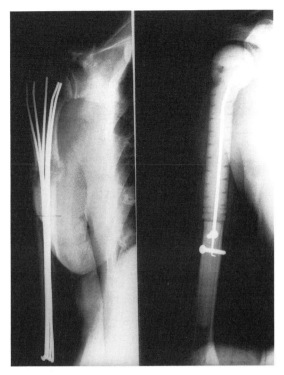

Figure 14.12 Resection of the proximal humerus and isoelastic humerus prosthesis insertion. In this patient 6 weeks before, a pathological proximal humerus fracture was treated with intramedullary rods and radiotherapy. The arm could not be used at all and caused severe pain.

standard total hip prosthesis can then be implanted. Only in selected cases with a favorable prognosis is inner hemipelvectomy and reconstruction with an individual pelvic prosthesis indicated (Enneking and Dunham, 1978).

SHOULDER GIRDLE

Clavicle

Clavicular shaft metastases are resected and stabilization performed with a small DC plate compound osteosynthesis. It is important, as in all other compound osteosyntheses, that

the intramedullary space is evacuated and filled with bone cement. Intramedullary rods as proposed by some authors are less valuable in the clavicle as this bone performs rotational movements of up to 60 degrees with each elevation of the arm.

Scapula

Metastases of the scapula are usually treated with radiotherapy. If radiotherapy is not effective and the tumor growth disables the patient, resection of the affected part of the scapula without replacement is performed. Preservation of the acromion is preferable, but, when this is not possible, the humerus can also be fixed to the thoracic wall with a synthetic material, such as Goretex.

SPINAL COLUMN

Where the expected surgical time is over 3 to 6 months, metastasis resection should be performed. Dorsal decompression alone is not indicated because these operations increase the instability of the spinal column.

Thoracolumbar spine

When the vertebral body is affected, a ventral retroperitoneal approach is indicated. In metastases of the distal thoracic and first two lumbar vertebral bodies a retropleural, retroperitoneal and transdiaphragmatic approach is performed. A transperitoneal approach is indicated only for metastases of the 5th lumbar vertebra. This is necessary because the implant must be fixed ventrally onto the sacrum.

The vertebral body is resected along with the intervertebral discs so that the spinal canal can be revised and all tumor masses evacuated. Stabilization should be performed with bone cement and appropriate internal fixation. We use the Wolter plate fixator system because it is relatively flat and

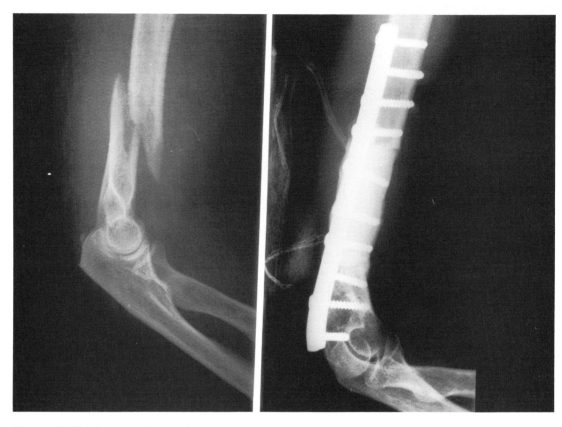

Figure 14.13 Segmental resection in a patient with pathological humerus shaft fracture and stabilization with a simple plate compound osteosynthesis.

smooth. Bone cement, as compared to cancellous bone blocks, has the advantage that tumor infiltration is not possible. Before the bone cement is applied the spinal canal is closed with a collagen sponge. We have never seen thermal damage to the spine.

If the dorsal columns of the spine are also infiltrated by the metastasis, resection of the dorsal parts of the vertebral segment and transpedicular stabilization with an internal fixator system is also necessary (Figure 14.15). Resection and stabilization can bridge one or more affected vertebral segments.

In patients with a short life expectancy only dorsal decompression with laminectomy and some form of posterior stabilization should be performed. For rotational stabilization of the system, a transverse bar should be placed between the two fixator systems.

Thoracic and cervical spine

Upper thoracic pathological fractures are very rare due to the stabilization by the chest skeleton. Stabilization can usually be performed by an anterolateral thoracotomy alone but, if extended dorsal infiltration is present, additional dorsal resection and plate

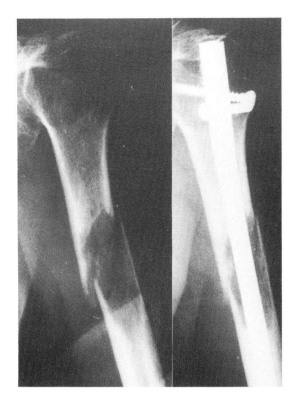

Figure 14.14 In a patient with advanced brochial carcinoma and pathological fracture of the humerus no resection and stabilization with a locked humerus nail was performed.

fixation is required. Because of the size of the implants, internal fixation systems such as Harrington rods are not ideal at this site.

Cervical metastases occur mainly in the vertebral body. Using the easier ventral approach, the vertebral body and discs are resected. Stabilization is performed with bone cement and a Cramer plate, Orozco plate or with the Morscher cervical plate. If dorsal tension force transmission is interrupted, dorsal stabilization is also necessary. This is best performed with two small plates with screws placed in the articular processes.

STERNUM

Sternal metastases can easily be detected by ultra-sonography. Surgical management is recommended in large metastases with the possibility of skin ulceration. Partial sternal defects must not be replaced. Larger defects can be closed by Marlex or Goretex patches. The soft tissue coverage can be effected with muscle flaps, like pectoralis major, or by omentumplasty.

HYPERCALCEMIA IN PATIENTS WITH BONE METASTASES

Hypercalcemia is a frequent paraneoplastic syndrome. Hypercalcemia is caused by osteoclast activation by tumor cells. Bone metastases are not necessarily present in patients with hypercalcemia, although in advanced metastatic disease, tumor cells can directly destroy the bone tissue (Krempien and Manegold, 1992). Bone metastases are the most frequent cause of hypercalcemia except hyperparathyroidism.

Because hypercalcemia and local bone destruction are mainly caused by osteoclast activation, biphosphonate therapy is indicated. Because of the low enteral resorption rate, parenteral bisphosphonate therapy as clodronat (OstacR300mb in 500 ml saline infusion over 2 hours per day = 4mg/kg/day), or similar, should preferably be used. In osteolytic bone metastases oral long-term biphosphonate therapy (400–3200 mg/day) is effective in preventing the development of new bone metastases. Prophylactic use would be desirable to avoid the formation of osteolytic bone metastases in tumors with a high bone metastasis rate like breast cancer but because of the high costs of this therapy this is rarely practicable (Friedl, 1992).

Malignant hypercalcemia, characterized by very high calcium plasma levels, is caused in over 50% of cases by metastatic carcinoma. The mortality of malignant hypercalcemia is

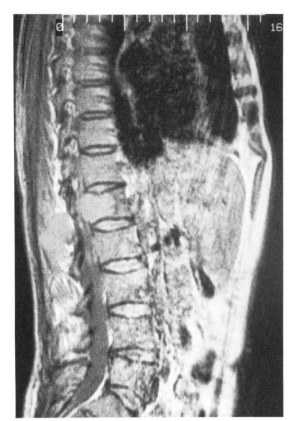

Figure 14.15 When the dorsal parts of the vertebra are also affected, additional dorsal resection and stabilization with two internal fixators is indicated.

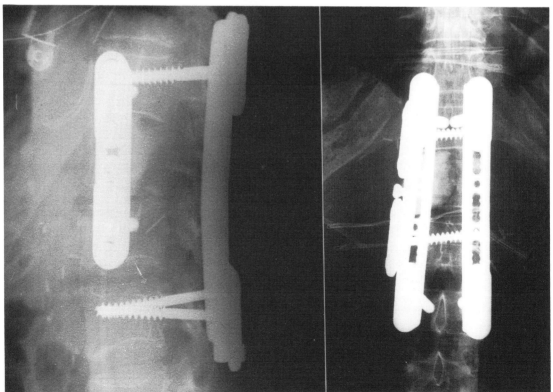

very high. Biphosphonates, calcitonin and hemofiltration are used for therapy.

REFERENCES

Becker, W. (1992) Surgical management of bone metastases of the upper extremity, in *Surgery for Bone Metastases* (German) (eds V. Everbeck and W. Friedl), Springer Verlag, Heidelberg, pp. 201–13.

Chao, E.Y.S., Sim, F.H., Shives, T.C. and Pritchard, D.J. (1988) *Management of Pathologic Fracture in Diagnosis and Management of Metastatic Bone Disease. A Multidisciplinary Approach*, Raven Press, New York.

Dittel K, and Marklin, H. (1985) Results of compound osteosynthesis. (German-Engl Abst.) *Akt. Traumatol.*, **15**, 115–119.

Enneking, W.F. and Dunham, W.K. (1978) Resection and reconstruction of primary neoplasms involving the innominate bone. *J. Bone Joint Surg.*, **60A**, 731–46.

Everbeck, V. (1992) Operative management of spinal metastases, in *Surgery for Bone Metastases*, (German) (eds V. Everbeck and W. Fried), Springer Verlag, Heidelberg, pp. 77–110.

Fasno, F.J. Jr., Olysav, D.J. and Stauffer, E.S. (1988). Intramedullary stabilisation in neoplastic destructive disease involving the subtrochanteric region of the femur. *Orthopaedics*, **11**, 1699–1704.

Fidler, M. (1981) Incidence of fracture through metastases in long bones. *Acta Orthop. Scand.*, **52**, 623–31.

Friedl, W. (1990) Indications, management and results of surgical therapy of pathological fractures in patients with bone metastases. *Europ. J. Surg. Oncol.*, **16**, 380–96.

Friedl, W. (1992) Surgical management of bone metastases and pathological fractures of the leg, in *Surgery for Bone Metastases* (German), (eds V. Everbeck and W. Friedl), Springer Verlag, Heidelberg, pp. 171–89.

Friedl, W., Ruf, W. and Krebs, H. (1986) Functional results of operative and nonoperative management of bone metastases (German – Engl Abstr), *Langenbecks Arch. Chir.*, **386**, 185–96.

Friedl, W., Ruf, W. and Mischkowsky, T. (1986) Double plate compound osteosynthesis in pathological subtrochanteric fractures (German-Engl Abstr), *Chirurg.*, **57**, 713–18.

Friedl, W. (1992) Double plate compound osteosynthesis versus tumour prosthesis in the management of pathological fractures and reversed inter- and subtrochanteric femur fractures in patients with severe osteoporosis. *Proceedings of the Congress Osteosynthesis International*, G. Kunscherkreis 1991, Budapest.

Galasko, C.S.B. (1974) Pathologic fractures secondary to bone metastases. *J.R.Coll. Surg. Edinb.* **19**, 351–62.

Gulenchyn, K.Y. and Papoff, W. (1987) Technetium 99mMdp scintigraphy. An insensitive tool for the detection of bone marrow metastases. *Clin. Nucl. Med.*, **12**, 45–6.

Harrington, K.D. (1981) The management of acetabular insufficiency secondary to metastatic malignant disease. *J. Bone Joint Surg.* **63**, 653–64.

Hecht, L., Beck, H. and Hecht-Zilch, E. (1979) Bone metastases: diagnosis, therapy and prognosis. (German–Engl. Abstr.) *Med.Klin.*, **74**, 349–52.

Heisel, I., Schmitt, E. and Mittelmeier, H. (1983) Indication and results of hip tumour prosthesis. (German–Engl. Abstr.) *Akt. Traumatol.* **13**, 164–70.

Herrmann, R. (1992) Indication and results of hormone- and chemotherapy of bone metastases (German), in *Surgery of Bone Metastases* (eds V. Everbeck and W. Fried), Springer Verlag, Heidelberg, pp. 61–6.

Krempien, B. and Manegold, C. (1992) Pathogenesis and diagnosis of bone metastases and tumour osteopathies (German), in *Surgery for Bone Metastases* (eds V. Everbeck and W. Fried), Springer Verlag, Heidelberg, pp. 5–20.

Lies, A. and Rhen, J. (1984) Pathological fractures of the hip. (German, Engl. Abstr) *Akt. Traumatol.* **14**, 79–84.

Manegold, C., Krempien, B., Kaufmann, M. *et al.* (1988) The value of bone marrow examination for tumour staging in breast cancer. *J. Cancer Res. Clin. Oncol.*, **114**, 118–24.

Mansi, J.L., Berger, U., Easton, D. *et al.* (1987) Micrometastases in bone marrow in patients with primary breast cancer: evaluation as an early predictor of bone metastases. *B.M.J.*, **295**, 1092–7.

McBroom, R.J., Cheal, E.J. and Hayes, W.C. (1988) Strength reduction from metastatic cortical defects in long bones. *J. Orthop. Res.*, **6**, 369–78.

Menck, H., Schulze, S. and Larsen, E. (1988) Metastasis size in pathological femoral fractures. *Act. Orthop. Scand*. **59**, 151–4.

Mende, U., Everbeck, V., Krempien, B. *et al.* (1992) Sonography in the diagnosis and follow up of primary bone and soft tissue tumours. (German, Engl. Abstr) *Bildebung*, **59**, 4–14.

Mirels, H. (1989) Metastatic disease in long bones. A proposed scoring system for diagnosing impending pathological fractures. *Clin. Orthop.*, **249**, 256–64.

Monnypenny, I.J., Grieve, R.J., Howell, A. and Morrison, J.M. (1984) The value of serial bone scanning in operable breast cancer. *Br. J. Surg.*, **71**, 466–8.

Mutschler, W., Sabo, D. and Schulte, M. (1992) Surgery for bone metastases of the acetabulum and of the proximal femoral end (German), in *Surgery for Bone Metastases* (ed. V. Everbeck and W. Fried), Springer Verlag, Heidelberg, pp. 191–9.

Peiss, J. and Bohndorf, K. (1992) MRI in the diagnosis of bone metastases (German), in *Surgery for Bone Metastases* (eds V. Everbeck and W. Fried), Springer Verlag, Heidelberg, pp. 33–50.

Richter, G.M., Roeren, T. Noeldge, G. and Kaufmann, G.W. (1992) Bone metastases – interventional radiology. Embolisation in the surgical management of bone metastases (German), in *Surgery for Bone Metastases* (eds V. Everbeck and W. Fried), Springer Verlag, Heidelberg, pp. 67–73.

Rieden, K. (1988) *Knochenmetastasen – Radiological Diagnosis, Therapy and Follow Up* (German), Springer Verlag, Heidelberg.

Sim, E. (1990) Hip tumour prosthesis – indication and results in a trauma department. (German, Engl. Abstr.) *Unfallchirurgie*, **16**, 291–8.

Wannenmacher, M., Rieden, K. and Eble, M.J. (1992) Indication and results of primary radiotherapy in pathological and impending pathological fractures caused by bone metastases (German), in *Surgery for Bone Metastases* (eds V. Everbeck and W. Fried), Springer Verlag, Heidelberg, S. 53–60.

Windhager, R., Ritschel, P., Rokus, U. *et al.* (1989) Recurrence after intra- and extratumoral resection of bone metastases in long bones. (German, Engl. Abstr.) *Z. Orthop*, **127**, 402–10.

15

The geriatric amputee

COLIN STEWART

INTRODUCTION

The amputation of a major limb is not an uncommon surgical procedure. In the United Kingdom (population 55 000 000) there are over 5000 primary lower limb amputations per year. The majority of these amputations are of a lower limb with a small number of patients losing the upper limb. In the Western world this surgical event is usually performed on elderly individuals with long-standing vascular disease.

Historically amputation has occurred in war-related events and prosthetic history is similarly related to war injuries. It is likely that the military youth of the world represent the commonest amputee and as long as man insists on conflict with man they will remain the majority.

Prostheses are likely to have been available in one form for centuries but Ambroïse Parré, the 15th century naval surgeon, was the first to use the articulated metal prosthesis. These were probably first manufactured by military armourers, but by the nineteenth century willow and beechwood were commonly used, the Angelsey limb being the best known. This ingenious prosthesis was manu-factured for the Earl of Angelsey who lost his limb above the knee in the Battle of Waterloo. The prosthesis had leather cords running from the knee to the ankle so that on flexing the knee the foot dorsiflexed, easing swing during the gait cycle.

The renaissance of prosthetics occurred however in the late 1950s and early 1960s with the development of the patella tendon bearing (PTB) below knee prosthesis releas-ing the below knee amputee of any straps or suspension. This new thinking on prosthetics has led to the development of modular lightweight prosthesis for all levels and all ages of amputees.

The recent introduction of the ischial con-tainment socket with an Icelandic/Swedish/New York design (ICS with ISNY) has been a similar revolution for the above knee ampu-tee. The new prostheses are much easier to fabricate, maintain and use making the life of the amputee of all ages much easier.

Modern vascular surgical techniques have enabled the surgeon to attempt limb salvage in a way that was not possible a decade ago. As a consequence both the elderly patient and the young patient have a much greater chance of limb salvage.

Despite these advances the care of the amputee requires great consideration in both the amputation itself and in the post-amputation period. A closely integrated co-ordinated team is essential if all the elements required in the care of the amputee are to be drawn together, thereby ensuring the

Skeletal Trauma in Old Age
Published in 1994 by Chapman & Hall, London
ISBN 0 412 48750 0

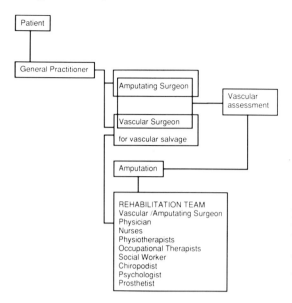

Patient

General Practitioner

Amputating Surgeon

Vascular assessment

Vascular Surgeon

for vascular salvage

Amputation

REHABILITATION TEAM
Vascular /Amputating Surgeon
Physician
Nurses
Physiotherapists
Occupational Therapists
Social Worker
Chiropodist
Psychologist
Prosthetist

Figure 15.1 A program allowing coordination between the surgeon and other team members.

patients regain as high a level of independence as possible.

PROGRAM DEVELOPMENT

A comprehensive program of care must be established if the amputee is to achieve his optimum level of independence after amputation. In many areas the vascular surgeon is the surgeon who eventually performs the amputation, in others it may be orthopedic or even the general surgeon.

Regardless of the basic training of the surgeon the individual must be conversant with vascular surgical techniques and their potential as well as modern amputation procedures, rehabilitation matters and a comprehensive up-to-date prosthetic knowledge. Ideally there should be a close working relationship between the surgeon and other team members. Figure 15.1 suggests a programe which allows this coordination and ensures that the best service is achieved for the patient. A fragmented service with no

integration can only lead to delayed inefficient rehabilitation with a disadvantaged patient.

In addition to the need for rehabilitation of the amputee there is a need for a comprehensive prosthetic service. Modern prosthetics may liberate the amputee from his disability, thereby reducing the degree of handicap. Efficient prosthetic care is an essential element in the overall provision of the amputee and for the prosthesis to be effective all team members must have a working knowledge of prosthetics and know their limitations. In particular, the surgeon who fashions the stump must understand that his handiwork will directly affect the ability of the patient to use these devices to the fullest.

ELDERLY AMPUTATION

In the Western World there is a degree of consistency in the pathologies leading up to major limb amputation.

The majority (approximately 90%) of amputations are due to peripheral vascular disease (PVD) with about 66% of these resulting from arteriosclerosis and 33% from diabetes mellitus. In addition to these pathologies a few amputations are as a result of neoplasm, trauma and other vascular causes such as painful varicose ulcers. In addition there are a few congenital cases. In recent years, however, the emergence of patients with failed knee replacements has resulted in some above knee amputations, and a few patients with long-standing renal disease on dialysis with accelerated arteriosclerosis have been referred from renal units.

The population in question is elderly with an average age of 70 and the vascular disease that has led to the amputation is often just one manifestation of a more widespread vascular problem.

At least 75% of all elderly amputees have at least one other significant pathology affecting them. These debilitating conditions add to the difficulty of operative recovery and rehabilitation.

In Dundee we have found that over 50% have significant cardiac pathology and 30% have some form of intracerebral disease at the time of surgery. These are in addition to the presence of osteoarthritis, deafness and visual difficulties, all of which are not uncommon in an elderly population.

The degree to which the widespread nature of generalized diseases are present can be seen when the survival of lower limb vascular patients is compared with the population as a whole. The average survival of a 70-year-old male from Dundee is 10.3 years (1988 figures), but that of the male vascular patient has been found to be just over 6 years for the 1980/89 decade (Stewart, Jain and Ogston, 1992). Cardiac disease has been found to be the commonest cause of death in these patients and significantly more than in similar national population studies. This latter figure is indicative of the more widespread nature of vascular disease, not purely affecting the lower limbs (Stewart and Jain, 1992). These facts need to be considered when deciding on amputation in an elderly person.

The average survival of 6 years is still a significant time and the surgeon must ensure that he provides his patient with the best residium possible; this must be as low a level of amputation as is surgically possible, ideally preserving the knee joint since this retains proprioception and stability enabling a light functional prosthesis to be fitted.

The surgery at any level should be a once-only event since repeated surgery is demoralizing and debilitating for the patient. At the same time it is essential to save the knee joint as often as possible.

LEVEL SELECTION

In some cases of amputation the level of amputation is predetermined, usually when the operation is for trauma, neoplasia or infection. The success of primary healing in vascular cases however requires careful preoperative evaluation if the optimum level in the patient is to be achieved.

Several laboratory procedures are available to the surgeon to help come to a complete clinical decision as to the optimum level of amputation.

Highly accurate prediction of the healing potential of skin is particularly valuable in below knee, through knee and Symes levels of amputation, and is possible with Doppler measurements, thermography or skin blood flow measurement (Spence *et al.*, 1984).

Doppler measurement of systolic blood pressure has become an accepted non-invasive method of evaluation. The ratio of brachial artery to posterior tibial artery pressures is of value in assessing whether or not tissues will heal.

Thermography, the method of mapping the infra-red image of the limb with accurate thermal calibration, can provide the surgeon with clear guidelines as to wound healing and flap construction.

^{134}I-4-iodoantipyrine subcutaneous injection with measurement of the skin washout of the radioactive dye, provides highly reproduceable and accurate measurement of skin blood flow. Skin fluroscein has also been used successfully as have transcutaneous oxygen measurements. All these techniques have been shown to be of value in allowing the surgeon to predict the likely healing potential of the skin. However the level of amputation must not be decided only on laboratory results.

The clinical decision must consider the patient as a whole and assess the effects of the amputation on the life of the patient and to the likely prosthetic outcome. The surgeon should consider the most recent lifestyle of the patient. Has the patient been walking independently and have they been able to go out and about in recent months? The mental state should be considered when considering their ability to cope with a prosthesis.

The presence of a cerebrovascular accident (CVA) resulting in hemiplegia on the same side as the patient's amputation may lead the surgeon to consider an above knee amputation even though a below knee amputation would heal. The loss of control of the knee in the CVA patient with a knee flexion deformity can make prosthetic fitting extremely difficult at the below knee level. An above knee or through knee amputation would in such cases be preferable, despite the high energy cost imposed by an above knee amputation and prosthesis. One might expect that in such circumstances the amputee would fail to regain their mobility, but it is our experience that many patients do manage remarkably well. There is however, evidence that amputations affecting the sound side will adversely affect the long-term ability of the patients to walk since they are relying on the hemiplegic side for their main stability.

The presence of a contralateral amputation should not deter the surgeon from considering a further below knee amputation since bilateral below knee amputees can walk remarkably well. Bilateral above knee or even an above knee/below knee combination generally do not use their prosthesis to any significant degree although there are of course notable exceptions.

PHYSIOLOGICAL CONSIDERATIONS

The body's ability to utilize oxygen declines as it ages (Figure 15.2). This reduces the respiratory reserve and as a consequence the patient's ability to cope with the added difficulty of a prosthesis.

Energy measurements have clearly shown that the lower the amputation the less additional energy is required to walk. The Symes and below knee amputations have been shown to require at least 25% more energy to walk than the normal subject, and the above

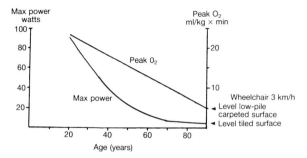

Figure 15.2 Graph of maximum power output of individuals of various ages and peak oxygen uptake. Subjects using wheelchairs on various surfaces. (After Grimby, 1983, from Sawka *et al.*, 1981).

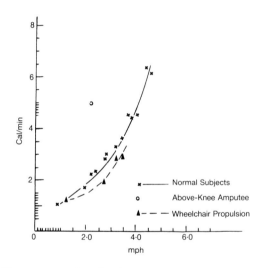

Figure 15.3 Graph of net energy costs of several locomotion modes (after Fishman *et al.*, 1962).

knee amputee may need twice as much energy to walk (Fishman, 1962) (Figure 15.3).

Those with an above knee amputation may be further compromised by the addition of a locked knee (Figure 15.4), which is necessary to stabilize the knee in the elderly patient. The younger patients frequently manage

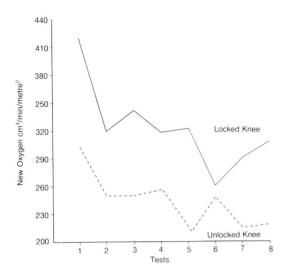

Figure 15.4 Graphs showing the energy costs of locked knee compared to unlocked knee prostheses (from Murdoch, 1970).

Table 15.1 Speed and oxygen consumption in peripheral vascular disease related amputees compared with normal individuals (Waters *et al*. 1976)

Level	Speed	Oxygen consumption/ metre
Normal	82 m/min	16 ml/kg metre
Symes	57 m/min	21 ml/kg metre
Below knee	47 m/min	26 ml/kg metre
Above knee	36 m/min	35 ml/kg metre

with a unlocked knee gaining even greater benefit.

Waters *et al*. in 1976 showed that the higher the amputation level then the slower the walking and the greater the oxygen consumption (Table 15.1). It is clear that with higher amputations and advancing age, the reduced oxygen utilization and increasing energy requirements, make it increasingly difficult to walk efficiently. This further emphasizes the need to consider and strive

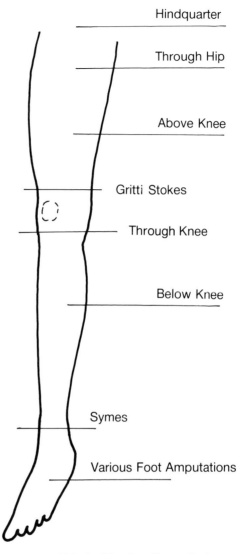

Figure 15.5 Principal levels of lower limb amputation.

for lower levels of amputation since this will help the patient greatly.

LEVEL OF AMPUTATION

Figure 15.5 lists the main lower limb amputation levels and Table 15.2 describes the levels and some of the prosthetic solutions.

205

Table 15.2 Amputation level in elderly patients

Level	Surgical	Prosthetic replacement	Comments
Toes	Commonest level	Toe blocker on insole	Common in diabetes mellitus and trauma
Partial feet	Lisfranc Chopart	Bootee prosthesis	Distal end of stump – metatarsals – often develop hyperkeratosis. Trauma and diabetes mellitus
Symes	Transmalleolar	Openback Plunge Fit Tukker Canadian	(Choice for congenital deformed feet in children) Trauma Diabetes mellitus Poor cosmesis of prosthesis – Less useful for women patients Good for elderly patients as they can stand on the stump, e.g. to go to the toilet at night
Below knee	Burgess surgical technique of long posterior flap or medially skew flap	PTB Supracondylar cuff suspension, or thigh corset side steel and metal shin	Amputation of choice for elderly amputee 25% more energy to walk than non amputee Good cosmesis Functional limb Thigh corset limb heavy, noisy but functional
Through knee	Knee disarticulation	Plunge fit Canadian 'type' thigh corset side steel and metal shin	Trauma – PVD Poor cosmesis of prosthesis Good end bearing
'Gritti Stokes'	Transcondylan	Ischial bearing above knee type	No end bearing Very poor cosmesis Poor suspension Rarely indicated
Above knee	Mid-thigh	Socket material: plastic metal wood Design quadrilateral Ischael containment Prosthesis Knee lock commonest	Cosmesis good Reasonably comfortable, 75% more energy to walk Prosthesis heavy and inefficient Vascular disease
Through hip	Hip disarticulation	Plastic socket (various materials) Leather socket	Heavy, energy consuming prosthesis Commonest for neoplasm Uncommon amputation

In summary the below knee amputation is the amputation of choice although the Symes amputation provides a useful stump if the patient rises at night and forgets or does not wish to don the prosthesis. Full weightbearing is possible from the distal end of the Symes amputation. Despite this advantage it is often difficult to heal when arteriosclerosis is the main cause of amputation.

In the case of a female Symes patient the poor cosmesis can for some be a major disadvantage and a below knee amputation may be a suitable compromise. The below knee stump provides good weightbearing characteristics, less psychological trauma for the patient and the ability to use a light functional prosthesis. The knee joint is intact and provides stability, proprioception and the normal knee musculature. Healing is slower however at this level than above the knee.

The above knee amputee requires 75% more energy to walk than a normal person and this results in a slow gait since the optimum walking pace is reduced. There is significantly less muscle to use when walking and as a result the effort to walk can therefore be quite considerable. Most patients require some additional support to help walk whether a single stick, a quadrilateral stick or a Zimmer frame. The mechanical knee used in an above knee prosthesis is more frequently of the locked variety, only being flexed when sitting. The need for this is the degree of control that the free knee prosthesis requires, which in an elderly person may be impossible. Healing is however more assured and rapid than at lower levels.

Levels even higher than this are uncommon and require even more energy for walking. The prostheses are more complex, sometimes with a hip joint, knee joint and ankle joint for the patient to contend with. Greater psychological trauma results from the high levels of amputation and this can have a significant effect on the overall success of rehabilitation.

AMPUTATION TECHNIQUE

The lower limb amputation is a major procedure and requires all the care and consideration one would expect from an event that will immeasurably change the patient's lifestyle. The surgeon must be experienced and meticulous in his technique if the patient is to achieve his full potential. He must have the fullest knowledge of the modern prosthetic techniques so that his stump can be readily fitted with as efficient a prosthesis as possible. The patient must also be as fit as possible for surgery with attention paid to the nutritional state, cardiac state, renal condition and diabetic control.

The affected limb should be prepared by dousing in a betadine solution (unless iodine sensitive) preoperatively. The long posterior flap is the generally accepted procedure as popularized by Burgess in 1968 for the below knee amputation. The surgeon must aim for as little handling of the critically ischemic tissues as possible, with careful ligation of blood vessels and nerves, careful cutting and shaping of the bone and meticulous close apposition of skin edges to allow rapid epithelialization.

Post-operative prophylaxis with penicillin for seven days is recommended to counteract any problem with *Clostridium welchi*, and subcutaneous heparin is used to minimize the incidence of deep venous thrombosis.

STUMP MANAGEMENT

The essential outcome of the surgery is to provide the patient with a well healed, comfortable, mature stump which allows fully functional pain-free early mobilization and a return to life in the community as soon as possible.

Jain and Stewart (1992) state that four basic principles are involved:

1. relief of pain;
2. reduction of edema or swelling;

3. prevention of joint contractures;
4. early ambulation.

The surgeon's skill at achieving all four objectives by performing the operation will be lessened if the dressing applied to the stump does not encourage primary healing. Significant physical and psychological morbidity will result if this is not achieved.

There is considerable debate about the most appropriate dressing for the amputation stump. In Dundee where a fully integrated amputation service exists it is the policy to use the technique as recommended by Burgess, Ramaro and Zettel (1969). This follows the pattern of rigid dressings for through knee, below knee and Symes, with elastoplast adherent dressing being used for the above knee and higher amputations. With the below knee stump a rigid dressing (Figure 15.6) is applied in theatre with a vacuum drain, which is removed in 48 hours if no excess drainage occurs. This primary plaster of Paris cast remains for approximately seven days. Replacement at this time is considered advisable since it allows the operator to view the stump to ensure that healing is taking place and allows a new plaster of Paris to be fitted to take up any of the space which has occurred after resolution of the surgical edema. This rigid dressing now remains on for a further 14 days being finally removed 21 days postoperatively. During this period records are kept of the temperature and pulse. If the patient complains of tightness and excessive pain under the POP, or if there is considerable seepage of blood or serous material then the POP is removed and if possible, replaced. Overt infection is treated accordingly.

One of the most significant aspects of this technique is that often after the first 24 hours following surgery opiates are rarely needed and simple analgesics such as paracetamol and codeine mixtures are all that is frequently required.

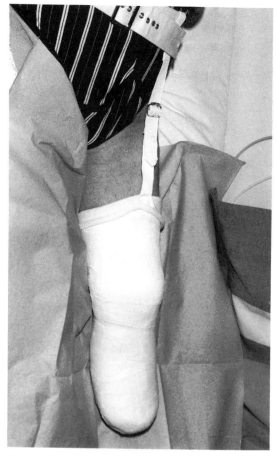

Figure 15.6 A rigid dressing for the below knee stump.

As a result of this technique well healed stumps can be consistently achieved (Figure 15.7).

The through knee and Symes procedures are similar, although weight bearing at seven days postoperatively may be by way of an immediate post operative fitting, with a tube fitted to the bottom of a through knee POP or in a case of the Symes a rubber rocker being fitted at the distal end of the plaster.

Mobilization with weight bearing through the rigid dressing can commence at seven to ten days, either with an early walking aid as

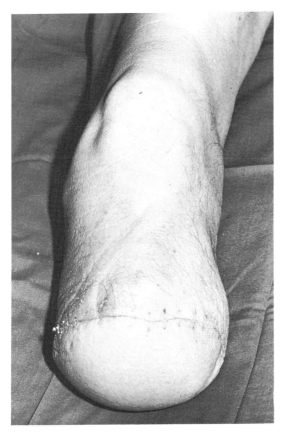

Figure 15.7 A well healed stump.

described below or by fitting an immediate postoperative device as outlined above.

Measurement for the definitive prosthesis can proceed on the 22nd postoperative day, and is fitted two to three days later provided the stump is healing well and there is minimal edema. Sufficient maturation of the stump has taken place by this time for this first prosthesis to last over seven months before a new socket is required.

The elastoplast above knee dressing is removed on day seven postoperatively and a simple gauze dressing with crepe bandage is then applied. Similar early walking aids are used at this time and prosthetic fitting commences at 14 days when the stitches come out.

In circumstances where excessive edema is present it is the Dundee experience that the removal of the rigid dressing and the application of the Flowtron air system can be of significant benefit. This can continue even after delivery of the prosthesis, to ease early maturation. Mooney *et al.* (1971) advocated POP as a dressing noting the reduction in postoperative pain, prevention of edema and more rapid healing with reduction of infection and early comfortable mobility. These findings are echoed in the Dundee experience.

Surgeons not familiar with a rigid dressing are reluctant to use it, and prefer to use soft gauze and crepe dressings. These certainly allow wound observation but comparative experience has shown a greater requirement for opiates and an increase in wound infection, edema and a delay in the maturation of the stump with a consequent delay in prosthetic fitting.

The skill of rigid dressing application is easily acquired but requires practice. It must be questioned whether the surgeon who does only a few amputations per year should use a rigid dressing. The argument could similarly be used to ask whether he should perform the amputation at all since he is unlikely to have sufficient experience or skill to ensure the optimum outcome. In circumstances where amputation is infrequent, the surgeon must realize his patient may acquire more morbidity than is necessary and consider referring his patient to a skilled operator, which may be in the best interests of the patient rather the surgeon's personal pride.

Indeed the specialization of surgeons in this major surgical event should ensure that the patient enjoys the rest of his life in as mobile a state as possible.

In a comparison of two amputation environments, one with a comprehensive amputation service (using POP) and the other without such integrated provision (using soft dressing) it was found that the time taken to discharge with the definitive prosthesis was 57 days (integrated service) and 77 days (non-integrated). In addition, and more significantly, the AK:BK ratio was 1: 4.6 with the integrated service and only 1:1.2 in the other less organized service. This latter ratio is in keeping with the national UK level and is depressingly low (Jain and Stewart, 1992).

POSTOPERATIVE MANAGEMENT AND REHABILITATION

The patient is often tired from peripheral vascular disease and opiate modified pain, they are demoralized from the amputation especially if vascular surgery has failed, they are frightened of the prospects of a limbless life. A team working closely together must combat all these elements allowing the patient to regain physical and psychological strength, recover motivation and look forward to a mobile useful life.

TEAM MEMBERS

The clinician plays a vital role in coordinating the team and ensuring that the patient is medically fit. The overall clinical status of the patient will affect the ultimate outcome of rehabilitation. The surgeon who performs the amputation may well be this clinician or he may complement the rehabilitation specialist's expertise depending on local circumstances.

The clinician should be responsible for pre- and postoperative counseling of the patient, with an explanation of the expectations and an outline of future care. The full explanation of phantom phenomena should be discussed since this can be a very frightening experience, especially phantom pain, which may occur in upwards of 30% of patients. This feeling that the absent limb is still present is common, affecting about 90% of all amputees. The phantom pain can be short and stabbing, or of a long duration and severe. It is difficult to treat, with dozens of attempted remedies. These range from simple analgesics (e.g. Paracetamol) to antidepressants (e.g. amitryptiline), anti-convulsants (e.g. sodium valproate) and the use of TENS devices. The origin of the phenomenon is unclear with cerebral, spinal and peripheral theories being used to explain it. It may improve with time but although in many cases it does not, it may change in character. No predictions are possible as to which patients' feeling or pain will go, so reassurance is often all we can offer.

The nursing staff are responsible for the daily care of the patient and clearly should have a knowledge of the surgical techniques and postoperative management requirements of the amputee. They provide the day-to-day continuity of care for the patient. The psychological wellbeing is often the nurses' responsibility with counselling both for the patients and the relatives who may need reassurance as to the individual's future needs and immediate problems.

The care of skin is especially important in diabetic cases, particularly the prevention and treatment of debilitating pressure sores which may well delay mobilization and reduce the quality of life for the patient. The nurse should also be aware of the need for chiropody since these patients have already lost one limb, possibly due to ulcers of the feet and the intervention of a chiropodist may be a vital part in the prevention of a further amputation.

The physiotherapist may see the patient preoperatively but also in the immediate postoperative phase to encourage chest expansion and early mobilization. The overall physical state of the elderly patient often needs improving with both upper limb and lower limb strengthening exercises.

The visit by the physiotherapist and surgeon preoperatively to explain the postoperative phase can be of value in certain

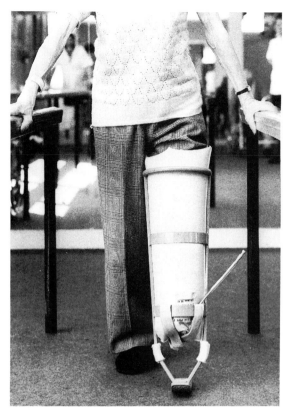

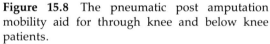

Figure 15.8 The pneumatic post amputation mobility aid for through knee and below knee patients.

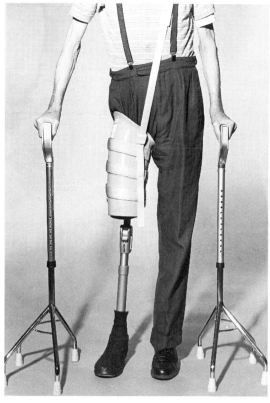

Figure 15.9 The Femoret, for above knee amputation patients.

circumstances but often the patient who is in such distress about his amputation does not necessarily take in all that is said, so unless the situation allows for elective amputation such preoperative counselling in our experience is not as useful as might be thought.

Early standing, in parallel bars, and hopping will encourage the patient to see that they will walk again and will also strengthen the remaining limb. Mobilization with appropriate early walking aids plays an important part in early gait training. The through knee and below knee patients can use the pneumatic post amputation mobility aid (PPA-

Maid) (Figure 15.8) and the above knee group can use the Femoret (Figure 15.9). In some centers the PPAMaid is also used for above knee amputees but it is not as stable as the Femoret.

Close cooperation with the prosthetist is valuable, enabling gait training to be continued under the care of both specialists with early completion of the prosthesis and subsequent discharge. The prosthetist is therefore also a member of the team. Their involvement in a rehabilitation process will ensure the provision of a well fitting, well aligned prosthesis and in the early stages they can be alert to any immediate changes in the prosthesis that are needed.

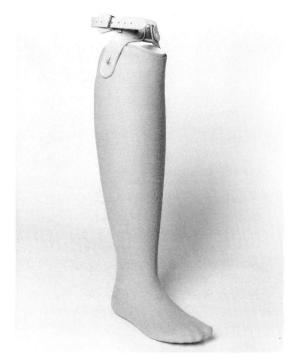

Figure 15.10 The standard prosthesis for the below knee amputation patient.

A wide range of prostheses are available for the amputee (Table 15.2). For the below knee patient the standard prosthesis is a patella tendon bearing one. This has a socket to allow full weight bearing on the stump, partly over the patella tendon, on either side of the tibial crest and in particular on the calf area (Figure 15.10). The prosthesis can be self suspending, reasonably lightweight and cosmetic in appearance.

The above knee prosthesis has the need for a mechanical knee. These are now endoskeletal with modular components covered with a foam faring to look cosmetically acceptable (Figure 15.11). The knee can be self locking (locked in extension for walking, normally unlocked to sit and usually provided for the older patient), or free swinging with the added options of various swing phase devices to provide smooth swing-through for the younger patient.

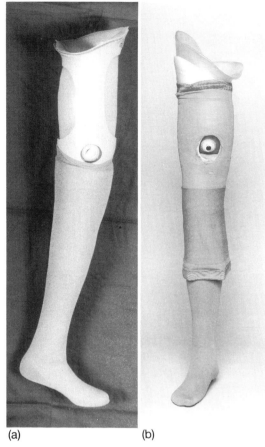

(a)   (b)

Figure 15.11 The above knee prosthesis; (a) ISNY, (b) ICS. Both can be fitted with a suction socket.

Since the late 1940s, the use of a quadrilateral shaped socket has been popular. A recent American socket, the ischial containment socket, which is more intimate in its fit has been introduced. The Icelandic fenestrated frame, which is much cooler and dynamic, has made the fit of the prosthesis more comfortable for the majority of patients. Suspension can be by way of a leather belt or an elastic belt (TES Belt). For the younger amputee or the fitter elderly amputee a suction socket can be very successful as shown in Figure 15.11. The latter socket is very close fitting with the stump in total contact. There is a valve sited at the bottom of the socket. The patient puts the stump in by way of a light bandage wrapped round the stump and then pulled out through the valve hole. A one way valve is placed in the hole and air can leak out but not in, providing a vacuum which holds the socket on to the stump. This can be difficult for the elderly patient.

The choice of prosthesis naturally depends on the level of amputation but also on the projected activity of the amputee and should usually be decided by discussion with the team. The correct selection of prosthesis will ensure a smooth transfer from immobility to mobility.

The occupational therapist provides the vital link with the community. The needs relating to the activities of daily living require close attention. These include dressing, toileting and kitchen assessment. In addition the occupational therapist's knowledge of psychology can be of help and alert team members to possible counseling needs. The occupational therapist spends a considerable amount of time on home visits both with and without the patient prior to discharge. A home assessment allows the future needs of the patient to be catered for. These visits can often be with the domiciliary occupational therapist whose responsibility the patient will become after discharge.

In this context close links with the social worker are essential. The social worker ensures the coordination of the community services once the discharge has been achieved. In a few centres a psychologist is attached. Addressing the significant psychological trauma associated with amputation can be of benefit to the patient helping them to come to terms with their disability and resulting handicap. Any involvement where phantom pain is a problem as distinct from the almost inevitable phantom sensation can be helpful.

Finally the general practitioner who will care for the amputee once discharge has taken place should be involved. The doctor should be aware of potential problems that could arise from wearing a prosthesis and also be aware of the fact that the patient can be referred back to the limb fitting center for an early appointment.

COSMETIC LIMBS

For some patients it may be decided that it is inappropriate to provide limbs for the amputee to walk with. Those with severe respiratory or cardiac pathology may find that they cannot walk with a prosthesis and the provision of a functioning limb may be detrimental to the overall health of the individual. In these circumstances a self-propelling wheelchair is essential for independent living. Appropriate training of the amputee in the use of the wheelchair is necessary as well as the assessment of the house for a wheelchair existence.

In a few cases the provision of cosmetic limbs may be considered. These are lightweight, non-weightbearing prostheses. Their use is limited since they cannot take any weight at all. However the improved appearance can be of significant value to the wellbeing of the patient, who can feel 'whole again'. Cosmetic limbs are more often used for bilateral above knee amputees for whom prosthetic fitting is often inappropriate.

WHEELCHAIRS

A significant number of amputees, especially the elderly, benefit from the provision of a wheelchair. For many the Transit type which is propelled by an attendant is all that is needed. This will allow the amputee to be taken out and about without exhausting the patient by walking. In some the use of a selfpropelling chair may be of use. This may

213

however discourage the patient from walking and this is not to be encouraged unless medically important. In some circumstances however, for example to go to the toilet at night, the use of a selfpropelling chair may be of great value. Comprehensive assessment prior to discharge will identify those who would benefit from such a provision.

POST DISCHARGE MANAGEMENT

The amputee remains a patient for the rest of his or her life. Prosthetic care is needed to ensure the stump's integrity and that the continuing mobilization of the patient is maintained.

Limb fitting centers continue to see patients at regular intervals and treat problems as they arise. Amputees need free access to this service.

The elderly amputee remains at risk of losing the contralateral limb. About 18% of all amputees are bilateral and further vascular surgery to salvage the other limb should be borne in mind. Further surgery to the stumps of existing amputees is uncommon once initial healing has occurred.

CONCLUSION

The elderly amputee is in a group of patients who require very specialized and careful consideration. Total care is needed if they are to minimize their disability.

Only with a dedicated team will the amputee achieve as distal an amputation as possible, followed by primary healing, early mobilization, rapid discharge home and as low a morbidity as possible. The social reintegration of the patient should be the aim of all rehabilitation teams.

The amputee should have his lifestyle marginalized as little as possible by the surgery.

214

REFERENCES

Burgess, E.M., Ramano, R.L., and Zettel, J.H. (1969) *The Management of Lower Extremity Amputation* published for the Prosthetic and Sensory Aids Service Veterans Administration, Washington.

Fishman, S. (1962) *Metabolic Measures and Evaluation of Prosthetic and Orthotic Devices*, Research Division of the College of Engineering New York University, New York.

Grimby, G. (1983) Energy costs in achieving mobility. Lawrence Pool Price Lecture on Rehabilitation. First European Conference on Research and Rehabilitation, Edinburgh.

Jain, A.S. and Stewart, C.P.U. (1992) Comparison on integrated amputee service. Proceedings of Joint Meeting between Scottish Orthopaedic Association and Irish Orthopaedic Association, April, 1992.

Mooney, V., Harvey, J.P., McBride E. and Snelson, R. (1971) Comparison of post operative stump management plaster versus soft dressing. *J. Bone Joint Surg.*, **53a**, 241–9.

Murdoch, G. and Donovan, R.G. (1988) *Amputation Surgery and Lower Limb Prosthetics*. Blackwells Scientific Publications, Edinburgh.

Murdoch, G. (1970) *Prosthetic and Orthotic Practices*, Edward Arnold, London.

Swaka, M., Glaser, R.M., Lambach, L.L. *et al.* (1981) Wheelchair exercise performance of young, middle-aged and elderly. *J. Appl. Physiol. Respirat. Environ.*, Exercise Physiology, **50** (4), 824–8.

Spence, V.A., McCollum, P.T., Walker, W.F. and Murdoch, G. (1984) Assessment of tissue viability in relation to the selection of amputation level. *Prosth. Ortho. Int.*, **8**, 67–75.

Stewart, C.P.U., Jain, A.S. and Ogston, S.A. (1992) Lower limb amputee survival. *Prosth. Ortho. Int.*, **16**, 11–18.

Stewart, C.P.U. and Jain, A.S. Causes of death in lower limb amputees. *Prosth. Ortho. Int.*, **16**, 124–132.

Troup I.M. and Wood, M.A. (1982) *Total Care of the Lower Limb Amputee*, Pitman Press, Bath.

Waters, R., Henry, R., Antonelli, D. and Hyslop, H. (1976) Energy cost of walking amputees: the inference of level of amputation. *J. Bone Joint Surg.*, 58a(1), 42–6.

Index

Page numbers appearing in **bold** refer to figures and page numbers appearing in *italic* refer to tables.